General Principles in the Basic Sciences

2nd edition

◄ Board Simulator ►

DEVELOPED BY

NATIONAL MEDICAL SCHOOL REVIEW®

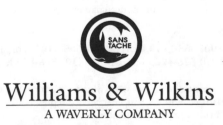

Williams & Wilkins

A WAVERLY COMPANY

BALTIMORE • PHILADELPHIA • LONDON • PARIS • BANGKOK
BUENOS AIRES • HONG KONG • MUNICH • SYDNEY • TOKYO • WROCLAW

Editor: Elizabeth A. Nieginski
Managing Editors: Amy G. Dinkel, Darrin Kiessling
Development Editors: Melanie Cann, Beth Goldner, Carol Loyd
Manager, Development Editing: Julie Scardiglia
Editorial Assistant: Lisa Kiesel
Marketing Manager: Rebecca Himmelheber
Production Coordinator: Danielle Hagan
Text/Cover Designer: Cotter Visual Communications
Typesetter: Port City Press
Printer/Binder: Port City Press

Copyright © 1997 Williams & Wilkins

351 West Camden Street
Baltimore, Maryland 21201-2436 USA

Rose Tree Corporate Center
1400 North Providence Road
Building II, Suite 5025
Media, Pennsylvania 19063-2043 USA

Accurate indications, adverse reactions, and dosage schedules for drugs are provided in this book, but it is possible that they may change. The reader is urged to review the package information data of the manufacturers of the medications mentioned.

Printed in the United States of America

First Edition,

Library of Congress Cataloging-in-Publication Data
General principles in the basic sciences / developed by National
   Medical School Review. — 2nd ed.
      p.   cm. — (Board simulator)
   ISBN 0-683-30296-5
   1. Medicine—Examinations, questions, etc.   I. National Medical
School Review (Firm)   II. Series.
   [DNLM: 1. Medicine—examination questions.   2. Biological
Sciences—examination questions.   W 18.2 G326 1997]
   R834.5.G46   1997
   610′.76—dc21
   DNLM/DLC
   for Library of Congress   97-6903
                                                                     CIP

The publishers have made every effort to trace the copyright holders for borrowed material. If they have inadvertently overlooked any, they will be pleased to make the necessary arrangements at the first opportunity.

To purchase additional copies of this book, call our customer service department at **(800) 638-0672** or fax orders to **(800) 447-8438.** For other book services, including chapter reprints and large-quantity sales, ask for the Special Sales department.

Canadian customers should call **(800) 665-1148**, or fax **(800) 665-0103.** For all other calls originating outside of the United States, please call **(410) 528-4223** or fax us at **(410) 528-8550.**

Visit Williams & Wilkins on the Internet: http://www.wwilkins.com or contact our customer service department at **custserv@wwilkins.com.** Williams & Wilkins customer service representatives are available from 8:30 am to 6:00 pm, EST, Monday through Friday, for telephone access.

97 98 99 00
1 2 3 4 5 6 7 8 9 10

DEDICATION

This book is dedicated to the loving memory of Dr. Richard Swanson: 1954–1996. Rick was an inspiration as an author, teacher, and physician. Rick led by example, and his death is a loss to all of us whose lives he touched.

Rick is survived by his wife Stella, daughter Heidi, and sons Eric and Jason.

CONTENTS

EDITORS AND CONTRIBUTORS

GERALD D. BARRY, Ph.D.
Professor of Physiology and Director of the MA/MD
    Biomedical Program
Touro College School of Health Sciences

GRACE BINGHAM, Ed.D.
President and Educational Consultant
Bingham Associates, Inc.
Toms River, NJ
Coordinator of Cognitive Skills
National Medical School Review

GEORGE M. BRENNER, Ph.D.
Professor and Chairman
Department of Pharmacology
Oklahoma State University
College of Osteopathic Medicine

BARBARA FADEM, Ph.D.
Professor, Department of Psychiatry
University of Medicine and Dentistry
New Jersey Medical School

EDWARD F. GOLJAN, M.D.
Associate Professor and Chairman of Pathology
Oklahoma State University
College of Osteopathic Medicine

DAILA S. GRIDLEY, Ph.D.
Professor
Department of Microbiology and Molecular Genetics
Department of Radiation Medicine
Loma Linda University
School of Medicine

KENNETH H. IBSEN, Ph.D.
Professor, Emeritus
Department of Biochemistry
University of California at Irvine
Director of Academic Development
National Medical School Review

KIRBY L. JAROLIM, Ph.D.
Professor and Chairman
Department of Anatomy
Oklahoma State University
College of Osteopathic Medicine

KATHLEEN KEEF, Ph.D.
Professor
Department of Physiology and Cell Biology
University of Nevada
School of Medicine

JAMES KETTERING, Ph.D.
Professor and Assistant Chairman
Department of Microbiology and Molecular Genetics
Loma Linda University
School of Medicine

RICHARD M. KRIEBEL, Ph.D.
Professor
Department of Anatomy
Philadelphia College of Osteopathic Medicine

WILLIAM D. MEEK, Ph.D.
Professor
Department of Anatomy
Oklahoma State University
College of Osteopathic Medicine

STANLEY PASSO, Ph.D.

Associate Professor
Department of Physiology
New York Medical College

JAMES P. PORTER, Ph.D.

Associate Professor
Department of Physiology and Biophysics
University of Louisville
School of Medicine

VERNON REICHENBECHER, Ph.D.

Associate Professor
Department of Biochemistry and Molecular Biology
Marshall University
School of Medicine

DAVID SEIDEN, Ph.D.

Professor
Department of Neuroscience and Cell Biology
University of Medicine and Dentistry
Robert Wood Johnson Medical School

PREFACE

Since its establishment in 1988, the goal of National Medical School Review® (NMSR) has been to provide medical students and physicians with the information they need to know to pass their national licensing examinations. During this period, NMSR has developed a national reputation for high-quality programs delivered by the best teaching faculty available in United States and Canadian medical schools. Nearly 12,000 participants in NMSR programs have had access to outstanding faculty lectures as well as to diagnostic and practice examinations and high-yield notes that can be kept as learning tools. As a result, NMSR students have achieved an impressive level of success on the United States Medical Licensing Examination (USMLE) Steps 1, 2, and 3.

With the development and publication of the *Board Simulator Series* (BSS), NMSR ushered in a truly innovative new educational experience for medical students and physicians preparing for Step 1 of the USMLE. This five-volume series' unique format was designed to follow the content guidelines published by the National Board of Medical Examiners (NBME) for the USMLE, Step 1, rather than being organized strictly by isolated basic science discipline (for example, volumes dealing only with biochemistry or anatomy). Therefore, just as they appear on the real Step 1 examination, many questions in this series are preceded by a clinical vignette that often integrates two or more disciplines and can require the student to perform a multi-step reasoning process to arrive at a correct answer. Thus, students are challenged not only to recall a particular fact or principle, but to analyze and apply that information to the situation defined by the clinical vignette.

One proven way to increase the likelihood of answering these questions correctly is to practice with questions that are at a similar level of difficulty and that have a similar emphasis. The BSS series provides students with just such an experience. In fact, it is NMSR's belief that this series gives most second-year medical students attending a United States medical school the essential information and test-taking experience required to pass the USMLE, Step 1. This series could also serve as an adjunct to students who feel they would benefit from attending a structured review program.

Furthermore, the BSS series provides far more than simulated Step 1 examinations, because each question is answered with a full and detailed explanation. A student can use these explanations to clarify why the right answers are correct choices and the wrong answers are incorrect choices. In the process of doing this evaluation the student will have performed a comprehensive review of the material covered on the Step 1 examination.

To make this process even more effective, this second edition of the BSS contains 770 questions in each volume, 120 more than in the first edition. Each of the tests in each volume, with the exception of the introductory 50-question diagnostic test, contains 180 questions, which reflects the new USMLE examination booklet's length. This edition also includes a subject item index, allowing students who wish to use these books in a subject-based fashion to do so with greater ease. NMSR believes that as an educational tool this series can help maximize a student's opportunity to make reviewing for the USMLE, Step 1 both a successful and rewarding experience.

Victor Gruber, M.D.
Founder and Executive Director
National Medical School Review®

ACKNOWLEDGMENT

NMSR would like to recognize Edward F. Goljan, M.D., for his valuable contribution to the development and unique organization of topics in this series.

ACKNOWLEDGMENT

GUIDE TO USING THIS BOOK

During the past 10 years, a number of changes in curriculum organization have occurred in many U.S. and Canadian medical schools, particularly within the first 2 years of education. A number of meaningful innovations have been implemented, such as more self-directed learning, de-emphasis of lectures as the dominant instructional mode, earlier introduction of clinical experiences, and increases in the proportion of problem-based learning.

Today, regardless of which curriculum a medical school adopts, one trend exists even in those schools that have maintained a traditional stance: a loosening of the boundaries that organized basic science material into large territorial "subject" courses. The move is toward synthesizing domains of medical knowledge into more flexible cross-disciplinary patterns believed to approximate interactions that characterize medical practice today.

From a student's perspective, all the attention given to the number and variety of medical school curriculum reforms may have highlighted only the differences among the curricula and neglected to underscore the important similarities remaining. Regardless of the specific curriculum followed at any school, medical students are still expected to:

1. Read and understand large quantities of material. Whether the access mode is texts, handouts, specialized print materials, or computer modules, the reading demands remain significant.

2. Organize information in meaningful ways. No matter how well written a concept may appear in a text, or how well explained in a lecture, the students should *generate* the pattern of meaning that makes the most sense to them.

3. Develop relationships among experiences. All medical students are expected to engage in higher order thinking processes. New information about a topic will need to be *encoded* and *synthesized* with prior knowledge; *compared* with a lab experiment; *evaluated* through discussion with a colleague; or *solved* as a problem.

4. Store, retrieve, and remember information dependably. Historically, the demands on memory for medical personnel have been exceptional. The rapidity with which new technological advances in diagnosis and increases in treatment options are becoming available makes it more difficult than ever to learn and stay up to date in the field. Distinguishing between what needs to be mastered and recalled readily and what does not is a professional decision with which medical practitioners will struggle for the rest of their careers.

5. Demonstrate achievement through various forms of evaluation. Regardless of their curriculum model, all medical schools still require high levels of performance of their students. Evaluators can choose from a large range of methods to assess students, from the traditional instructor-designed examinations to oral evaluations, on-site observations, behavioral checklists, and product evaluations (e.g., written reports, research papers, problem solutions). Whatever the method, students will need to give evidence of competency.

6. Demonstrate competency on national standardized examinations. To qualify for licensure, students need to be successful on Steps 1, 2, and 3 of the USMLE. After further graduate training, students need to demonstrate success on specialty examinations to qualify for Board certification.

Series Design

Some of the more positive changes that characterize medical learning today are already reflected in the design of current instructional materials. One such change is the design of the five books in this series. The organization differs from the traditional subject-oriented subdivisions of basic science in that it conforms more closely to the content outline of USMLE Step 1 as presented in the *General Instructions* booklet. In Step 1, basic science material is organized along two dimensions: system (consisting of general principles and individual organ systems) and processes, which divide each organ system into normal development, abnormal processes, therapeutics, and psychosocial and other considerations.

Book I: General Principles in the Basic Sciences
Book II: Normal and Abnormal Processes in the Basic Sciences
Book III: Body Systems Review I: Hematopoietic/Lymphoreticular, Respiratory, Cardiovascular
Book IV: Body Systems Review II: Gastrointestinal, Renal, Reproductive, Endocrine
Book V: Body Systems Review III: Nervous, Skin/Connective Tissue, Musculoskeletal

Each book contains five examinations: a condensed 50-question diagnostic test and four tests containing 180 questions each for a total of 770 questions per book. The distribution of questions within each test in books III, IV, and V approximates subcategory percentages as follows: normal development, 10%–20%; normal processes, 20%–30%; abnormal processes, 30%–40%; principles of therapeutics, 10%–20%; psychosocial, cultural, and environmental considerations, 10%–20%. By comparing your performance on the diagnostic test in each volume, you will be able to prioritize your use of the books.

Questions in each test are presented using the two multiple-choice formats that appear in USMLE Step 1: One Best Answer (including negatively phrased items) and Matching Sets, with the largest number of questions of the One Best Answer type.

Who Can Use These Questions?

The group likely to use the questions in this series of books most frequently is students preparing for USMLE Step 1. However, other student groups who can benefit from these questions are medical students in years I, II, III, and IV. These students may turn to individual books in the series or use the entire set of books as a supplemental self-testing resource.

Students Preparing for USMLE Step 1

Students preparing for the Step 1 exam will use these books as a **diagnostic tool,** as a **guide to focus further study,** and as a **self-evaluation device.**

Specific instructions about how to use the question sets for each purpose will be described in the next section.

Students in Years I and II

Students in years I and II will use these books for **periodic self-testing.** Students in the first 2 years of medical school take a large number of examinations that evaluate their performance on material covered in their courses or other learning experiences. Those tests are usually compiled by the instructors and reflect the intructors' choice of emphasis. The questions in the five books in this series provide a sampling of the wide range of material typically taught in the first 2 years of medical school. For students who want to practice with questions that go beyond the scope of their specific school's course, these question sets provide another level of testing, one that approximates more closely the expectations of the Step 1 exam. These questions also offer opportunities for practice to those students in medical school courses that use Board shelf exams as one of their required evaluations. The section How to Use These Practice Exams provides guidance on their use.

Students in Years III and IV

Students in years III and IV will use these books for **reactivating and assessing prior learning.** During their third and fourth years, students may find during clinical situations that they have forgotten some material they learned during the first 2 years. One way to stimulate, reactivate, and supplement that knowledge is by responding to questions. The content and organization of the questions in each book of the series make it possible for students in the clinical years to select and use specific segments for review.

How to Use These Practice Exams

The practice questions in this book assess knowledge of principles in ten major topics: (1) biochemistry and molecular biology, (2) biology of cells, (3) human development and genetics, (4) tissues and their responses to disease (e.g., inflammation, repair and regeneration, neoplasias), (5) psychosocial, cultural, and environmental influences on behavior, health, and disease processes, (6) multisystem processes (e.g., nutrition, temperature regulation), (7) pharmacodynamic and pharmacokinetic processes, (8) microbial biology and infection, (9) immune responses, and (10) quantitative methods. Questions in this book focus on **General Principles,** whereas the questions in book II concentrate on normal and abnormal processes related to each of the preceding ten topics. These ten topics are cross-referenced via the subject item index to the seven traditional academic disciplines in which the topic might have been taught or may be found in other NMS or BRS review books.

Whereas the specific information to be assessed in each topic and its subtopics differs, there are certain *categories* of knowledge organization that recur regardless of differences, as can be noted in the small sampling from topics in this book:

— Structure and composition of. . . (cell membranes; ion channels and pumps; endocytosis)
— Structure and function of. . . (proteins; ribosomes; tRNA)
— Characteristics of. . . (endothelium, epithelium, mesothelium)
— Regulation of. . . (transcription factors; translation; energy metabolism)
— Mechanisms of. . . (vasoconstriction; biosynthesis and degradation)
— Concepts of. . . (measurement; study design; statistical significance)
— Issues related to. . . (medical ethics; patient participation in research; professional behavior)

These question sets may be used in a number of ways: (1) as a diagnostic tool (pretest), (2) as a guide and focus for further study, and (3) for self-evaluation. The least effective use of these questions is to "study" them by reading them one at at time, and then looking at the correct response. Although the questions have been compiled to be representative of the domains of information found in USMLE Step 1, simply knowing the answers to these particular 770 questions does not ensure a passing grade on the exam. The questions are intended to be an integral part of a well-planned review, rather than an isolated resource. If used appropriately, the four sets can provide self-assessment information beyond a numeric score.

As a diagnostic tool. It is possible to use each set of questions as a screening device to gather diagnostic information about relative performance across the 10 large topics presented in this book. For those who have been away from basic science study for awhile and have no other recent performance data, using a practice exam in this manner provides a form of feedback before beginning review. This method also allows students to respond to Board-type questions similar to those on the examination so they can experience the structure and complexity of such questions and acquire a sense of what the questions "feel" like.

1. Select any one of the four complete tests in this book. It does not matter which one you choose, since they are all approximately equal in terms of topics represented and question difficulty.

2. Allow yourself the same amount of time as will be allowed on the Board exam (approximately 60 seconds per question).

3. Use a separate sheet of paper for your answers (instead of writing in the book). This will make it easier for you to score, analyze, and interpret the results.

4. Score your responses (but do not read the correct answer to the question or record the correct response next to your incorrect one). Compute an accuracy level by counting the number of correct responses and dividing by the total number of questions to get the percent correct. Note your score, but be careful not to overreact to this initial score. Remember that this type of sampling provides only a rough indication of how familiar or remote this basic science material seems to you before review. Not reading the correct answer to these questions may seem a bit strange at first, but by not doing so now, you will be able to use these questions again later in your review as a posttest to check progress.

5. Know your distribution of errors across the topics. To find out, categorize each error (e.g., biochemistry, cell biology, genetics; tissue biology, pharmacokinetics, multisystem processes). If in doubt about how to categorize a particular question, check the reference listed in the answer and use that to make your decision.

6. Arrange topics in a hierarchy from relatively strong (few errors) to relatively weak (many errors). Did you do well in those topics you thought you would do well in, and vice versa, or were there some unexpected highs or lows?

To guide further study. After reviewing the material of the major areas noted previously and giving the information a complete "first pass," it is time to test yourself using another question set in this book. Your purpose is to check your estimates of which topics and subtopics have been learned well, which are still shaky, and which are quite weak. To do that:

1. Follow the first five steps described previously.

2. Analyze errors using the guidelines described in the section "Monitoring Functions for Consolidating Information."

3. Focus your follow-up study on the content areas or specific subtopics noted to still be weak. Pay particular attention to whether a pattern of errors has emerged (e.g., questions requiring understanding of genetic principles; questions requiring knowledge of repair and regenerative processes; or questions requiring knowledge of metabolic pathways and associated diseases).

There is another possible use for these questions. If you already know from experience the two or three major topics in this book that cause you the greatest concern, you can:

1. Select from *two* question sets only those questions that deal with those specific topics. (You can identify them easily because each answer is topically keyed.)

2. If the number of questions is large, you may want to divide the number in half and reserve one half for a later test.

3. Follow steps 2 to 4 from the diagnostic testing section.

4. In conducting error analysis, try to pin down more specifically your within-topic errors, so that in follow-up study you can concentrate on strengthening weaknesses that remain.

5. When you feel you have firmed up your information base, test yourself with the other half of the questions and note your progress, as well as any remaining subtopics for follow-up study. The questions not used in the first two sets of questions, as well as the two full sets, can be used as your review progresses.

For self-evaluation. As the last few weeks before the exam approach, some students begin to experience feelings of "approach/avoidance"; they would like to know if they are close to, or even beyond, the minimum needed to pass, but they also fear that if they find a large discrepancy, it may deplete their efforts during the final phase of their review. This situation is less likely to occur with students who have engaged in self-testing throughout their preparation. These students have been collecting and analyzing test data all along and adjusting their study agenda accordingly. The last level of evaluation is not likely to give them any surprises about strengths and weaknesses, but will identify areas in which they can continue to fine-tune.

There are a few different ways to handle the last round of self-testing. Some students feel less anxious if they do the final round of self-evaluation in the first few days of the last week and reserve the rest of the time for last-minute follow-up study. Other students prefer to start the week with a composite test, continue with further study, and then take another practice test 2 or 3 days before the exam.

1. If you have used one full question set as a pretest, it would now be informative to start with those questions as a posttest. Follow the steps described previously and compare performance (both total score and the score across each large basic science topic).

2. The four remaining tests can be used as individual question sets, or they can be combined into one large composite set.

3. If none of the tests has been used for pretesting, you might take every other question from all five tests (385 questions) and follow up later with the remaining 385 questions.

4. If you are using other books in this series, you can select a set from each of the other four books to form a comprehensive final evaluation.

Score Interpretation

Keeping in mind that the percentage of items needed to pass the USMLE Step 1 is between 55% and 65% should help you interpret accuracy levels from your self-testing. The practice test samples suggested here (usually 180 questions) provide useful feedback to chart your progress. On your tests, percentages between 55% and 60% are minimal, but encouraging. Percentages between 60% and 75% show you are moving beyond the bare minimum needed for passing. Scores of 75% and above are indicators of substantial strength.

EXAM PREPARATION GUIDE

USMLE Step 1: What to Expect

USMLE Step 1 is the first examination of the three-step sequence required for medical licensure, so it is not surprising that its approach engenders apprehension in many students. Successful performance is particularly consequential in those medical schools that require successful passage of Step 1 before permitting students to proceed to third year. The "new" Step 1 has been in effect since 1991, and although most people are now familiar with its general contours, some "myths" still circulate.

The sources that contain the most complete and specific information about the examination are those distributed to students when they register to take Step 1: *Bulletin of Information* and *USMLE Step 1— General Instructions, Content Outline, and Sample Items*. **Both books should be read in their entirety before taking the examination.** What follows is a brief summary of what can be found in much more detail in those materials.

Description. The purpose of the Step 1 exam is to assess students' understanding and application of important concepts in the basic biomedical sciences: anatomy, behavioral science, biochemistry, microbiology, pathology, pharmacology, and physiology. Emphasis is placed on **principles and mechanisms underlying health, disease, and modes of therapy.**

A "blueprint" in the Guidelines booklet shows how basic science material is organized for the examination. Two dimensions are used: system and process. The first dimension includes a section on General Principles and ten Individual Organ Systems. The second dimension is divided into normal development; normal processes; abnormal processes; principles of therapeutics; and psychosocial, cultural, and environmental considerations. Also shown are the percentages of questions across categories of the two dimensions. The percentages are rather close between General Principles, 40%–50%, and Individual Organ Systems, 50%–60%. Of the categories in dimension 2, abnormal processes has the largest percentage (30%–40%). A more detailed breakdown of content can be found in the *Step1 Content Outline*, but not all the topics listed are included in each test administration.

Students are expected to respond to some questions that require straightforward basic science knowledge, but the majority of questions require application of basic science principles to clinical situations. There are also questions that require interpretation of graphic and tabular data and identification of gross and microscopic specimens. There seems to be more coverage of content typically taught in the second year, but interdisciplinary topics such as Immunology, which is usually taught in the first year, receive quite a bit of attention.

Format. The 2-day examination consists of four books with approximately 180 items in each book (total, 720 questions). Two books are given on each of the days. Three hours are allowed to complete each book, or approximately 60 seconds per question.

Question types. Two types of questions are on the exam: single best answer and matching sets, which begin with a list of a certain number of response options used for all items in the set.

Scores. Passing is based on the total score. Raw scores are converted to a standard score scale with a mean of 200 and a standard deviation of 20. A score of 176, or 1.2 standard deviations below the mean, is needed to pass.

Examinees will receive a total test score, a pass/fail designation, and a graphic performance "profile" depicting strengths and weaknesses by discipline and organ system. No individual subscores are reported. A two-digit score is also reported, in which a score of 75 corresponds to the minimum passing score and 82 is equivalent to the mean of 200.

A Framework for Successful Preparation

By the time you reach medical school, you have been a student for most of your life. You have learned in a variety of settings and have achieved a number of personal goals. There is probably little that you have not observed about your own learning. Despite this, you may still approach medical studies with some degree of apprehension and have questions about the effectiveness of your study strategies, specific skills, and attitudes.

After experiencing medical courses during their first year or two, most students accommodate well and, if necessary, make whatever adjustments in their study patterns seem warranted. But, even the most competent student, given the pressure of frequent and demanding examinations, will have occasional doubts regarding the efficiency of a particular study method. For those planning to take USMLE Step 1, many questions occur about how best to proceed. "How much time is adequate for review?" "What materials should I use?" "What should I study and in what order?" In discussions with other students, you will hear about approaches they took and what worked for them. But, eventually, you will need to make important decisions for yourself about how to *initiate* and *sustain* a preparation plan that results in success on the exam.

This preparatory guide selects and summarizes, from many different areas of cognitive and educational psychology, those findings that have most applicability to a medical learning context. Strategies, skills, and functions are organized according to their potential utility for students as they move progressively from initial encounter with new learning at stage I, acquiring information, to stage II, consolidating information, and finally to the goal of self-confident achievement, stage III, reaching mastery. In the sections that follow, the conceptual framework shown in Figure 1 will be used to discuss specific suggestions and activities.

FIGURE 1. Medical learning framework.

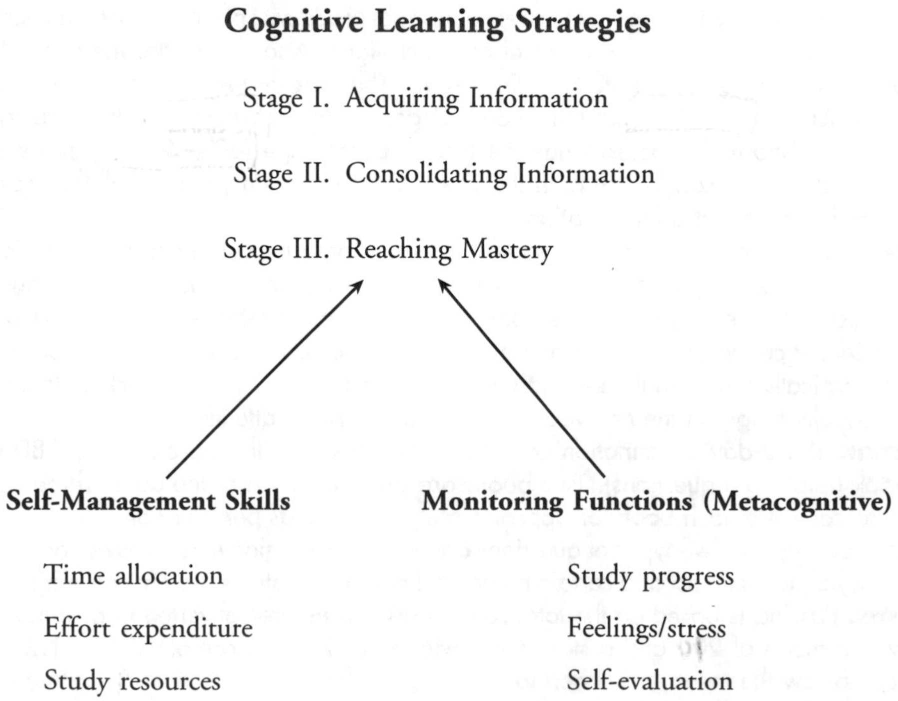

Cognitive Learning Strategies

Stage I. Acquiring Information

Stage II. Consolidating Information

Stage III. Reaching Mastery

Self-Management Skills

Time allocation

Effort expenditure

Study resources

Monitoring Functions (Metacognitive)

Study progress

Feelings/stress

Self-evaluation

Three main subdivisions are represented in this Medical Learning Framework: cognitive learning strategies, self-management skills, and monitoring functions.

Cognitive learning strategies. These strategies can be used to acquire, retain, and master a massive amount of information in the basic sciences. The strategies will be arranged according to which ones are appropriate at each stage in the learning sequence.

Self-management skills. At each stage of learning noted previously, there are skills that can help students allocate time efficiently, expend effort productively, and use study resources effectively.

Monitoring functions. In addition to the cognitive dimensions, medical learning requires metacognitive functions—the ongoing self-regulation that helps students track their progress and decide whether they need to modify or fine-tune any behaviors. Students also need to monitor and try to control potentially interfering negative feelings and stress.

Cognitive Learning Strategies

Any learning experience a student engages in, whether listening to a lecture, reading a text, observing a demonstration, or viewing a video presentation can be said to move through three stages as the learner proceeds from initial enounter to eventual mastery. Many factors influence the progression from one stage to another, among them the characteristics of the student, such as ability, motivation, attitudes, and interests. Also influential are the characteristics of the material, its conceptual difficulty, its organization, and its relationship to the learner's prior knowledge. The specific study activities the student uses also will have an effect. Whether you are trying to learn medical material for the first time, or reviewing information you learned before and need to reactivate and strengthen, the three-stage concept of how learning takes place offers a handy scheme for deciding which study strategies to use when.

Strategies for Acquiring Information

In this first stage, as you read or listen to a lecture, the main task is consciously and intentionally to generate as much *meaning* (understanding) as you can. Because studies have shown that strong initial *encoding* influences to a large extent what will be stored in long-term memory, there is a payoff for being *active* at this stage. The ongoing task is to decide if what you are reading or hearing is unfamiliar information, somewhat familiar, or already part of your fund of knowledge. Rarely will you encounter something that is completely new, but some topics will seem more remote than others if your previous experience with them has been limited. As you move through the information, do so at as brisk a pace as you can without sacrificing meaning. Following are some productive strategies that can be used at this stage:

1. Preview. Before starting to read, notice how a topic or other chunk of material has been organized. Use external arrangements such as titles and subheadings to get an idea of how the topic has been segmented. One technique is to convert these subdivisions into questions. Study any pictorial material such as figures and diagrams. Read the introduction, summary, and questions, if available. Read anything that is printed in different type, such as italic, or highlighted. Notice unfamiliar terms and look them up. Remember that the purpose of previewing is to give you a preliminary cognitive "map" that should help you extract more meaning from your subsequent reading.

2. Read actively. When reading a text, handouts, and notes, some parts will trigger recollection from your previous learning. When you encounter familiarity, try *prompting*: Pause and look away from the page, anticipate what will be coming, and try to bring forth from your memory whatever you can recall about that topic. Also, try to read as if on a *search*. Having looked at the subheading of a section and raised questions in your mind about what to expect, read to see if you can find responses to your questions.

3. Link information. Many medical students acknowledge that this is an important and useful strategy for enhancing understanding, yet few actually implement it. As you read, stop periodically and (a) summarize in your own words, (b) draw relationships to other knowledge by comparing and contrasting, (c) make an educated guess (inference), and (d) raise questions (What would happen if. . .?). If you are wondering whether you have time to think about the material given the usual pressures, remind yourself that these are the very thinking processes that are built into the questions of the Step 1 exam.

4. Construct notes. You probably have been taking notes in class since your earliest school days, and you may have developed a system for reducing and compacting lecture information that has served you well in the past. If so, continue using it. If, however, you are still trying to listen and write as much as you can, and as fast as you can, then perhaps you want to try a different method. When an instructor has provided a handout or other type of script before a lecture, preview it ahead and "cue" the sections that are obscure and need more elaboration. Then, you can limit note taking to what is essential to make sense of that script. Use whatever symbols you wish as cues (e.g., stars, circles, triangles) and assign a particular meaning to each. When you return to that handout after the lecture, you can translate your cues into further study activities (e.g., rewrite a particular section, supplement from a text, memorize a procedure).

One activity you might find helpful to institute fairly early is a last-minute study list consisting of those topics, mechanisms, procedures, and details that you find particularly problematic. Record either a brief explanation or the page and reference source where the information can be found. This list is particularly useful toward the end of your exam preparation sequence when you will want to make the most effective use of whatever time remains.

Self-Management Skills

At this early stage there are certain activities related to time, effort, and resources that are appropriate to carry out.

Time

Form a realistic study plan. Before plunging in, give some thought to how you want to organize your plan of study and which factors you need to consider. What is the amount of time you can reasonably allocate to preparation for the exam? If you are preparing for Step 1, it might be 3 or 4 months. If your experience with basic science material goes back a number of years, you will be doing more than simply activating former learning. There will be chunks of recent scientific knowledge that will require more intensive processing and more study time to reach a level of familiarity.

There are a few principles worth observing regardless of the total time actually allocated: (a) Use whatever diagnostic information you have (data-based, if possible) to assign time on the basis of relative strengths and weaknesses. Your review should be comprehensive, but some topics should be given more time than others. (b) Draft a long-range, tentative plan across the time you have available and estimate approximately how much you want to assign to each segment of content. Even a rough plan written down will reduce concern about whether you can fit everything in. You will be able to observe whether you underestimated the number of hours needed and increase them as you implement your plan. (c) Leave the last 2 weeks unscheduled so that you can return to areas that need a second pass. (d) At the end of each week, look at your plan and make changes based on your experiences during that week.

Effort

Get started. Perhaps what takes the most effort at this stage is just "lifting off" and getting into some type of study routine. You may find yourself putting off the actual start until you can finish other "essential" things, but you are probably procrastinating. It may help if you begin by studying something that you are strong in because a feeling of success will encourage you to continue. Gradually, shift to a topic that is less familiar and requires a little more intentional effort.

Select conditions conducive to study. Find a place where you can sustain a study block with few or no distractions. Put yourself in an active study posture, sitting upright, not lying on a couch or bed. Make yourself go to your study place as part of your routine. Staying in your apartment may be convenient, but it also makes it tempting to give in to other distractions.

Establish a reasonable, steady pace. If you are highly motivated, you may be tempted to work for exceptionally lengthy stretches, particularly during the early days of your review. Try, instead, to establish a reasonable routine that allows you to get a return from each study block. Know what your peak work periods are and do your most difficult studying at those times. Pay attention to whether you are getting fatigued and losing your ability to concentrate. Build in breaks that will reenergize you and help you feel refreshed when you return to studying.

Resources

Select effective study materials. Whether you are studying for a class exam or USMLE Step 1, finding just the right study material often can prove frustrating. Although quite a number of study resources are available in bookstores, each differs in purpose, format, depth, and comprehensiveness of coverage. For review, your own notes, charts, and handouts are good sources if you still have them available. They are familiar and have personal associations helpful for recalling information. To initiate review, look for publications that summarize or "compact" information, are not excessively wordy, but still provide enough narrative for you to make sense of the topic. The purpose of such books (e.g., Williams & Wilkins' *Board Review Series*) is to stimulate recall of material learned previously. Finally, have a reliable text available in each of the basic sciences so that you can use them selectively as a supplemental resource, if needed.

Monitoring Functions

Since you are just beginning to get into your study routine, this is the time to:

Initiate self-observations. These are the "informal" impressions, thoughts, and reactions that you form as you experience certain learning activities. For example, as you listen to a lecture, everything is making sense and fitting in with what you already know. Or, you feel some discomfort because the lecture is moving at too rapid a pace for you to process material meaningfully. Your reactions may be telling you that all is going well, and you should continue without change, or they may be signaling the need for some attention and possible adjustment in your study strategies.

Monitor emerging negative thoughts. If in reviewing you are reactivating without difficulty material you studied previously, you will feel productive and have a sense of accomplishment. But, there will be times when the proportion of understanding will seem relatively meager, and some discouragement will be felt. Try to confine your discouragement to the specific event that prompted the feeling without letting it generalize to *all* study activities.

Strategies for Consolidating Information

After you have listened to lectures or have read sections of material, you probably have acquired a reasonable percentage of the meaning. But, you also know that to *retain* what you understood, you will need to engage in other study activities. Of the multitude of activities from which you could choose, the following have been found to be effective to *maintain, consolidate, integrate,* and *synthesize* your knowledge.

1. Fill in gaps in your understanding. As soon after a lecture as is practical, follow up any of the "cued" sections in your notes or handouts by filling in what was unclear or incomplete. You can use another reference book, discuss the lecture with a peer, or ask for clarification from the instructor. Whatever action you take will make your learning stronger and move the information to long-term memory.

2. Reorganize for recall. Most students are familiar with the devices that can be used to reorganize information for better retrieval and recall: outlines, charts, index cards, concept maps, tree diagrams, and so forth. Following are guidelines for whether you should bother restructuring information and, if so, when it should be done.

If the material being used for study is already well organized, little if any restructuring may be needed. Sometimes, however, a different schematic format may make even well-organized material easier to recall.

If you reorganize, arrange the information so that *meaning* is emphasized. Note prototypes such as the most common and least common disease for a category, and the most frequent and least frequent treatment. In a set of diseases sharing similar symptoms, note particularly the differentiating feature(s).

If you decide to use one or more of the preceding devices, remember to do so during this stage, rather than close to the exam deadline, so you will have sufficient time to incorporate what you have restructured into your memory.

3. Synthesize from multiple sources. Avoid studying the same topic in three or four different sources. Use one substantive source as your "road map" and check other sources if you think yours is not comprehensive enough. Notice what needs to be added to make yours more complete, but end up with one dependable "script" that you can use for any subsequent study.

4. Rehearse to strengthen recall. Many students read things over and over. Rereading alone is not likely to be effective. The following habits could lead to more durable learning because they involve more active processing:

Use visual imaging. Visualize what you are trying to learn by "seeing" it in the form you will use when you want to retrieve it later (e.g., an anatomic structure as you saw it in lab, or as a schematic representation from the text, or as the instructor detailed it on a transparency).

Form analogies. Wherever possible, try to associate a new concept to a similar and simpler one that is already familiar to you.

Elaborate verbally. Talk about what you want to remember. Say it either to yourself or to others, but in your own words. "Stretch" beyond the script in the book or handout and develop inferences (make reasonable guesses about other relationships or applications).

Use mnemonics. These mental cues can be used to associate a wide range of medical information. Many can be found in student resources, or you can construct your own. Although you can be creative and even bizarre, avoid complexities that make the mnemonic harder to remember than the material itself. Using the first letter of each word to **form acronyms** is a common mnemonic device. For example, the causes of coma are AEIOU TIPS, which means *alcoholism, encephalopathy, insulin excess or deficiency, opiates, uremia, trauma, infection, psychosis, syncope.* **Method of loci** is one of the oldest mnemonic devices. You "place" mentally what you want to remember in certain familiar locations, such as rooms in your house, or locations within a room.

5. Establish patterns of practice. Certain "essentials" may need to be memorized and recalled almost verbatim. For such learning, **distribute the practice** so that you rehearse for a number of short periods, with breaks and other activities interspersed, rather than trying to sustain one lengthy period. Try **cumulative practice** by learning a few "chunks" at one session; then at a subsequent session, review those and add a few more. Continue the same pattern until all you want to memorize has been incorporated.

6. Study with others. This can be an effective study activity if used properly. An initial exploration of material by each student in the group will make group discussion more valuable. Discussion can then focus on clarifiying material and confirming and extending understanding. Studying with others works best if the group is small so everyone participates, and if some ground rules are established about how the sessions will be conducted.

7. Self-test periodically. The purpose of self-testing at this stage is **to guide further study.** Self-testing can help you decide which topics need more intense study, which are fairly close to being learned, and which have been learned well. Resources to use for this purpose and the sequence to follow will be described in later sections.

Applying Effective Testing Skills

Following are suggestions that will increase the likelihood that what you have learned and can recall from your study will translate into correct responses on multiple-choice examinations.

General test-taking skills

Read carefully for comprehension, not speed and respond to questions in sequence. Mark every item on your answer sheet as you go along, even if you are not completely sure of your choice. Cue the questions to which you want to return if there is time.

Be positive. Suppose the first question you see as you open the test book is a particularly difficult one, and you can feel yourself getting anxious. After giving it a try, go to the second question and respond to that one, which in all likelihood will feel more manageable.

Avoid mechanical errors. At the end of each page of questions, before going to the next page, check to make sure the **number of the question** you just finished **matches the number on your answer sheet.**

Be alert to key terms in the question stem such as "most," "least," "primarily," "frequently," "most often," and "most likely." Notice transition words that signal a change in meaning, such as "but," "although," and "however."

Let your original response stand unless you have thought of additional information.

Pace yourself. You will have approximately 60 seconds per question. Avoid dwelling on any one question, or rushing to finish. Set up checkpoints in your test booklet of where you want to be at the end of the first hour, second hour, and so on. You will know before you get close to the end whether you need to adjust your pace.

Analyzing questions

When you first read a question and look at the options, the answer may not be immediately apparent. Although you may be uncertain, don't just pick an answer arbitrarily. You can apply systematic skills of logic and deduction to narrow the five options to two or three possibilities.

Search for key information. As you read the question stem, notice key information (e.g., age, symptoms, lab results, chronic or acute condition, history). Highlight the key information by underlining or circling. **Notice particularly the request of the question** in phrases such as "the most likely diagnosis is," "the most appropriate initial step in management is," "which initial diagnostic evaluation is most appropriate." Take a quick look at the last line of the stem before reading the specific information in the remainder of the stem, especially if it is lengthy.

Analyze options. As you read each option, **try to eliminate** those that are inconsistent with the information you highlighted in the stem. For example, if a question concerns a 65-year-old woman, you would eliminate a procedure that you know applies only to children.

Cue each option. As you consider each option, mark down your initial reaction. In a "one best answer" question there are four "false" options and one "true" answer. For negative one best answer questions, the reverse applies. As you read each option, cue those you are sure of with a symbol such as "F," "N," or a minus sign. Cue true responses with a "T," "Y," or a plus sign. Cue those options you are uncertain about with the symbol you are using and a question mark.

Analyze structural clues in words. Pay attention to the meaning of prefixes, suffixes, and root words, which can sometimes help you decide whether to eliminate an option.

Approaching questions strategically. The following examples show how you might approach questions found in the books of this series.

Example: Amikacin is ordered for a patient with pyelonephritis due to *Klebsiella pneumoniae*. The clearance and volume of distribution of amikacin in this patient are 50 ml/

min and 20 L, respectively. What dose should be administered every 8 hours to obtain an average steady-state plasma concentration of 20 mg/L?
A. 125 mg
B. 400 mg
C. 480 mg
D. 760 mg
E. 1000 mg

Analysis: This is a basic pharmacokinetics question. I can compute the dose needed to reach steady-state plasma concentration by using the information given. Both clearance and the volume of distribution are provided. I remember that only one of them is used in calculating the dose, but which one? My inclination is to use clearance and to multiply by plasma level and time. In that case, my choice is C.

Comment: Although this is a fairly elementary pharmacokinetics question that is probably part of most students' fund of knowledge by the time they take Step 1, it illustrates the possibility of making an error if volume of distribution rather than clearance is used in the computation.

Example: Which of the following individuals has the highest risk of developing schizophrenia?
A. The brother of a patient with schizophrenia
B. The child of one parent with schizophrenia
C. The child of two parents with schizophrenia
D. The monozygotic twin of a patient with schizophrenia
E. A child raised in an institutional setting

Analysis: I know this question has to do with the genetics of mental illness and the chances that relatives of people who have schizophrenia will develop the disease. I can eliminate E because there is no genetic relationship there. The likelihood is greater for a child of two parents with schizophrenia than one, so B can be eliminated. Although I don't remember specific rates associated with the remaining options, from what I know of hereditary patterns in general among monozygotic twins, I am inclined to choose D.

Comment: Although this question, too, may not be particularly difficult, the strongest possibility for making an error is in misjudging the genetic pre-eminence of one relationship over another, and thereby choosing A or C instead of D. Students may be unable to remember specific concordance *rates* for the disease, but from their knowledge of genetic principles, they can infer which relationship presents the highest risk.

Relying on test question cues

The ability to use the characteristics or the formats of the test itself to increase your score is sometimes referred to as "test wiseness." It is possible to make use of idiosyncrasies in the way the questions are constructed to decide on the correct choice. This technique should be used only if you are unable to answer the question based on direct knowledge or reasoning. The following are examples of the principles of test wiseness, but you may have little opportunity to use them on USMLE Step 1, because the experts who construct the questions eliminate these cues.

Length of an option. If an option is much longer or much shorter than the others, it is more likely to be correct.

Grammatical consistency. Options that are not grammatically aligned with the stem are probably false.

Specific determiners. Options that contain words such as "all," "always," and "never" overqualify an option and are likely to be false.

Overuse of the same words or expressions. Some test makers have a tendency to repeat words or phrases in the options. If you are unsure of an answer, select from the options with the repeated words or phrases. Another variation of this principle is to select an option in which a key word from the stem is repeated.

Numeric midrange. When all options can be listed in numeric order (e.g., percentages), the correct choice will most often be one of the two middle values.

Guessing

The following are "last resort" strategies, but you should be aware of them.

1. If you have eliminated one or two options, but have no idea about the remaining ones, choose the first in the list.

2. If you are unable to eliminate any options, choose A, B, or C.

3. If you have a number of questions left to do and time is running out, **do not leave blanks.** Choose A, B, or C, and fill in the same letter for all remaining questions.

Self-Management Skills

Time

Study in blocks. Assuming you plan to study 4 to 5 hours each night, you might consider dividing those hours into two study blocks. This allows you to study two areas, one that is weaker and therefore requires more time, and another that is relatively strong and can be allocated less time. The advantage of studying two sciences concurrently is that you will move through your strong science with ease and feel a sense of accomplishment, even if the weaker science does not reach the same level of confidence.

Set goals for each study block. Begin by identifying a few goals you think can be accomplished within that block of time. The goals need not be elaborately stated. Identifying what you think is important to study increases the chances that you will study *actively* (with heightened awareness) since you are controlling the purpose, direction, and rate of the studying.

Set realistic deadlines. Although your accuracy in estimating how long it takes you to complete a study agenda will vary, observe whether you habitually overestimate. Arbitrary deadlines are self-defeating if you have little or no chance of meeting them. Set more realistic targets and attempt to meet them most of the time.

Use record-keeping devices. Calendars and appointment books will help you schedule your study agenda and permit you to look ahead and adjust plans to meet deadlines.

Control distractions. There are many kinds of distractions, some of which are self-imposed. Others, such as telephone calls, can interrupt concentration and make it harder to get back to work. If a call is not urgent, decide on a response within the first 30 seconds (e.g., "I'll call you back later. I'm in the middle of something important."). When you do call later, use it as a reward for having worked well, and enjoy it. Also, learn to say "No" to requests that take time and distract you from your schedule.

Effort

Avoid activities that dissipate effort. Be aware of whether there are things you do each day that reduce your total energy, and particularly the energy you want to give to studying. Think about which of the "nonessential" tasks you can delegate to other family members, or to friends who want to be helpful. Give them some direction about what kind of help you would appreciate most.

Try to anticipate crises. There are disruptive life events that happen to all of us that we cannot anticipate but must deal with as best we can. But, there are other events of a less traumatic nature that, if they occur, can interrrupt the flow of a study plan and throw you off course (e.g., the car breaking down and needing immediate repair, a relative who wants to come and stay with you, or a friend who needs your advice on a troublesome problem).

Anticipate crises that may happen during the span of your preparation and have alternative plans ready that permit you to be a part of what is going on but do not derail you completely.

Reward yourself for good effort. After having sustained a stretch of "heavy duty" studying, reward yourself by doing something that for you is pleasurable. A phone call to or from a friend that might be a distraction if it happens when you are trying to study can be a source of pleasure if you can defer it until you have completed your agenda for that day.

Resources

The following testing materials are appropriate for self-testing to guide further study. Their use is described in the next section.

Instructor content tests. These tests consist of questions prepared by the instructor who taught a particular segment of content. Some medical schools retain former course exams on file for student practice. Although the questions may not be structured as they appear on the Step 1 exam, they are good for pinpointing specific gaps or confusions in your knowledge base. Keep records of each practice test result and note relative performance across sciences and across topics in each science. For example, in pathology, note if one system (e.g., respiratory, cardiovascular, endocrine) is notably weaker than another. Cue topics that will need more sustained study. Take advantage of the instructor's presence to seek help, if needed.

Published books of practice questions. The books in this series arrange basic science content into "principles" (one book), "normal and abnormal processes" (one book), and "body systems" (three books).

Monitoring Functions

Monitor study progress

During this phase, when you are strengthening your learning, you will want to get **data-based feedback** using numeric scores to chart your progress.

Use questions to monitor progress

The pattern that works best is study, test, follow-up. Although there are times when it is appropriate to use questions before study to stimulate motivation or trigger recall, at this stage the best use of questions is after preliminary study. When you believe you have learned a segment of material, try a batch of questions. If time permits, you might want to test yourself on each major topic after completing its study, and before testing yourself on a mixed batch of topics in a science. However, if time is limited, select those topics about which you feel the most uncertainty, and use the feedback to guide additional study.

Select a representative sample of questions and complete them using the same time limits as will be used on your class exam or Board exam (approximately 60 seconds per question). Record your answers on a sheet of paper rather than in the question book or on the class practice exam. A separate sheet will allow you to do error analysis (described later) and keeps the book "clean" for future question retakes. **Do not do questions one at a time and then read the answer.** The purpose is not to learn a particular question, but to find out which topics require follow-up.

Score your responses, but do not read answers immediately since you may want to give some questions a second try. After performing error analysis, decide which topics need further study and the type of study needed.

Compute an accuracy percentage by dividing the number correct by the total number of questions. Keep a record of your scores and note whether your accuracy level is approaching the percentage required for passing (for Board exams, between 55% and 65%). For class exams, the percentage may be higher.

Analyze for errors. It is important to analyze more specific aspects of your study and test-taking behavior to direct further study and make it more focused and productive.

1. Were patterns of errors noted (e.g., questions related to DNA principles, or questions about immune responses, or questions regarding quantitative methods)?
2. Did you misread or misinterpret the question?
3. Were questions missed because, although you understood the concept, you forgot important details?
4. Did you note errors in addressing the *decision* required by the question? For example, although you knew much about the disease process described, you could not differentiate a likely diagnosis, or you were unable to form a judgment about a mechanism involved, draw an inference about the appropriate next step in management, or make a prediction about which drug would cause an adverse effect. In other words, you were unable to transform your conceptual and factual knowledge to meet the request of the question.

Monitor test anxiety

One aspect of self-testing that you should be monitoring is whether you are experiencing *inordinate* anxiety when dealing with test questions. It is not unusual to feel some elevation in anxiety when facing a comprehensive and consequential examination such as Step 1. But, if the amount of worry and the physiologic aspects (rapid breathing, sweaty palms, increased heartbeat) become so preoccupying that they interfere with productive studying, then some professional attention may be needed. If, however, test anxiety is of reasonable proportion, then remember what many studies have found. The best defense against test anxiety is a combination of strong review of subject matter, practice on tests similar to the target test, and positive self-reinforcement throughout the preparation process.

Combat negative self-statements

Part of your monitoring should include awareness of your moods and general state of being. Be sensitive to when you are about to give yourself a negative self-evaluation and combat it with an accurate, but positive one. "What if I don't. . ." statements will intrude periodically and, if permitted, can change your mood and distract you from your study. Start practicing self-talk by having a positive statement ready to use to redirect yourself back to your agenda ("I've been studying well and my scores show I'm making progress. . . I just need to keep going!" or "I can't afford the time to worry now; maybe late tonight; back to the topic now").

Strategies for Reaching Mastery

By the time you reach this stage you should feel more confident that your knowledge is firmer and that you can retrieve information dependably. The tasks of this stage deal with refining, or fine-tuning, for increased accuracy.

1. Focus on follow-up study. Your study agenda at this stage should be based on findings from your error analysis of questions you practiced, as well as any behavioral observations you noted from monitoring your performance.

If there are topics you need to reinforce, check your resources to note if those explanations are adequate, or if confusions still remain that may need to be clarified through use of another text or discussion with a peer.

If details are eluding you, engage in some of the memory strengthening activities noted in the previous stage, particularly use of mnemonics, and cumulative practice.

If you misread information in questions, remember to highlight pertinent cues as you read, to focus on comprehension and avoid regressions, and to vary your rate to emphasize meaning.

If one of the patterns you noted is that errors were made on questions with very long stems, practice by first reading the "request" at the end of the question stem. You may then be able to interpret the direction and relevance of the information in the question more quickly and accurately.

If you found that you were unable to translate your knowledge to the specific *thinking* requirement of the question (form a judgment, integrate information to form a conclusion, draw an inference), first check to make sure you know the principles or mechanisms the question assumes you know (e.g., biosynthesis and degradation, dose–effect relationships, alterations in immunologic function). Then, analyze the question through a "think aloud" procedure, with a peer if possible, and try to identify why your thinking is inaccurate.

2. Engage in comprehensive self-evaluation. If you have practiced questions topically, and through a systems approach, as in this series, and followed up with focused review, you should be ready to test yourself with comprehensive question sets. These sets will contain questions that sample most of the domains of information represented on the target exam. The procedure in using those questions, scoring them, and analyzing errors is the same as described previously. Since the question sets are likely to be longer (approximately 150–200 questions), schedule them during the last 2 or 3 weeks, with time between each to benefit from the feedback. Some students end self-evaluation before the last week because further testing too close to the exam date heightens their anxiety.

3. Deal with interfering test-taking behaviors and attitudes. If your self-observations have noted any test-taking behaviors that need improvement, this is the time to correct them.

Impulsive responding. Do you find yourself getting annoyed if the answer to a question is not immediately apparent, and simply choose an option impulsively? Try to curb your impatience, and remind yourself that some questions are designed to engage you in an internal dialogue before deciding on a response.

Inability to move on. Are you unable to disengage from a particularly troublesome question and move on to the next one? This is especially bothersome when you have that tip-of-the tongue feeling that the answer is something you know, but seems just a little out of reach. Difficult as it seems, try not to allow yourself to become irritated and get "stuck" to that question. Choose an answer and move on. It is likely that if you return to it later on, something may trigger recall.

Carrying over previous unsuccessful testing experiences. If comprehensive multiple-choice exams have been problematic for you in the past, and particularly if a recent attempt has not been successful, you may be tempted to see yourself as a "poor test-taker" and allow a defeatist attitude to permeate your self-testing activities. It would be better to start by asking yourself, "Why do I not do as well as I would like on multiple-choice exams?" Then, through your self-observations and data-based assessments, note any interfering behaviors you would like to change and implement activities that are more effective and can lead to success on such exams.

Self-Management Skills

Time

Set and maintain study priorities. One of the biggest problems experienced by some medical students at any level of training is approaching an exam deadline realizing that there is still so much to learn that they will not reach the stage of "mastery." After some last minute cramming they may even "pass," but the feeling of personal accomplishment eludes them. Although this has happened to all of us at one time or another, if it occurs as an ongoing pattern, then some change is needed. Make a list at the beginning of the week of all the study activities you want to accomplish and rank them in order of *importance* and *urgency*. At the beginning of the next week look at any low-priority items left undone and decide where to arrange them in that week's list. Make a record of each time you procrastinated or gave in to other distractions. Also note how often you kept to your schedule—it can motivate and encourage you to stay with it.

Schedule time for self-testing. Avoid deferring your first self-testing until just before an exam deadline. Build it into your schedule as part of your ongoing study activities and benefit from the feedback. You can then do "last minute" testing to aim for greater accuracy.

Effort

Avoid excessive fatigue. It is expected that you will work hard to be ready for an exam, but allowing yourself to get excessively tired and sleep deprived sabotages your goal. Respond to your body's need for rest instead of pushing for another hour's study with little to show for it. Try to pace yourself so that you have energy left to think clearly when you take the exam.

Keep motivation high. One of the possible pitfalls toward the end of your review is a reduction in your level of attention and concentration, because of either fatigue or emerging apprehension about the imminence of the exam. If you have done some record keeping during the preparation sequence, it is now helpful to look back and acknowledge how far you have come from the point where you started. Reward yourself for progress by planning a pleasurable activity following a block of concentrated study, and enjoy it without guilt.

Resources
Comprehensive question sets. For USMLE Step 1, materials such as Williams & Wilkins' *Review for USMLE Step 1* (NMS series), which provides five practice exams with approximately 200 questions in each exam, will be useful for comprehensive evaluation.

Monitoring Functions

As the exam deadline approaches, you may find that you are experiencing frequent mood shifts. When things are going well, your spirits may be high, but after a disappointing day you may feel blue, gloomy, or even angry. Recent research has found that some techniques work better than others to escape from a bad mood:

1. Take some action. If possible, do something to solve the problem that is causing the bad mood.
2. Spend time with other people, particularly to shake sadness. Focus on something other than what is getting you down.
3. Exercise. The biggest boost comes to people who are usually sedentary, rather than the already aerobically fit.
4. Pick a sensual pleasure, such as taking a hot bath or listening to a favorite piece of music. Be careful of using eating for this purpose; it may work in the short run, but may backfire, leaving you feeling guilty. Drinking and drugs are to be avoided for obvious reasons.
5. Try a mental maneuver such as reminding yourself of previous successes to help bolster your self-esteem.
6. Take a walk. Cool down before confronting whatever gave rise to your negative feelings.
7. Try to see the situation from the other person's point of view—why someone might have done whatever provoked your anger.
8. Lend a helping hand to someone in need. If you are studying, offer to help someone understand a science topic in which you feel very competent.
9. Use stress reduction techniques. Among the most effective are progressive relaxation, which uses tension and tension release in the body's muscle groups; mental imagery, which is putting yourself mentally in a location that evokes feelings of calm and peacefulness; and meditation, which aims for a state of relaxed alertness.

Grace Bingham, Ed.D.

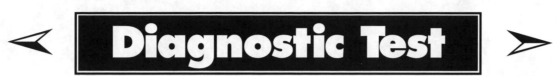

Diagnostic Test

QUESTIONS

DIRECTIONS:

Each of the numbered items or incomplete statements in this section is followed by answers or by completions of the statement. Select the ONE lettered answer or completion that is BEST in each case.

Questions 1-2

A researcher isolates messenger RNA (mRNA) from a rat's liver. He uses this material as the template for the production of complementary DNA (cDNA), and then clones the product to construct a cDNA library.

1. Which one of the following enzymes is used to synthesize cDNA from an mRNA template?

(A) DNA polymerase I
(B) DNA polymerase-α
(C) Terminal transferase
(D) Reverse transcriptase
(E) RNA polymerase

2. The cDNA library is most likely to contain which one of the following?

(A) Exons
(B) Promoters
(C) Introns
(D) TATA sequences
(E) Enhancers

3. Assuming the use of two standard deviations to establish the reference interval of a test, what is the approximate percent chance that a normal person could have at least one false-positive test result if two tests are ordered?

(A) 5%
(B) 10%
(C) 15%
(D) 20%
(E) 30%

4. The trace metal that is a cofactor for mitochondrial superoxide dismutase and glycosyl transferase in mucopolysaccharide synthesis is

(A) manganese
(B) selenium
(C) molybdenum
(D) fluoride
(E) chromium

5. A 7-year-old child whose parents divorced 1 year ago has been getting into her mother's bed each night at 2 A.M. for the past 3 months. She often complains of a headache on weekday mornings and seems reluctant to go to school. The best diagnosis for this child is

(A) specific phobia
(B) separation anxiety disorder
(C) social phobia
(D) post-traumatic stress disorder
(E) somatization disorder

6. Which of the following amino acids is a precursor of melatonin?

(A) Tyrosine
(B) Tryptophan
(C) Histidine
(D) Isoleucine
(E) Phenylalanine

Questions 7-8

Study the following hemagglutination inhibition (HI) assay pattern. Circles 1 through 7 represent test tubes in which increasing dilutions of a serum-containing antibody have been added to influenza virus, followed by constant amounts of influenza virus, and finally red blood cells (RBCs). The controls contain RBCs plus saline (8), RBCs plus serum (9), or RBCs plus virus (10).

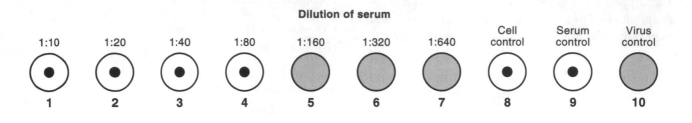

7. Which of the test tubes demonstrate hemagglutination inhibition (HI)?

(A) 1, 2, 3, 4, 8, 9
(B) 5, 6, 7, 10
(C) 8, 9
(D) 5, 6, 7
(E) 1, 2, 3, 4

8. What is the titer of the serum assayed in the hemagglutination inhibition (HI) test?

(A) Less than 10
(B) 80
(C) 120
(D) 160
(E) Greater than or equal to 640

9. Which of the following trace metals is a cofactor for the enzyme that is inhibited by allopurinol?

(A) Selenium
(B) Zinc
(C) Molybdenum
(D) Copper
(E) Manganese

10. A woman tells her primary care physician that she cannot urinate in a public restroom because she is embarrassed. Because of this problem, she can rarely leave home. The best diagnosis for this patient is

(A) specific phobia
(B) separation anxiety disorder
(C) social phobia
(D) post-traumatic stress disorder
(E) somatization disorder

11. A patient has maple-syrup urine disease. Enzymes of the branched-chain α-keto acid dehydrogenase complex are isolated by biopsy and have a higher than normal K_M value for a cofactor. Which of the following vitamins has the greatest probability of allaying the patient's disease symptoms when administered in pharmacologic doses?

(A) Thiamine
(B) Folate
(C) Ascorbate
(D) Pyridoxine
(E) Niacin

12. Middlevillage, New York is a city of 100,000 people. During 1990, there were 1000 deaths from all causes. There were a total of 300 patients with AIDS, of which 200 were men and 100 were women. During 1990, 50 of 60 deaths from AIDS occurred in men. What is the sex-specific mortality rate for men given these data?

(A) 50 per 60
(B) 50 per 200
(C) 50 per 100,000
(D) 110 per 100,000
(E) It cannot be calculated from the data given

13. An assay from the liver biopsy from a patient with high serum levels of phenylalanine shows that the phenylalanine hydroxylase activity is within normal limits. Which of the following cofactors is most likely to be deficient in vivo?

(A) Coenzyme Q
(B) Flavin adenine dinucleotide (FAD)
(C) Flavin mononucleotide (FMN)
(D) Lipoic acid
(E) Tetrahydrobiopterin

14. A married, 35-year-old patient tells his physician that people at work have hated him for the past 10 years and have taken out a contract on his life because he filed a protest against them with the management 10 years previously. Although he is frightened because he believes he is going to be killed, his speech and behavior are otherwise normal. His wife tells the physician that aside from his belief about the people at work, he functions well in his job and participates in family life. The most likely diagnosis for this patient is

(A) schizophrenia
(B) major depressive disorder
(C) bipolar disorder
(D) delusional disorder
(E) brief psychotic disorder

15. Newborns with excessively high bilirubin levels are treated with blue fluorescent light. This treatment converts the bilirubin to more soluble isomers, which can then be excreted in the urine. Before receiving this treatment, these newborns fail to excrete sufficient quantities of bilirubin in the urine because they have a low activity of

(A) bilirubin glucuronyl transferase
(B) bilirubin albuminyl transferase
(C) bilirubin oxidase
(D) bilirubin dehydrogenase
(E) bilirubin glutathionyl-S-transferase

16. How do acyclovir and ganciclovir inhibit herpes-virus replication?

(A) They block capping of viral messenger RNA (mRNA)
(B) They inhibit reverse transcriptase activity
(C) They inhibit viral polymerase activity
(D) They block viral uncoating
(E) They inhibit viral induction of interferons

17. Dopamine hydroxylase converts dopamine to norepinephrine. The vitamin used as a cofactor in this reaction is

(A) A
(B) B_{12}
(C) C
(D) D
(E) E

18. The parents of a 3-year-old boy tell the pediatrician that although the child is toilet-trained during daytime hours, he wets his bed almost every night. What should the pediatrician do?

(A) Prescribe an antihistamine
(B) Prescribe amitriptyline
(C) Prescribe a mild benzodiazepine
(D) Advise the parents to restrict fluids after dinner each evening
(E) Speak to the child about the problem

19. A treatment that helps alleviate the symptoms of all the porphyrias is

(A) ingestion of carefully regulated levels of lead to inhibit δ-aminolevulinic acid (ALA) synthase
(B) avoidance of sunlight
(C) intravenous injection of hemin
(D) bleeding
(E) administration of barbiturates

20. Which organism listed below is regarded as the classic cause of atypical ("walking") pneumonia, characterized by an insidious onset, headache, nonproductive cough, and cold agglutinin formation?

(A) *Chlamydia psittaci*
(B) *Chlamydia trachomatis*
(C) *Klebsiella pneumoniae*
(D) *Mycoplasma pneumoniae*
(E) *Streptococcus pneumoniae*

21. Which of the following membranes has the greatest fraction of lipid?

(A) Mitochondrial outer membrane
(B) Liver cell plasma membrane
(C) Mitochondrial inner membrane
(D) Myelin
(E) Red cell plasma membrane

Questions 22-23

The data in the accompanying table were collected in a case-control study of the relationship between smoking and depression among 1,000 people.

	Level of Depression	
	Severe	Mild
Smokers	200	300
Nonsmokers	100	400

22. What is the prevalence rate of severe depression in this population?

(A) 10%
(B) 30%
(C) 40%
(D) 60%
(E) Cannot be computed from the information provided

23. What is the relative risk of severe depression among smokers compared to nonsmokers?

(A) 10%
(B) 30%
(C) 40%
(D) 60%
(E) Cannot be computed from the information provided

24. Which one of the following vitamins produces cofactors that are involved in glycolysis, ketone body synthesis, gluconeogenesis, and the pentose phosphate pathway?

(A) Niacin
(B) Thiamine
(C) Biotin
(D) Riboflavin
(E) Pantothenic acid

25. Why is it difficult to obtain a live, attenuated influenza virus vaccine?

(A) Antigen drifting results from major point mutations in the matrix protein

(B) The host immune response is poor

(C) Antigen shifts involving changes in hemagglutinin (H), neuramindase (N), or both occur

(D) It is not possible to serotype the viruses properly

(E) It is not possible to isolate the virus

26. The formula for calculating free-water clearance (C_{H_2O}) is: $C_{H_2O} = V - Cosm$, where V = the volume of urine in ml/min, and where $Cosm = (Uosm \times V) \div Posm$. If a patient has a V of 10 ml/min, a Uosm of 900 mOsm/kg, and a Posm of 300 mOsm/kg, you would conclude that

(A) the patient is excreting excess free water

(B) in this patient the diluting segment of the ascending limb is defective

(C) in this patient antidiuretic hormone (ADH) has been suppressed

(D) the patient must have hypernatremia

(E) the patient must be concentrating urine

27. Rhinoviruses differ from enteroviruses in that they

(A) are RNA viruses

(B) are inactivated at an acid pH

(C) must be inoculated into suckling mice to be isolated

(D) have the least number of serotypes

(E) are positive-strand viruses

28. In which of the following fluid derangements would the patient have pitting edema and a decrease in plasma osmolality (Posm)?

	Gain/Loss	TBNa	TBW
A	Loss	↓	⇓
B	Gain	↑	↑
C	Gain	↑	⇑
D	Gain	⇑	↑
E	Loss	⇓	↓

Abbreviations: ↓ = decrease; ↑ = increase; TBNa = total body sodium; TBW = total body water.

29. An American serviceman returns to the United States after service in the Persian Gulf. He was stationed in an area where sandflies and rodents are common. He makes an appointment with his physician because of a moist lesion on his skin. A leishmanial antigen skin test is positive. The serviceman is most likely infected with which organism listed below?

(A) *Leishmania donovani*

(B) *Leishmania major*

(C) *Leishmania braziliensis braziliensis*

(D) *Leishmania braziliensis guyanensis*

(E) *Leishmania aethiopica*

30. Which of the following vitamin:biochemical reaction relationships is correct?

(A) Biotin:Pyruvate → Acetyl CoA

(B) Thiamine pyrophosphate:Pyruvate → Oxaloacetate

(C) Riboflavin: NADPH + H^+ + Oxidized glutathione (GSSG) → $NADP^+$ + Reduced glutathione (GSH)

(D) Niacin:Alanine ↔ Pyruvate

(E) Pyridoxine:Malate ↔ Oxaloacetate

31. What is the term for bacteria that are human pathogens and grow preferentially at 37°C?

(A) Psychrophiles
(B) Thermophiles
(C) Mesophiles
(D) Protoplasts
(E) Spheroplasts

32. Which of the following correctly characterizes atrial natriuretic peptide (ANP)?

(A) Vasodilates peripheral and intrarenal vessels
(B) Enhances the release of antidiuretic hormone (ADH)
(C) Stimulates renin release
(D) Augments angiotensin II activity
(E) Is suppressed in left atrial failure

33. Which of the following organs is most affected in AIDS?

(A) Skin
(B) Brain
(C) Lungs
(D) Liver
(E) Bone marrow

34. The most common direct cause of death in anorexia nervosa is:

(A) a ventricular arrhythmia
(B) protein-energy malnutrition (PEM)
(C) negative nitrogen balance
(D) rupture of the stomach
(E) infection

35. Which one of the following organisms is responsible for the greatest number of cases of pelvic inflammatory disease (PID) in the United States?

(A) *Neisseria gonorrhoeae*
(B) *Chlamydia trachomatis*
(C) *Escherichia coli*
(D) Herpes simplex virus type II
(E) *Trichomonas vaginalis*

36. In protein-energy malnutrition (PEM), there is

(A) a decrease in cutaneous hypersensitivity to common antigens (anergy)
(B) a normal total lymphocyte count
(C) normal phagocytic function
(D) an increase in suppressor T cells
(E) a nitrogen balance approaching zero

37. A deficiency of aldosterone (e.g., Addison's disease) would be expected to have which of the following effects on the sodium/potassium pump in the distal and collecting tubules in the kidneys?

(A) Retention of sodium
(B) Retention of potassium
(C) Reclamation of bicarbonate
(D) Loss of hydrogen ions in the urine
(E) Metabolic alkalosis

38. "Zinc fingers" serve as binding sites for hormones that

(A) act rapidly
(B) effect cAMP levels
(C) liberate diacylglycerol
(D) alter transcription rates
(E) are proteinaceous

DIRECTIONS:

Each of the numbered items or incomplete statements in this section is negatively phrased, as indicated by a capitalized word such as NOT, LEAST, or EXCEPT. Select the ONE lettered answer or completion that is BEST in each case.

39. All of the following statements concerning bacterial capsules are true EXCEPT

(A) most capsules are polysaccharide capsules, but some bacteria have polypeptide capsules
(B) loss of the ability to produce capsules has no effect on viability
(C) capsule production is not influenced by environmental conditions
(D) both gram-negative and gram-positive bacteria can produce capsules
(E) capsules interfere with normal phagocyte function

40. All of the following statements concerning animal viruses with RNA genomes are true EXCEPT

(A) the genomes can be segmented
(B) the nucleocapsids can be icosahedral
(C) the nucleocapsids can be helically symmetric
(D) the genomes must use the host cell's RNA polymerase II to produce viral messenger RNA (mRNA)
(E) the genomes may be single stranded or double stranded

Questions 41-42

A teacher complains that an 8-year-old student cannot pay attention and is often disruptive in class.

41. All of the following characteristics are probably true EXCEPT that this child

(A) is more likely to be male than female
(B) has a very low IQ
(C) cried excessively as an infant
(D) will have problems paying attention in adulthood
(E) has an alcoholic parent

42. All of the following statements are correct regarding the condition described in the preceding question EXCEPT that it

(A) is treated with psychostimulants
(B) has a genetic component
(C) is usually due to disease of the right hemisphere
(D) can coexist with conduct disorders
(E) occurs in 3% to 5% of children ages 5 to 12

43. All of the following are true statements concerning poliovirus infection EXCEPT

(A) the incidence is highest during the summer months
(B) the virus destroys anterior horn cells to produce lower motor neuron paralysis
(C) infection can be associated with fever and myalgias
(D) the virus proliferates in lymphoid tissue within the gastrointestinal tract
(E) infection is more likely to produce death in children than in adults

44. Which one of the following mechanisms is LEAST likely to be operative as a host defense against tumors?

(A) The formation of immune complexes leading to activation of the complement system
(B) Activation of natural killer (NK) cells
(C) Activation of macrophages
(D) Activation of cytotoxic CD8 T cells
(E) Activation of antibody-dependent cell-mediated cytotoxicity

DIRECTIONS:

Each set of matching questions in this section consists of a list of four to twenty-six lettered options (some of which may be in figures) followed by several numbered items. For each numbered item, select the ONE lettered option that is most closely associated with it. To avoid spending too much time on matching sets with a large number of options, it is generally advisable to begin each set by reading the list of options. Then for each item in the set, try to generate the correct answer and locate it in the option list, rather than evaluating each option individually. Each lettered option may be selected once, more than once, or not at all.

Questions 45-47

For each clinical description, select the most likely diagnosis.

(A) Pernicious anemia
(B) Goodpasture's syndrome
(C) Grave's disease
(D) Hashimoto's disease
(E) Myasthenia gravis
(F) Rheumatoid arthritis
(G) Systemic lupus erythematosus (SLE)
(H) Insulin-dependent diabetes mellitus

45. During a visit to her physician, a 48-year-old executive shows signs of excessive irritability, nervousness, and heat intolerance. She has weight loss in spite of a good appetite.

46. The mother of an 11-year-old boy with a recent history of mumps brings her son to the pediatrician because of frequent, copious urination, excessive thirst, and weight loss. The mother relates that her son has had visual disturbances and constantly complains of being tired.

47. A 30-year-old woman presents with fever, weight loss, and painful joints. Laboratory tests show that the patient has a direct Coombs'-positive hemolytic anemia, a high-titered serum antinuclear antibody with a "rim pattern," and a low C3 level.

Questions 48-50

For each characteristic, select the most likely mediator.

(A) Prostaglandin D_2
(B) Leukotriene C_4
(C) Histamine
(D) Platelet-activating factor
(E) Eosinophil chemotactic factor of anaphylaxis

48. It is the major preformed mediator in immediate hypersensitivity reactions.

49. Nonsteroidal anti-inflammatory drugs (NSAIDs) act primarily by blocking its synthesis.

50. Its action may indirectly down-regulate immediate hypersensitivity reactions.

ANSWER KEY

1. D	10. C	19. C	27. B	35. B	43. E
2. A	11. A	20. D	28. C	36. A	44. A
3. B	12. E	21. D	29. B	37. B	45. C
4. A	13. E	22. B	30. C	38. D	46. H
5. B	14. D	23. E	31. C	39. B	47. G
6. B	15. A	24. A	32. A	40. D	48. C
7. E	16. C	25. C	33. C	41. B	49. A
8. B	17. C	26. E	34. A	42. C	50. E
9. C	18. D				

ANSWERS AND EXPLANATIONS

1-2. The answers are: 1-D, 2-A. *(Biochemistry)*
Reverse transcriptase, an enzyme isolated from retroviruses, uses RNA as a template for the synthesis of a complementary strand of DNA (known as complementary DNA or cDNA). This enzyme is commonly used in recombinant DNA work as a step in the generation of a cDNA library. DNA polymerase I, isolated from bacteria, and DNA polymerase-α, isolated from eukaryotes, both synthesize DNA from a DNA template. RNA polymerase synthesizes RNA from a DNA template. Terminal transferase is an enzyme that synthesizes DNA without using a template; therefore, it produces random sequences based on whatever deoxynucleotides are available.

The entire pool of clones produced from a cDNA population is known as a cDNA library. Because cDNA is produced from messenger RNA (mRNA), it will contain exons, or coding regions. Promoters, TATA sequences, and enhancers are all regulatory elements found in DNA, usually outside the transcribed region. Introns, or intervening sequences, are found in mRNA precursors, but they are removed by splicing before mature mRNA is produced.

3. The answer is B. *(Pathology)*
The more tests that are performed on a patient, the greater the chance of obtaining a false-positive result, which is called an outlier (value outside the normal range). The formula to calculate the chance of this happening is: $100 - (0.95^n \times 100)$, where n = the number of tests performed on the patient. Therefore, if two tests are ordered $(100 - [0.95^2 \times 100] = \approx 10\%)$, there is a 10% chance that one of the tests will result in an outlier.

4. The answer is A. *(Biochemistry)*
Manganese is a cofactor for mitochondrial superoxide dismutase and glycosyl transferase, which is used in the synthesis of mucopolysaccharides. Selenium is a cofactor for the enzyme glutathione peroxidase, which is an antioxidant located in the cytosol. Molybdenum is a cofactor for xanthine oxidase. Fluoride is incorporated into bone and enamel, hence strengthening bone and preventing dental caries, respectively. Chromium enhances insulin activity.

5. The answer is B. *(Behavioral science)*
This 7-year-old child is probably suffering from separation anxiety, which occurs most commonly in children 7–8 years of age. It is characterized by excessive concern about separation from parents, reluctance to go to school and sleep alone, and vague physical symptoms. There is no evidence in this child of either a specific phobia (i.e., an irrational fear of something) or a social phobia (i.e., an irrational fear in a social situation). Somatization disorder is characterized by multiple physical complaints in a patient with no physical illness. In post-traumatic stress disorder, symptoms of anxiety occur following a stressful event that most people would consider catastrophic (e.g., an earthquake).

6. The answer is B. *(Biochemistry)*
Melatonin, 5-acetyl-5-methoxytryptamine, is released from the pineal gland in a cyclic fashion; its secretion is stimulated by decreasing light levels and inhibited by light. This hormone is a popular over-the-counter sedative; some 20 million individuals are estimated to have used melatonin products in 1995. It is synthesized from tryptophan according to the following schema:

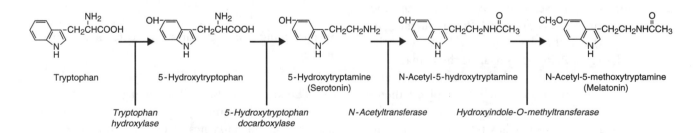

The decrease in light perceived by the retina is passed to sympathetic fibers that innervate the pineal gland via a route through the suprachiasmatic nucleus of the hypothalamus, to the reticular system, to cervical sympathetic ganglia, and finally to the postganglionic sympathetic fibers. The sympathetic-induced release of norepinephrine binds to a β_1 receptor, which raises pineal cAMP levels through the mediation of a G_s protein. The cAMP activates a protein kinase, which phosphorylates and activates the N-acetyltransferase that converts serotonin to N-acetyl-5-hydroxytryptamine, leading to the synthesis and secretion of melatonin. By interfering with this sequence, β-blockers may induce disturbances in the normal sleep pattern.

The role of melatonin has not been fully elucidated in humans, but it is a potent hormone that plays a crucial role in regulating sleep patterns and perhaps, either directly or indirectly, mood and even depressive disorders, such as seasonal affective disorder (SAD). In the United States, melatonin is regulated as a dietary supplement rather than as a drug, which means that its production is not scrutinized by the government and studies have shown that the purity of commercial melatonin products vary greatly. Purity of dietary supplements can be a critical parameter with respect to both potency and safety. L-tryptophan supplements, which were also widely used as sedatives in the 1980s, were removed from the market after several deaths occurred due to a contaminant in some preparations. The effects of tryptophan, no doubt, are related to the fact that it is a serotonin and melatonin precursor.

7-8. The answers are: 7-E, 8-B. *(Microbiology)*
Influenza viruses attach to chicken and guinea pig red blood cells (RBCs), by means of the viral hemagglutinin, to receptors on the RBCs. The virus–RBC combination forms complexes that become aggregant and attach to a surface that is contacted. Positive hemagglutination (HA) is a thin layer of virus RBCs over the bottom of a tube. Antibodies against the hemagglutinin block the attachment of the virus to the RBC and prevent hemagglutination from taking place; therefore, tubes 1, 2, 3, and 4 contain antibody against the viral hemagglutinin, which has prevented HA from occuring. The cell control (tube 8) has only RBCs and saline. No HA is expected. The serum control (tube 9) checks for the presence of nonspecific agglutinins. No HA is expected in this control. Tube 10 is

the virus agglutination positive control. It demonstrates that the virus used is capable of producing HA with the RBCs in the test system.

The titer (measure) of the antibody against the influenza antibody was sufficient to cause hemagglutination inhibition (HI), even when diluted 1:80. There was not sufficient antibody to allow HI at the 1:160 dilution. The definition of HI titer is the last dilution of the patient's serum causing HI to occur. The titer, in this example, would be tube number 4 (1:80 dilution).

9. The answer is C. *(Biochemistry)*
Molybdenum is a cofactor for the enzyme xanthine oxidase in purine metabolism. This enzyme is also inhibited by allopurinol, hence decreasing the synthesis of uric acid. Selenium and vitamin E are important antioxidants in the cytosol and the cell membrane, respectively. Zinc is a cofactor for many different enzymes (e.g., superoxide dismutase, carbonic anhydrase, collagenase, alkaline phosphatase, RNA and DNA polymerases, thymidine kinase). Copper is involved with enzymes that catalyze oxidation–reduction reactions involving oxygen (e.g., cytochrome *c* oxidase in the electron transport system). Manganese is a cofactor for superoxide dismutase.

10. The answer is C. *(Behavioral science)*
The woman who cannot urinate in a public restroom because of embarrassment is probably suffering from social phobia. In social phobia, aspects of the social situation cause irrational fear in the individual. There is no evidence in this woman of separation anxiety disorder or of a specific phobia (i.e., an irrational fear of something). Somatization disorder involves multiple physical complaints in a patient with no physical illness. In post-traumatic stress disorder, symptoms of anxiety occur following a stressful event that most people would consider catastrophic (e.g., an earthquake).

11. The answer is A. *(Biochemistry)*
Thiamine, as thiamine pyrophosphate, serves as the cofactor for four enzymes or enzyme complexes: the pyruvate and α-ketoglutarate dehydrogenase complexes, transketolase, and the α-keto acid dehydrogenase complex. Because the aberrant enzyme from the affected individual has a low affinity for this cofactor,

saturating the body with thiamine may help alleviate the symptoms of the disease. There is no evidence that the other vitamins have any effect on the activity of the α-keto acid dehydrogenase complex.

12. The answer is E. *(Behavioral science)*
The mortality rate is the number of deaths divided by the number of people in the population per year. The sex-specific mortality rate is the number of male deaths or female deaths divided by the number of men or women in the population. Because the number of men in the total population is not given, it is not possible to calculate the sex-specific mortality rate given these data.

13. The answer is E. *(Biochemistry)*
Tetrahydrobiopterin is a cofactor required for phenylalanine hydroxylase, tyrosine hydroxylase, tryptophan hydroxylase, and nitric oxide (NO) synthase. Normally, bihydrobiopterin is synthesized in a reaction catalyzed by bihydrobiopterin synthetase, using guanosine triphosphate (GTP) as a cofactor. Once formed, bihydrobiopterin is reduced to, and maintained as, tetrahydrobiopterin by bihydrobiopterin reductase. A deficiency of either bihydrobiopterin synthetase or bihydrobiopterin reductase leads to lower than normal levels of tetrahydrobiopterin, which in turn reduces the activity of the four enzymes for which it is a cofactor. These variants account for almost half of the cases of phenylketonuria and differ from the classical form, due to phenylalanine hydroxylase deficiency, in that all four tetrahydrobiopterin-requiring enzymes are affected. Therefore, restricting dietary phenylalanine cannot alleviate all symptoms.

14. The answer is D. *(Behavioral science)*
The married 35-year-old patient who believes that people at work have been conspiring against him for the past 10 years is suffering from delusional disorder. Individuals with delusional disorder have one fixed delusional system, but are otherwise relatively functional. Schizophrenic patients also have delusions, but are dysfunctional in other ways as well. There is no evidence of a mood disorder (e.g., major depressive disorder, bipolar disorder) in this patient. This individual is not suffering from brief psychotic disorder because he has had the problem for over 10 years.

15. The answer is A. *(Biochemistry)*
Formation of the water-soluble glucuronide of bilirubin, which is catalyzed by bilirubin glucuronyl transferase, permits the conjugate to be excreted via the bile and in the urine. This enzyme is synthesized late in development, and many newborns have a deficiency that causes jaundice. The other enzymes listed do not exist. Glucuronyl transferases and glutathionyl-S-transferases have the common function of being used in many "detoxification" reactions.

16. The answer is C. *(Microbiology)*
Acyclovir and ganciclovir are variants of acycloguanosine and are used to treat herpes simplex virus and cytomegalovirus infections, respectively. Both agents are viricidal and act by interfering with viral polymerase activity. In the case of herpes simplex virus infection, the virally-coded thymidine kinase monophosphorylates the acyclovir. Cellular kinases then add two more phosphates, creating a nucleotide that is accepted by the virally-coded DNA polymerase. The structural analog is incorporated into the growing DNA chain and elongation is terminated. Ribavirin, used to treat paramyxovirus (respiratory syncytial virus) infection, works by interferring with viral messenger RNA (mRNA) capping. Amantadine, used to treat influenza A infections, blocks viral uncoating. It is most effective when given before viral infection occurs. Reverse transcriptase inhibitors (e.g., azidothymidine, didioxycytocine, didioxyinosine) directly interfere with normal enzyme activity. These agents are virostatic, and virus growth occurs when the agents are removed. Interferons are induced as a result of viral infection of a cell. Products of viral nucleic acid replication activate genes that code for interferons, which directly prevent virus growth by inducing an antiviral protein within virus-infected cells.

17. The answer is C. *(Biochemistry)*
Vitamin C (ascorbate) serves as a cofactor in several hydroxylation reactions, for example, dopamine hydroxylase. In this reaction, the vitamin is used to reduce copper on the enzyme, thereby activating it. Vitamin C has also been implicated as a cofactor required for the hydroxylation of steroids, and it aids in the absorption of iron by reducing it to the ferrous state in the stomach. Its roles in monoamine and

corticosteroid synthesis probably account for its high concentration in the adrenal gland and its rapid use in times of stress. The importance of the vitamin as a cofactor in the formation of collagen, where it is used to hydroxylate proline and lysine, is usually stressed because the most dramatic effect of ascorbate deficiency is scurvy. At higher concentrations, it also plays an important function as a scavenger of toxic free radicals. This nonenzymatic role may help retard development of heart and lung disease, as well as cancer, and may even slow the aging process.

18. The answer is D. *(Behavioral science)*
Enuresis cannot be diagnosed in children younger than 5 years of age. Bedwetting is a normal occurrence in 3-year-old children. The most effective way to reduce bedwetting in this 3-year-old would be to restrict his fluid intake after dinner each evening. Medications are not appropriate for a child this young and speaking to the child about the problem will have little effect because children of this age do not have total control over their bladders.

19. The answer is C. *(Biochemistry)*
Hemin, a compound derived from heme by the oxidation of Fe^{2+} to Fe^{3+}, is an inhibitor of δ-aminolevulinic acid (ALA) synthase, the committed and normally the rate-limiting reaction in porphyrin synthesis. The porphyrias are a group of diseases in which the rate-limiting reaction is one of the intermediary steps in heme synthesis, occurring after the step catalyzed by ALA synthase. The four porphyrias are acute intermittent porphyria, in which uroporphyrin I synthetase is deficient; congenital erythropoietic porphyria, in which uroporphyrin III cosynthetase is deficient; porphyria cutanea tarda, in which uroporphyrin decarboxylase is deficient; and hereditary coproporphyria, in which coproporphyrinogen oxidase is deficient. The clinical symptoms of the porphyrias are due to the accumulation of products behind the step catalyzed by the deficient enzyme, which has now become the rate-limiting one. Using hemin to inhibit ALA synthase, the initial step in the sequence, reduces the accumulation of these intermediary products and alleviates the symptoms. Lead inhibits the second enzyme in the sequence, δ-aminolevulinic acid dehydrase, and in theory should also help alleviate the porphyrias,

but is too toxic to use in therapy. Accumulation of any of the porphyrin ring structures causes the patient to become photosensitive. Therefore, photosensitivity is a symptom of all of the porphyrias except acute intermittent porphyria, in which the block occurs before the ring is formed. Avoiding sunlight does not alleviate symptoms in patients with this disease. Barbiturates accentuate the symptoms of all the porphyrias.

20. The answer is D. *(Microbiology)*
Mycoplasma pneumoniae infection is the classic cause of primary atypical pneumonia, characterized by an insidious onset, headache, nonproductive cough, and cold agglutinin formation. Immunity appears complete, but second episodes of the disease can occur. Autoantibodies against red blood cells (cold agglutinins) are produced, as well as antibodies against brain, lung, and liver cells. Mycoplasma do not have cell walls, but can be grown on complex agar medium. The colony morphology is a small, "fried egg" morphology. *M. pneumoniae* accounts for 5%–10% of community pneumonias and is treated with erythromycin or tetracycline. *Chlamydia trachomatis* respiratory tract involvement is usually seen in 2- to 12-week-old infants. Infection is characterized by a paroxysmal cough, absence of fever, and eosinophilia. Radiographic examination may demonstrate lung consolidation and hyperinflation. Systemic erythromycin is an effective treatment. *Chlamydia psittaci* infections cause a patchy inflammation of the lungs in which consolidated areas are sharply demarcated. An exudate containing mononuclear cells is usually present. The sudden onset of illness in a person exposed to birds is suggestive of psittacosis, which presents with fever, anorexia, a sore throat, and severe headache. Tetracyclines are the drugs of choice. *Klebsiella pneumoniae* causes approximately 3% of bacterial pneumonias and produces an extensive hemorrhagic necrotizing consolidation of the lung. Sensitivity testing is necessary for effective antibacterial treatment. *Streptococcus pneumoniae* causes 75%–80% of bacterial pneumonias and produces disease by multiplying in the lung. The polysaccharide capsule resists phagocytosis, and infection causes an outpouring of fibrinous edematous fluid into the alveoli, followed by red blood cells and leukocytes,

resulting in consolidation of the lung. Eventually, antibody production against the capsules and mononuclear phagocytosis eliminate the infection. Expectoration of bloody sputum and a high fever are characteristic of early disease. Penicillins are the drugs of choice, but recently some resistance has been seen. None of these organisms, except *M. pneumoniae*, causes cold agglutinins to be formed.

21. The answer is D. *(Biochemistry)*

The amount of lipid in a membrane correlates with its function; for example, myelin acts as an insulator. Therefore, it has to be very nonpolar; and, indeed, it contains a very high lipid/protein ratio. In contrast, the inner membrane of a mitochondrion serves as a barrier to most substances, but it has many transporters, each for a specific substance. Therefore, it has approximately 10 times more protein than myelin. Plasma membranes and the outer mitochondrial membrane also permit selective transport, but not to the same degree as the inner membrane of the mitochondria. They, therefore, have an intermediate amount of protein, about 30% of that of the inner membrane of the mitochondria.

22-23. The answers are: 22-B, 23-E. *(Behavioral science)*

The prevalence rate is the number of cases of a condition existing divided by the total population. Because a total of 300 people have severe depression, prevalence rate is calculated as 300 divided by 1,000.

Relative risk cannot be obtained for this case-control (retrospective) study design. Relative risk is obtained for cohort (prospective) studies. The measure of increased risk of severe depression to individuals who smoke is obtained using the odds ratio for case-control studies.

24. The answer is A. *(Biochemistry)*

Niacin produces the cofactors nicotinamide adenine dinucleotide (NAD^+) and nicotinamide adenine dinucleotide phosphate ($NADP^+$), which are involved in oxidation/reduction reactions throughout the body. In glycolysis, NAD^+ and NADH catalyze the glyceraldehyde 3-phosphate to 1,3-diphosphoglycerate reaction and the lactate to pyruvate reaction. In gluconeogenesis, the same pair of cofactors convert malate to oxaloacetate. The conversion of acetoacetate to beta-hydroxybutyrate in ketone synthesis is also catalyzed by the NAD^+/NADH pair. In the pentose phosphate pathway, NADPH is produced, which is involved in the synthesis of glutathione, fatty acids, and cholesterol. Riboflavin is important in the synthesis of flavin mononucleotide (FMN) and flavin adenine dinucleotide (FAD), which are important in oxidative phosphorylation reactions in the mitochondria. Thiamine is involved in the pyruvate dehydrogenase complex (pyruvate conversion to acetyl CoA), α-ketoglutarate complex (conversion of α-ketoglutarate to succinyl CoA), transketolase reactions in the pentose phosphate pathway, and long-chain keto acid decarboxylases. Biotin is a cofactor for pyruvate carboxylase (pyruvate conversion to oxaloacetate). Pantothenic acid is a cofactor in the fatty acid synthase complex and is a component of coenzyme A (transfers acyl groups).

25. The answer is C. *(Microbiology)*

Influenza viruses (orthomyxoviruses) are classified as A, B, or C, based on the protein antigenicity differences found in the capsid coats. Influenza A virus is the most significant for causing frequent epidemics. The viruses can be isolated fairly easily in the diagnostic laboratory on primary monkey kidney cells and identified with monoclonal antibodies. The two main glycoproteins on the viral envelope are the hemagglutinin (H) and neuraminidase (N) proteins. The H protein is the viral receptor molecule; 14 subtypes are known. The N protein aids in the release of the virus from the host cell and exposes cellular receptors by lowering the viscosity of the mucous film in the respiratory tract; nine subtypes are known. Antibodies to these two proteins are the main mechanisms that protect against reinfection by the virus. Antigenic shift is a major, sudden change in the antigenic type of the H protein, N protein, or both (for example, H1 to H2 or N2 to N3). Antigenic shift is most likely caused by a process known as genetic reassortment, which occurs in the growth cycle of viruses with segmented genomes. (For example, the influenza virus has eight pieces of single-stranded, negative-sense RNA.) Coinfection of a single host cell by two such related, but different, viruses can result in up to 256 progeny types with various combinations of RNA genome segments, allowing for a sudden change in antigenicity of the H or N proteins, or both. Such changes produce a new virus that may cause a new epidemic, due to the absence of protecting antibodies in the population. Because major antigenic changes are not predictable, a live, attenuated vaccine would be difficult to develop. Such a vaccine would have to encompass all 14 H and all 9 N proteins. Such viruses simply do not exist, even in this day of genetic manipulation. Antigenic drift represents a minor change in the H or N protein, caused by point mutation. Such changes would not cause a new epidemic. A live, attenuated vaccine is preferable to a killed virus vaccine because live, attenuated vaccines mimic natural infection and elicit a more complete immune response (i.e., humoral and cell-mediated immunity).

26. The answer is E.   *(Physiology)*
Free water is generated in the thick medullary segment of the ascending limb of the nephron when the sodium/potassium/2 chloride cotransport pump transports these electrolytes out of the urine into the medullary interstitium. The formula for calculating free-water clearance is: $C_{H_2O} = V - Cosm$, where V = the volume of urine in ml/min, and where Cosm = (Uosm × V) ÷ Posm. Free water is not bound to solute in the urine and differs from water that must accompany solute, which is called obligated water and is calculated using osmolar clearance (Cosm) as indicated in the formula for free-water clearance. When free water is lost in the urine (absence of antidiuretic hormone) normal dilution occurs, and when it is reabsorbed from the urine (presence of antidiuretic hormone) concentration occurs. Loss of free water is called a positive–free water clearance ($+C_{H_2O}$), whereas reabsorption of free water is called a negative–free water clearance ($-C_{H_2O}$).

Using the information given, the $C_{H_2O} = 10 - [(900 \times 10) \div 300] = -20$ ml/min. A negative C_{H_2O} indicates that normal concentration of urine is occurring in the patient. A defective diluting segment would not result in the generation of free water, hence interfering with normal dilution. Hypernatremia per se would have no direct effect on C_{H_2O}.

27. The answer is B.   *(Microbiology)*
Rhinoviruses, agents of the common cold, and enteroviruses (e.g., poliovirus, coxsackievirus, and echoviruses) are both members of the *Picornaviridae* family.

Rhinoviruses differ from enteroviruses in that they are inactivated at an acid pH. Because enteroviruses must survive the acid in the stomach as part of the normal growth pattern, they do not lose viability if exposed to a pH of 3–5 for 1–2 hours. Rhinoviruses, however, normally reside only in the upper respiratory tract and are acid-sensitive. All picornaviruses have positive-sense, single-stranded RNA. Coxsackieviruses may be classified as belonging to either group A or group B, based on the paralysis pattern that devlops in 1- to 2-day-old suckling mice that have been inoculated intracerebrally with the virus. There are three polioviruses, 29 coxsackieviruses, 32 echoviruses, and more than 120 serotypes of rhinoviruses. Enteroviruses can be easily isolated in the diagnostic laboratory and identified by a neutralizing test. Rhinoviruses can also be isolated, but would not be identified because no specific antibodies are included in the neutralization pools. Such identification, of course, is of little clinical interest, because common colds are recognized on the basis of patient presentation.

28. The answer is C.   *(Pathology)*
Pitting edema refers to excess sodium and water in the interstitial fluid compartment. This most commonly results from an alteration in Starling forces (e.g., increased hydrostatic pressure and/or decreased oncotic pressure). Because sodium is limited to the extracellular fluid compartment, an excess in total body sodium (TBNa) results in pitting edema caused by the greater volume of the interstitial space compared to the vascular compartment. Therefore, to reduce plasma osmolality (2 sodium + glucose/18 + blood urea nitrogen/ 2.8) and produce pitting edema, there must be a greater gain in water than in sodium (dilutional hyponatremia; choice C). Choice A produces an increase in plasma osmolality (Posm; hypernatremia), resulting from a greater loss of water than sodium. A reduction in TBNa leads to poor skin turgor, or dehydration. Choice B results in a normal Posm caused by an isotonic gain of both sodium (pitting edema) and water. Choice D produces an increase in Posm (hypernatremia) with pitting edema. Choice E leads to a low Posm (hyponatremia) and dehydration, resulting from the loss of sodium.

29. The answer is B. *(Microbiology)*
The American serviceman is most likely infected with *Leishmania major*, which has a wide distribution in rural areas of Iran and the Middle East, including the Arabian peninsula. *L. major* causes the moist type of cutaneous leishmaniasis. Humans become infected when they are bitten by sandflies (*Phlebotonus*). Normally transmission of *L. major* is zoonotic, between desert rodents and sandflies, which live in rodent burrows. Many species are members of the *Leishmania donovani* complex, which causes visceral leishmaniasis (e.g., kala-azar, Oriental sore, and mucocutaneous leishmaniasis). In Ethiopia, *Leishmania aethiopica* causes a nonulcerating, blistering, spreading leishmaniasis. The two *Leishmania braziliensis* subspecies (*L. b. braziliensis* and *L. b. guyanensis*) are New World leishmanial organisms. *L. b. braziliensis* causes mucocutaneous leishmaniasis in Amazonian South America, whereas *L. b. guyanensis* infects individuals in other areas of South America. These infections frequently spread along lymphatic routes.

30. The answer is C. *(Biochemistry)*
Riboflavin (B_2) is a component of flavin mononucleotide (FMN) and flavin adenine dinucleotide (FAD), which are important in oxidative phosphorylation reactions in the mitochondria. In addition, riboflavin is a component of glutathione reductase, which produces glutathione, a potent antioxidant that neutralizes peroxides in the cytosol. The pyruvate to acetyl CoA reaction requires thiamine pyrophosphate, which is part of the pyruvate dehydrogenase complex. Biotin is responsible for the conversion of pyruvate to oxaloacetate by acting as a cofactor with pyruvate carboxylase. Pyridoxine (B_6) is involved in transamination reactions, where amino acids are converted into α-keto-acids (e.g., alanine ↔ pyruvate) and α-ketoacids into amino acids. Niacin, formed by nicotinamide adenine dinucleotide (NAD^+) and its reduced form NADH + H^+, is responsible for the conversion of malate to oxaloacetate by malate dehydrogenase.

31. The answer is C. *(Microbiology)*
Bacteria can be classified according to their preferred temperature for growth. Psychrophilic bacteria prefer to grow at low temperatures (10°C), whereas bacteria capable of growing at temperatures of up to 100°C are known as thermophiles. Human pathogens have a temperature preference of 37°C and are called mesophiles. Mesophilic bacteria may be aerobic, anaerobic, or facultative. Removal of the bacterial cell wall by hydrolysis with lysozyme or by blocking peptidoglycan biosynthesis with penicillin produces bacteria that are at risk of lysis because of osmotic pressure situations. Such organisms may survive in an osmotically protective medium. Under these conditions and in a protective medium, protoplasts are produced from gram-positive bacteria, whereas spheroplasts (which retain some outer membrane peptidoglycan components) are produced from gram-negative cells.

32. The answer is A. *(Pathology)*
Atrial natriuretic peptide (ANP) is a counterregulatory factor that offsets an increase in extracellular fluid volume. It is released from the left atrium in response to atrial distention (e.g., left atrial failure). ANP suppresses the hypothalamic release of antidiuretic hormone, inhibits the effect of angiotensin II on stimulating thirst and aldosterone secretion, acts as a vasodilator in the peripheral resistance and intrarenal vessels, directly inhibits sodium reabsorption in the kidneys, and suppresses the release of renin.

33. The answer is C. *(Microbiology)*
Overall, the lungs are the most frequently involved organs in AIDS. The first opportunistic infection is most commonly *Pneumocystis carinii*. Cytomegalovirus and *Mycobacterium avium-intracellulare* are also common pulmonary pathogens. In the brain, AIDS-related dementia and primary malignant lymphomas may occur. Kaposi's sarcoma is the most common cancer in AIDS and often presents first on the skin. Hepatitis A, B, and C are frequently encountered in AIDS patients. Various cytopenias (e.g., thrombocytopenia) and anemia of inflammation are common hematologic manifestations.

34. The answer is A. *(Pathology)*
Ventricular arrhythmias are the most common direct cause of death in anorexia nervosa. In this disease that most commonly afflicts young, intelligent women, a distortion of the body image manifests itself with self-induced weight loss. Once the body fat drops below

15% of the normal weight for the patient, gonadotropin-releasing hormone production drops off, producing gonadotropin deficiency and secondary amenorrhea. Protein-energy malnutrition (PEM) with an associated negative nitrogen balance also occurs, but it is not the most common direct cause of death. Cellular immunity is impaired in PEM, thereby predisposing patients to infection. Bulimia nervosa is more frequently associated with rupture of the stomach (Boerhaave syndrome), owing to self-induced vomiting.

35. The answer is B. *(Microbiology)*
Pelvic inflammatory disease (PID) may include salpingitis, endometritis, and tubo-ovarian abscess and is most often caused by *Chlamydia trachomatis. C. trachomatis* (serovars D through K) causes sexually transmitted disease, especially in developed countries. A serious problem is that often these infections may be subclinical and remain undiagnosed for quite some time. The infection is communicable and may cause nongonococcal urethritis in men. Genital secretions of infected adults can be self-inoculated into the eye. *Neisseria gonorrhoeae* is the second most frequently seen cause of PID. In women, the primary infection is in the endocervix and extends to the urethra and vagina, possibly giving rise to a mucopurulent discharge. The infection may progress to the uterine tubes, with infertility occurring in 20% of women with gonococcal salpingitis. Chronic gonococcal infection may be asymptomatic. Gram-negative rods, such as *Escherichia coli*, are responsible for significant numbers of urinary tract infections in women. These infections are usually characterized by urinary frequency, dysuria, hematuria, and pyuria. The number of cases of PID caused by *E. coli* is relatively small. *Trichomonas vaginalis* infections are normally limited to the vulva, vagina, and cervix. The mucosal surfaces may be tender, inflamed, eroded, and covered with a frothy yellow or cream-colored discharge. Herpes simplex virus type II infection most often manifests as vesicular lesions and becomes latent in neural tissues. PID is usually not a complication of viral infection.

36. The answer is A. *(Biochemistry)*
In protein-energy malnutrition (PEM), impaired cellular immunity and a drop in the helper T-cell count (suppressor T cells are normal) result in problems with a cutaneous response to subcutaneous injection of common antigens. This condition is called anergy. All phases of phagocytic function (phagocytosis, killing, etc.) are impaired. The total lymphocyte count is decreased. In the negative nitrogen balance that occurs, endogenous amino acids derive from the breakdown of muscle. A nitrogen balance approaching zero is found in healthy individuals.

37. The answer is B. *(Pathology)*
Aldosterone deficiency (e.g., Addison's disease) would significantly reduce the activity of the sodium/potassium pump in the distal and collecting tubules. This reduced activity would result in the loss of sodium in the urine and retention of potassium. When potassium is depleted, hydrogen ions are used in the exchange with sodium. Therefore, hydrogen ions are retained (metabolic acidosis) and lose their important role in reclaiming bicarbonate.

38. The answer is D. *(Biochemistry)*
More than a hundred known proteins, including specific DNA binding proteins that have the "zinc finger" domain, require zinc as a cofactor for normal function. Proteins with the zinc finger domain bind to DNA at specific sites after they combine with a specific hormone. Such hormones include thyroid and the steroid hormones and the active forms of vitamins A and D. The interaction with DNA alters the transcription rate of proteins coded at the site where the hormone–protein complex binds. These hormones can thus affect metabolism through a change in the concentration of specific enzymes by altering their rates of synthesis. Because a new product is formed, or an old one is destroyed, as much as a few days may be required before the full effect of the change in concentration of these hormones is manifested. By contrast, hormones that change the activity of preformed enzymes, via effectors, such as cyclic AMP or diacylglycerol, exhibit their effects within seconds.

39. The answer is B. *(Microbiology)*
Capsules are protective devices for those bacteria that have the ability to produce them. Most capsules are polysaccharide, but *Bacillus anthracis* produces a polypeptide capsule. Capsules directly interfere with the

phagocytic function of white blood cells. The presence of capsules may be the primary reason why some microorganisms are pathogenic. *Streptococcus pneumoniae* is invasive because the well-defined polysaccharide capsules allow the bacteria to avoid phagocytosis and the body responds in such a manner that consolidation (pneumonia) of lung sections occurs. Natural recovery occurs coincidentally with the formation of antibodies against the capsular materials. Pneumococci can then be phagocytosed and destroyed. The ability to produce capsules is a genetic function. Like all genetic capabilities, this may be lost or altered by genetic mutation. If an organism loses the ability to produce a capsule, the organism can still survive in the environment or on an agar medium, but the outcome in the body may be less fortunate. When exposed to phagocytic cells, non–capsule-producing strains are efficiently phagocytosed and destroyed intracellularly. Both gram-negative and gram-positive bacteria can produce capsules. Because capsule production is under genetic control, environmental conditions have little or no effect on the production of capsules.

40. The answer is D. *(Microbiology)*

Negative-sense RNA genomes contain a virally-coded RNA-dependent RNA polymerase (transcriptase) that is responsible for viral messenger RNA (mRNA) production, as well as viral genome replication. By having such a necessary enzyme within the virion, these viruses do not depend on the host cell's RNA polymerase II enzyme to produce viral mRNA. (Positive-sense RNA has the same base composition as mRNA.) RNA viruses may have segmented genomes. The genomes may be single or double stranded. Picornaviruses, caliciviruses, reoviruses, and togaviruses all have icosahedral nucleocapsids. Orthomyxoviruses, paramyxoviruses, rhabdoviruses, and bunyaviruses all have helical capsids.

41-42. The answers are: 41-B, 42-C. *(Behavioral science)*

The 8-year-old student who cannot pay attention and is often disruptive in class is probably suffering from attention deficit hyperactivity disorder (ADHD). Children with ADHD have normal IQs and are more likely to be male than female. Alcoholism in parents is associated with ADHD and children with this condition often show excessive crying as infants. The problems associated with ADHD frequently persist into adulthood.

Although children with ADHD may have minor brain damage, there is no evidence of serious structural problems in the brain. ADHD occurs in 3% to 5% of children ages 5 to 12, has a genetic component, and can exist with conduct disorder. This condition is treated commonly with psychostimulant drugs, such as methylphenidate (Ritalin).

43. The answer is E. *(Microbiology)*

The case-fatality rate associated with poliovirus infection is highest in adults and may reach 5% 10%. When poliovirus epidemics occurred before vaccines were available, the vast majority of cases were observed during the summer months. Ingestion of virus-infected water (during swimming, for example) was the route of transmission. Abortive poliomyelitis is a mild, febrile illness characterized by headache, sore throat, nausea, and vomiting. A fever and stiff neck are symptoms of nonparalytic poliomyelitis, which usually resolves spontaneously. Approximately 1% of all infections are clinically apparent. Poliomyelitis occurs worldwide. In developing countries where hygiene and sanitation are poor, children are exposed at an early age and experience mostly asymptomatic infections. In more developed countries, there is an increase in the frequency of symptomatic infection among those who have not been vaccinated. In natural infection, the poliovirus replicates in the oropharynx and lymphoid tissue in the small intestine. The virus then spreads to the central nervous system (CNS) via a viremia or retrograde movement along nerve axons. In the CNS, the virus preferentially replicates in the motor neurons located in the anterior horn of the spinal cord. Death of these cells results in paralysis of the muscles related to those neurons (i.e., the paralysis does not result from the viral infection of muscle cells). The virus may also affect the brain stem, resulting in respiratory paralysis. A post-paralytic syndrome has been described that occurs years after acute illness. The post-paralytic syndrome is evidenced by a marked deterioration of function of affected muscles. The cause is unknown.

44. The answer is A. *(Microbiology)*
Activation of the complement system following the formation of immune complexes (a type III hypersensitivity reaction) is least likely to occur as a defense against tumor cells. Natural killer (NK) cells do not need antibodies to kill cells and can directly kill tumor cells by secreting cytotoxins called perforins, which damage the cell membrane. Macrophages, activated by γ-interferon, are able to attach to tumor cells, killing them by secreting cytolytic enzymes. Cytotoxic CD8 T cells are able to recognize altered class I antigens on neoplastic cells; they kill the neoplastic cells by secreting perforins. Activation of CD8 T cells is a type IV hypersensitivity reaction. Antibody-dependent cell-mediated cytotoxicity enhances the effectiveness of NK cells in destroying neoplastic cells. Complement is not required. The activation of antibody-dependent cell-mediated cytotoxicity is a type II hypersensitivity reaction.

45-47. The answers are: 45-C, 46-H, 47-G. *(Microbiology)*
Grave's disease is a relatively common autoimmune disorder with a peak incidence in the third and fourth decades of life. The female-to-male ratio is approximately 7:1. Major immunological features include autoantibodies against the thyroid-stimulating hormone (TSH) receptor. These autoantibodies stimulate the production of thyroid hormone and the expression of major histocompatibility complex (MHC) class II molecules by the thyroid cells. Goiter is caused by hyperplastic epithelium, the result of persistent TSH stimulation. Lymphocytic and plasma cell infiltration is much less than that seen in Hashimoto's disease. Clinical features of Grave's disease are typical of hyperthyroidism and include heat intolerance, nervousness, irritability, weight loss in the presence of a good appetite, tachycardia, and ophthalmopathy (lid stare, bulging eyes).

Insulin-dependent diabetes mellitis (type I diabetes) is seen most often in children and frequently follows infections with mumps virus, influenza virus, coxsackievirus, cytomegalovirus, or rubella virus. Almost all patients are younger than 30 years of age; the highest incidence is in patients between the ages of 10 and 14 years. An autoimmune etiology has been established in nearly all cases of this disease. The characteristic immunological finding is the presence of autoantibodies against pancreatic beta cells in the islets of Langerhans. These autoantibodies activate complement and destroy the beta cells, resulting in reduced insulin levels and an increase in blood glucose levels. Although it has not been proven yet, the consensus is that similarities between the amino acid sequences of viral proteins and those of beta islet cells leads to attack by complement-activating autoantibodies (and perhaps also self-reactive CD8+ T cytotoxic cells). Lymphocytic infiltration is evident in pancreatic islets, sometimes even before symptoms of glucose intolerance become evident.

Systemic lupus erythematosus (SLE) is the prototype of all autoimmune diseases. It is thought to be caused by a generalized breakdown in immune tolerance. Many organs and organ systems can be affected, including the musculoskeletal system, skin, lungs, heart, kidneys, central nervous system (CNS), gastrointestinal tract, and hematopoietic system. In the young woman described in the question, the clues all point to SLE, especially the diversity of organ systems involved, the "rim pattern" (which represents anti–double-stranded DNA antibody, the most common autoantibody seen in SLE), and the Coombs'-positive hemolytic anemia. Additional support for a diagnosis of SLE is the fact that the patient is female (80%–90% of SLE patients are female) and the low level of C3 (complement is being used up because of extensive immune complex formation).

48-50. The answers are: 48-C, 49-A, 50-E. *(Microbiology)*
Histamine is a very potent preformed mediator found in the granules of mast cells and basophils. In mast cells, it is tightly bound to heparin (which dissociates from it when the complex is released into the extracellular mileu). It is derived from histidine by the action of histidine decarboxylase.

The effects of most nonsteroidal anti-inflammatory drugs (NSAIDs) are similar. They inhibit the production of prostaglandins by inhibiting cyclooxygenase. Prostaglandin D_2 (PGD_2) is a product of arachidonic acid metabolism, via the cyclooxygenase pathway, and is generated during anaphylactic reactions. It is the major prostaglandin produced by mast cells (basophils do not produce PGD_2). It promotes dilatation of blood vessels and increases vascular permeability, but is less potent than histamine in this respect. It also attracts neutrophils. PGD_2, together with histamine, mediates the "wheal-and-flare" reaction seen after skin testing for type I hypersensitivity.

The leukotrienes (LTB_4, LTC_4, LTD_4, and LTE_4) are generated from arachidonic acid by the lipoxygenase pathway. Their activity is not decreased by NSAIDs. LTB_4 is an extremely potent chemoattractant and adhesion agent for neutrophils. LTC_4, LTD_4, and LTE_4 (sometimes referred to as slow-reactive substance of anaphylaxis or SRS-A) induce a slow, sustained contraction of smooth muscle, bronchoconstriction, and mucus secretion. They are among the most important mediators of asthma. The leukotrienes are several hundred times more potent than histamine, when compared on a molecule-to-molecule basis.

Platelet-activating factor (PAF) is a low molecular weight phospholipid that is derived from alkyl phospholipids in platelets, mast cells, and other cell types. The stored inactive form of PAF contains arachidonate, which is excised (upon cell activation) and replaced by acetate to make the bioactive version of the molecule. Activated platelets aggregate and release the contents of their granules, including PGE_2, PGH_2, thromboxane A_2, bioactive amines, and various enzymes.

The proinflammatory effects of PAF include activation and degranulation of neutrophils and eosinophils. In addition, it is the most potent chemoattractant for eosinophils ever identified.

Eosinophil chemotactic factor of anaphylaxis (ECF-A) is a small tetrapeptide that is present in preformed state in the granules of mast cells. It is released during IgE-mediated (type I hypersensitivity), mast cell degranulation, and when certain other molecules (e.g., C3a, C4A, and C5a) bind to the cells. Eosinophils release a variety of substances upon arrival at the site of ECF-A production, including histaminase and arylsulfatase, which degrade histamine and the leukotrienes, respectively. Thus, it has been proposed that eosinophils may be important in down-regulating allergic responses.

The role of eosinophils in allergic reactions remains somewhat controversial. The cells have potential to cause extensive tissue damage, because they contain peroxidase, superoxide dismutase, and numerous acid hydrolases. In addition, they release mediators that can induce degranulation of mast cells and basophils. Large numbers of eosinophils are found in mucous plugs and bronchi of patients dying of asthma.

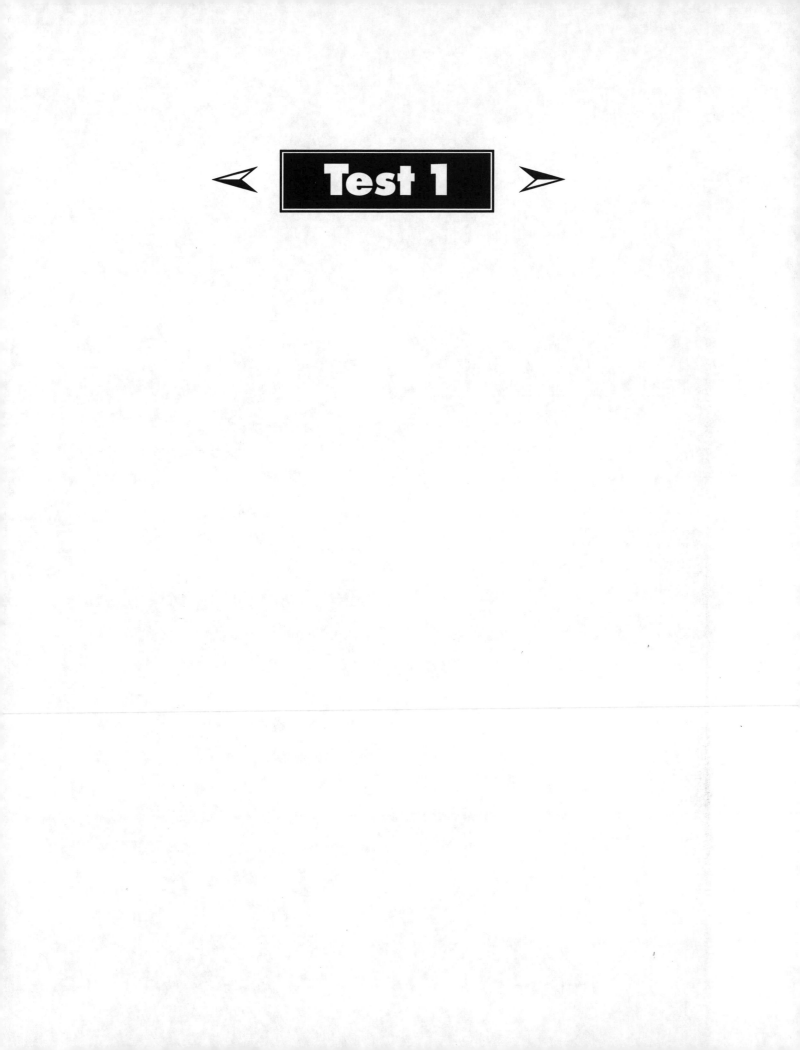

◄ **Test 1** ►

DIRECTIONS:

Each of the numbered items or incomplete statements in this section is followed by answers or by completions of the statement. Select the ONE lettered answer or completion that is BEST in each case.

1. In infants, the social smile develops at age

(A) 0–1 month
(B) 1–2 months
(C) 3–6 months
(D) 6–9 months
(E) 9–12 months

2. A prototroph, such as a wild-type *Escherichia coli*, is growing in a minimal salts and glucose medium. If the amino acid histidine is added to the growth medium, what would be the cell's most immediate response with respect to its biosynthesis of histidine?

(A) Histidine synthesis would be accelerated
(B) Histidine synthesis would be slowed following direct inhibition of enzymes essential to that particular pathway
(C) The enzymes involved in histidine synthesis would be inhibited by the added histidine
(D) The first enzyme in the biosynthetic pathway would be inhibited by histidine
(E) All biosynthetic pathways in the cell would be inhibited

3. Humans are unable to directly convert pyruvate to

(A) alanine
(B) oxaloacetate
(C) acetyl coenzyme A (acetyl CoA)
(D) lactate
(E) phosphoenolpyruvate

4. Some bacteria are pathogenic because they have acquired virulence factors following the incorporation of genetic material provided by the prophage of a bacteriophage. Loss of the prophage converts a pathogenic organism to a nonpathogenic strain. Which one of the following is an example of a virulence factor acquired via a prophage?

(A) The production of diphtheria toxin by *Corynebacterium diphtheriae* and erythrogenic toxin by *Streptococcus pyogenes*
(B) The production of endotoxin by *Escherichia coli* and toxic shock syndrome toxin by *Staphylococcus aureus*
(C) The ability of *Streptococcus pyogenes* to synthesize M protein and the ability of *Staphylococcus aureus* to synthesize protein A
(D) The acquisition of a polysaccharide capsule by *Bacteroides fragilis*
(E) The production of tetanus toxin and botulism toxin by *Clostridium* species

PATH

5. Which one of the following is more characteristic of autosomal recessive disease than autosomal dominant disease?

(A) Early onset of symptoms or signs of the disease T
(B) Variations in penetrance F
(C) Variable expressivity F
(D) Expression of the disease by heterozygotes
(E) Defects in structural proteins, receptors, or transport proteins T

6. Anaerobic organisms make up part of the body's normal flora. Which part of the body listed below has the largest population of indigenous anaerobic bacteria?

(A) Skin
(B) Mouth
(C) Vagina
(D) Lungs
(E) Colon

7. How are insulin and nitric oxide receptors similar?

(A) The interaction of the agonist with the receptor increases guanylate cyclase activity
(B) The interaction of the agonist with the receptor increases tyrosine kinase activity
(C) Both receptors have a rod-like transmembranal domain
(D) Both receptors are monomeric peptides
(E) The interaction of the agonist with the receptor increases adenylate cyclase activity

8. In which pair of disorders is edema related to an increase in vessel permeability?

(A) Right-sided congestive heart failure/minimal change disease
(B) Left-sided congestive heart failure/celiac disease
(C) Bee sting/adult respiratory distress syndrome (ARDS)
(D) Encephalitis/hyponatremia
(E) Pneumonia/cirrhosis

9. Which enzyme is found in muscle but not the liver?

(A) An active glycerol kinase
(B) An active aldolase B
(C) An active phosphocreatine kinase
(D) An allosterically regulated pyruvate kinase isozyme
(E) An active glucokinase

10. Primary cancer is more common than metastasis in which one of the following sites?

(A) Ovary
(B) Brain
(C) Bone
(D) Lung
(E) Liver

11. Which one of the following statements accurately describes the role of acetyl coenzyme A (acetyl CoA) carboxylase in fatty acid synthesis?

(A) It is activated by citrate in muscle
(B) It is inhibited by insulin and activated by glucagon
(C) It is activated by malonyl coenzyme A (CoA) in liver cells
(D) It is found in the mitochondrial matrix
(E) It is activated in the presence of activated biotin

12. Which one of the following is most abundant in secretions?

(A) Immunoglobulin G (IgG)
(B) Immunoglobulin A (IgA)
(C) Immunoglobulin M (IgM)
(D) Immunoglobulin D (IgD)
(E) Immunoglobulin E (IgE)

13. Sulfate groups contribute to the negative charge commonly associated with

(A) glycosaminoglycans
(B) glycogen
(C) proteins
(D) phosphosphingolipids
(E) lysosomal membranes

14. A 28-year-old man has multiple comminuted fractures of both femurs secondary to a motorcycle accident. On his second day in the intensive care unit, the patient develops alterations in his mental status, petechiae, and dyspnea. His arterial oxygen saturation is decreased, but the prothrombin time (PT) and partial thromboplastin time (PTT) are normal. What is the mechanism most likely responsible for this patient's clinical condition?

(A) Disseminated intravascular coagulation (DIC)
(B) Pneumonia
(C) Fat embolism
(D) Atelectasis
(E) Pulmonary embolism

Questions 15-16

At 5:30 A.M. on a Sunday, a febrile 55-year-old man is admitted to the emergency room complaining of acute pain in several joints. Examination of his left knee and right big toe reveals inflammation and exquisite tenderness. The man is recently divorced and had a date the previous evening. In an attempt to impress his date, he took her to an expensive French restaurant where he consumed most of a bottle of Bordeaux wine and a six-course meal, which included sweetbreads, liver pâté, and caviar. He awoke cold and in pain.

15. Which one of the following tests will most likely provide a definitive diagnosis?

(A) Radiography of the affected joints
(B) Magnetic resonance imaging (MRI) of the affected joints
(C) Synovial fluid analysis
(D) Radioimmunoassay to determine parathyroid hormone levels
(E) Serum rheumatoid factor assay

16. The patient is most likely afflicted by which one of the following enzymatic aberrations?

(A) Xanthine oxidase deficiency
(B) Phosphoribosyl-ribose-pyrophosphate (PRPP) synthetase excess
(C) Adenosine deaminase deficiency
(D) Glucose-6-phosphatase deficiency
(E) Complete hypoxanthine-guanine phosphoribosyltransferase (HGPRTase) deficiency

17. Which one of the following characteristics is representative of a venous clot rather than an arterial one?

(A) Predominantly composed of platelets
(B) Pale red in color
(C) Inhibited by aspirin
(D) Likely to occur in a setting of increased turbulence
(E) Composed of clotting factors, erythrocytes, and platelets

18. Digestion of proteins begins in the stomach by the proteolytic action of

(A) aminopeptidase
(B) chymotrypsin
(C) pepsin
(D) enteropeptidase
(E) trypsin

19. A bacterium has a lag phase of 40 minutes and a generation time of 20 minutes. How many cells will there be at the end of 120 minutes, if there are 4000 cells to begin with and there is no stationary phase?

(A) 4×10^{12}
(B) 2.56×10^5
(C) 6.4×10^4
(D) 3.2×10^4
(E) 1.6×10^4

20. Trypsin is likely to cleave the peptide shown below at which point?

A   B   C   D   E
↓   ↓   ↓   ↓   ↓
Leu – Phe – Gly – Arg – Met – Ser

21. The expected alteration in hemostasis is the same in which one of the following combinations?

(A) Postoperative state/aspirin therapy

(B) Disseminated malignancy/heparin therapy

(C) Antithrombin III deficiency/oral contraceptive use

(D) Polycythemia rubra vera/tissue plasminogen activator therapy

(E) Protein C deficiency/coumarin therapy

22. A 33-year-old man ruptures a tendon, restricting his activity. As a result, he gains 25 pounds and develops muscular weakness. His physician persuades him to watch his diet and to start an exercise program. Within a month, his muscular mass increases, but there is no change in weight. Which one of the following scenarios best describes what is happening in this patient?

(A) Before exercising, he was in negative nitrogen balance and his body fat content was increasing; now he is in positive nitrogen balance and his body fat content is constant

(B) Before exercising, he was in positive nitrogen balance and his body fat content was increasing; now he is in negative nitrogen balance and his body fat content is constant

(C) Before exercising, he was in negative nitrogen balance and his body fat content was increasing; now he is in positive nitrogen balance and his body fat content is decreasing

(D) Before exercising, he was in negative nitrogen balance and his body fat content was increasing; now he is in positive nitrogen balance and his body fat content is increasing

(E) Before exercising, he was in positive nitrogen balance and his body fat content was increasing; now he is in negative nitrogen balance and his body fat is constant

23. A teacher tells you that one of his students has tricked many fellow students into giving him their lunch money. The boy, who is 9 years old, rarely follows the school rules and shows little interest in the feelings of others. What is the most correct diagnosis for this child?

(A) Normal

(B) Attention deficit/hyperactivity disorder

(C) Oppositional defiant disorder

(D) Conduct disorder

(E) Antisocial personality disorder

24. Ketoacidosis is both a normal physiologic response to prolonged caloric restriction (e.g., during fasting or stringent dieting) and also an abnormal process associated with type I diabetes. Which one of the following sets of events best distinguishes the untreated diabetic process from the physiologic one of fasting? Relative to the fasting state, in type I diabetes, there is

(A) an increased glucagon–insulin ratio, a higher hepatocyte cyclic adenosine monophosphate (cAMP) level, and an equivalent blood glucose level

(B) an equivalent insulin level, a higher hepatocyte cAMP level, and a higher blood glucose level

(C) a lower insulin level, a higher blood glucose level, and a higher blood fatty acid level

(D) a lower insulin level, a higher blood glucose level, and an equivalent blood fatty acid level

(E) a lower insulin level, a higher blood glucose level, and a lower blood fatty acid level

25. The presence of catalase and superoxide dismutase enzymes in a bacterium indicates that

(A) it can grow under aerobic conditions
(B) it is an anaerobic organism
(C) it will not degrade hydrogen peroxide
(D) its growth will be inhibited by a lowered oxygen concentration
(E) its spores will not germinate in tissue

26. An outbreak of cholera occurs in a refugee camp in Africa. What is the most likely cause of the diarrhea?

(A) Adenosine diphosphate (ADP) ribosylation of elongation factor-2 (EF-2)
(B) ADP ribosylation of a G_s protein
(C) ADP ribosylation of a G_i protein
(D) Phosphorylation of cyclic adenosine monophosphate (cAMP) diesterase
(E) Phosphorylation of adenylate cyclase

27. The effect of changing urine pH on the renal clearance of three drugs is illustrated in the following table.

Drug	Renal Clearance at pH 8	Renal Clearance at pH 5
A	40 ml/min	40 ml/min
B	100 ml/min	35 ml/min
C	55 ml/min	110 ml/min

From this data, it can be concluded that

(A) drug C is a weak base
(B) drug C is a weak acid
(C) drug B is a weak base
(D) drug A is a weak acid
(E) drug A is a weak base

28. Choose the statement that most correctly describes protein and nitrogen metabolism.

(A) The rate-limiting reaction of the urea cycle is catalyzed by arginase
(B) The normal dietary requirement and the daily turnover of protein is approximately 50 grams per day
(C) Albumin serves as a storage form for amino acids in a manner analogous to the storage of glucose in glycogen
(D) The combined action of transaminases (aminotransferases) and glutamate dehydrogenase is responsible for most of the nitrogen in urea
(E) Alanine, the most abundant amino acid in muscle protein, is used as the primary carrier of carbons from muscle to liver for gluconeogenesis

29. The term selective toxicity refers to the fact that

(A) some microorganisms are killed only by large amounts of antibiotics
(B) gram-positive microorganisms are more sensitive to antibiotics than gram-negative organisms
(C) bacteria and their hosts will respond differently to the presence of an antimicrobial agent
(D) only pathogenic strains of a microorganism will be killed by an antibiotic
(E) both gram-positive and gram-negative bacteria will be killed by an antibiotic

30. In humans, which enzymes account for the majority of the nitrogen excreted as urea?

(A) D-Amino acid oxidase and carbamoyl synthetase II
(B) Glutamine synthetase and glutaminase
(C) Glutaminase and carbamoyl synthetase II
(D) Glutamate dehydrogenase and arginosuccinate synthetase
(E) Glutamine synthetase and urease

31. Which one of the following statements concerning phospholipase C is correct?

(A) Its activity is stimulated by hormone–receptor interactions coupled to a Gp protein
(B) It frees a fatty acid bound in an ester linkage to the carbon 2 of glycerol
(C) It initiates a cascade, resulting in the activation of protein kinase A
(D) It initiates a cascade, resulting in the activation of a tyrosine kinase
(E) It initiates a cascade, resulting in the activation of guanylate kinase

32. The inherited disorder cystinuria is caused by a defect in

(A) amino acid synthesis
(B) amino acid transport
(C) amino acid degradation
(D) disulfide bond formation
(E) disulfide bond cleavage

33. A young woman has a chronic gram-positive bacterial infection. Penicillin therapy has controlled successive outbreaks of infection, but a relapse always occurs within weeks of finishing the course of penicillin. The laboratory found no evidence of bacterial resistance to penicillin. Which of the following antibiotics would be the best for future treatment of the infection?

(A) Penicillin
(B) Bacitracin
(C) Cephalosporin
(D) Tetracycline
(E) Vancomycin

34. Five drugs are administered orally to a group of adult human subjects in whom the average rate of hepatic blood flow is 80 L/hour. Based on the data in the table below, which drug has the highest bioavailability?

Drug	Percent Absorbed	Hepatic Clearance
A	30	20 L/hour
B	40	20 L/hour
C	50	40 L/hour
D	50	60 L/hour
E	80	60 L/hour

(A) Drug A
(B) Drug B
(C) Drug C
(D) Drug D
(E) Drug E

35. Which one of the following cell types is most important in innate (natural) immunity?

(A) T lymphocytes
(B) B lymphocytes
(C) Neutrophils
(D) Plasmacytes
(E) Mast cells

36. Which one of the following statements concerning mineral ions is true?

(A) The majority of the calcium ion (excluding bone) in the body is intracellular and the majority of the magnesium ion is extracellular
(B) Magnesium ion induces relaxation and calcium ion induces stimulation
(C) Measurement of serum potassium or magnesium ion concentration provides a reliable index of total body levels
(D) Bone is an important reservoir of calcium ion, but lacks magnesium
(E) The adenosine triphosphate (ATP)-dependent sodium–potassium pump uses an inconsequential amount of energy

37. Which of the following cell types responds first to chemical mediators involved in adhesion, chemotaxis, and opsonization?

(A) Neutrophils
(B) Macrophages
(C) Mast cells
(D) B lymphocytes
(E) T lymphocytes

38. A patient was admitted to the hospital after the accidental ingestion of a large dose of phenytoin. The following plasma drug concentrations were measured.

Time after Drug Ingestion	Plasma Drug Concentration
2 hours	36 mg/L
6 hours	34 mg/L
10 hours	32 mg/L
14 hours	30 mg/L

These data indicate that

(A) first-order kinetics played a role in the elimination of the phenytoin
(B) the half-life of the phenytoin increased with time
(C) the elimination mechanism was saturated
(D) the elimination of the phenytoin was proportional to the plasma concentration
(E) acidifying the urine would accelerate phenytoin elimination

39. Which one of the following cell types is most important in mediating the acute inflammatory reaction seen in immune complex glomerulonephritis?

(A) Cytotoxic T lymphocytes
(B) Macrophages
(C) Neutrophils
(D) Eosinophils
(E) Natural killer (NK) cells

40. What is the leading cause of death in people 25–44 years old in the United States?

(A) Accidents
(B) Suicide
(C) Homicide
(D) AIDS
(E) Cancer

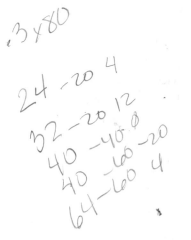

41. A 25-year-old man complains of a urethral discharge and painful urination. A Gram stain smear of the discharge shows many neutrophils but no bacteria. Of the following organisms, the one most likely to cause the discharge is

(A) *Treponema pallidum*
(B) *Neisseria gonorrhoeae*
(C) *Candida albicans*
(D) *Ureaplasma urealyticum*
(E) *Staphylococcus aureus*

42. The percentage of all health care costs incurred by the elderly in the United States is currently approximately

(A) 10%
(B) 30%
(C) 60%
(D) 80%
(E) 90%

43. Which one of the following statements regarding activated macrophages is true?

(A) They specifically destroy normal tissue
(B) They are major producers of interleukin-2
(C) They express antigen-specific receptors
(D) They lack major histocompatibility complex (MHC) class I and II molecules
(E) They are the epithelioid cells of granulomas

44. An individual is homozygous for a liver phosphofructokinase-1 that has a dissociation constant (K_d) for fructose 2,6-bisphosphate that is 10 times greater than normal. Relative to the normal individual, this person will have difficulty synthesizing

(A) fatty acids from glucose
(B) glucose from alanine
(C) glycogen from alanine
(D) glucose from fructose
(E) glycogen from glucose

45. Which of the following cell types is most important in early defense against a virus that has not been previously encountered?

(A) T cytotoxic lymphocytes
(B) Virgin lymphocytes
(C) Natural killer (NK) cells
(D) Plasmacytes
(E) Memory cells

46. Medicare was designed primarily for

(A) economically disadvantaged people
(B) minor children of economically disadvantaged people
(C) people eligible for Social Security
(D) people without health insurance
(E) people who require nursing home care

47. An elderly patient is placed on ampicillin and develops acute diarrhea with blood and mucus accompanied by fever and leukocytosis. Which one of the following organisms is the most likely cause of this patient's diarrhea?

(A) *Staphylococcus aureus*
(B) *Streptococcus pyogenes*
(C) *Clostridium difficile*
(D) *C. perfringens*
(E) *Bacillus cereus*

48. When compared to the number of visits made by patients to doctors in countries with systems of socialized medicine, the number of visits made by patients to doctors in the United States is

(A) lower
(B) the same
(C) twice as many
(D) three times as many
(E) four times as many

49. What is the elimination half-life of a drug with a volume of distribution of 40 L if the total body clearance is 7 L/hour? The hepatic extraction ratio of the drug is 0.5 and the T_{max} after oral administration is 2 hours.

(A) 2 hours
(B) 4 hours
(C) 6 hours
(D) 8 hours
(E) 12 hours

$$t_{1/2} = \frac{.7 \times V_d}{Cl}$$

50. A 75-year-old widow with $300,000 in savings develops Alzheimer disease and will require nursing home care for the rest of her life. Where will the money come from to finance the widow's nursing home care over the first few years?

(A) Medicare
(B) Medicaid
(C) A health maintenance organization (HMO)
(D) An independent practice association (IPA)
(E) The widow's savings

51. A student performs a Gram stain on a patient specimen, as well as on known gram-positive and gram-negative smears. The bacteria in all three preparations stain pink. What is the most probable reason for this finding?

(A) The student used too much acetone
(B) The organism in the patient specimen is not gram-positive or gram-negative
(C) The preparations were heat-fixed
(D) The student used too much iodine solution
(E) The student forgot to add acetone

52. Conscious, unconscious, and preconscious are terms closely associated with Freud's

(A) structural model of the mind
(B) topographic model of the mind
(C) research in neuroanatomy
(D) colleagues, Jung and Adler
(E) role model, Charcot

53. Which of the following are obligate intracellular parasites?

(A) *Mycoplasma* and *Mycobacterium*
(B) *Chlamydia* and *Rickettsia*
(C) *Chlamydia* and *Mycoplasma*
(D) *Chlamydia* and *Mycobacterium*
(E) *Mycoplasma* and *Rickettsia*

Questions 54-55

The 1994 United States census reported the following population data for a southern city: 500,000 fertile males; 450,000 fertile females; and 500,000 other residents. In the same year, there were 4000 live births, 3 fetal deaths, 4 deaths among children younger than 1 year of age, and 40 maternal deaths as a result of childbirth.

54. What was the crude birth rate in 1990?

(A) 0/500,000
(B) 4000/450,000
(C) 4000/950,000
(D) 4000/1,450,000
(E) 4003/450,000

55. What was the maternal mortality rate?

(A) 40/4007
(B) 40/4000
(C) 40/950,000
(D) 40/450,000
(E) 47/450,000

56. When compared to the infant mortality rate for white infants in the United States, the mortality rate for African-American infants is approximately

(A) 1.5 times higher
(B) 1.8 times higher
(C) 2.4 times higher
(D) 4.1 times higher
(E) the same

57. Which one of the following statements is true about the genetic basis of the affective disorders?

(A) The child of two parents with bipolar disorder has a 20% likelihood of having bipolar disorder in adulthood

(B) The concordance rate for unipolar disorder is higher than that for bipolar disorder

(C) The lifetime incidence of unipolar disorder is higher in men than in women

(D) Bipolar disorder has been linked to markers on the X chromosome

(E) The lifetime incidence of unipolar disorder is approximately 5% in women

58. Thirty minutes after a single intravenous injection of a drug, the plasma drug concentration is 400 mg/ml. Twelve hours later, the plasma concentration is 50 mg/ml. Assuming first-order kinetics, the half-life of the drug is

(A) 2 hours

(B) 4 hours

(C) 6 hours

(D) 8 hours

(E) 12 hours

59. At which age are children likely to form same-sex peer groups?

(A) 2–4 years

(B) 4–6 years

(C) 6–11 years

(D) 11–13 years

(E) 13–16 years

60. Which one of the following reactions is catalyzed by cytochrome P-450?

(A) Acetylation of isoniazid

(B) Hydrolysis of procaine

(C) Hydroxylation of phenytoin

(D) Glycine conjugation of salicylate

(E) Glucuronidation of chloramphenicol

61. The percentage of women who suffer from post-partum "blues" is approximately

(A) 5%–10%

(B) 15%–20%

(C) 35%–50%

(D) 75%–85%

(E) 90%–95%

62. In the United States, the infant mortality rate is lowest in which one of the following ethnic groups?

(A) Chinese-American

(B) African-American

(C) Native American

(D) Anglo-American

(E) Japanese-American

63. Which one of the following developmental theorists described the first month of postnatal life as the normal autistic phase?

(A) Mahler

(B) Freud

(C) Erikson

(D) Piaget

(E) Harlowe

64. Cimetidine may significantly prolong the prothrombin time and cause bleeding in patients who have been treated with warfarin by

(A) inhibiting the conversion of prothrombin to thrombin

(B) displacing warfarin from plasma proteins

(C) inhibiting renal tubular secretion of warfarin

(D) decreasing the hepatic clearance of warfarin

(E) increasing the oral bioavailability of warfarin

65. A 7-month-old boy who previously smiled at everyone begins to cry when he sees an individual he does not recognize. This behavior

(A) is normal
(B) is more likely to occur in infants who have multiple caregivers
(C) occurs primarily in anxious infants
(D) it is an indication that the child is not developing normally
(E) indicates that the child cannot distinguish between strangers and people that he knows

66. Amikacin is ordered for a patient with pyelonephritis caused by *Klebsiella pneumoniae*. The clearance and volume of distribution of amikacin in this patient are 50 ml/min and 20 L, respectively. What dose should be administered every 8 hours in order to obtain an average steady-state plasma concentration of 20 mg/L?

(A) 125 mg
(B) 400 mg
(C) 480 mg
(D) 760 mg
(E) 1000 mg

67. What is the most important strategy used in family therapy?

(A) Working with patients to uncover repressed events from early childhood
(B) Making the unconscious conscious
(C) Demonstrating how the patient's behavior is causing shame for the family
(D) Removing the focus from the identified patient
(E) Committing to daily 1-hour sessions

68. 2,4-Dinitrophenol is an effective weight-reducing agent. Unfortunately, it produces serious side effects, such as blindness, high fever, and even death, thus excluding it for clinical use. Its weight-reducing capacity is ascribed to its ability to

(A) inhibit reduced nicotinamide adenine dinucleotide (NADH) dehydrogenase
(B) uncouple substrate level phosphorylation in the cytosol at the level of glyceraldehyde 3-phosphate dehydrogenase
(C) lower the concentration of protons in the intermembranous space of the mitochondrion
(D) uncouple substrate-level phosphorylation at the level of mitochondrial succinylcoenzyme A (succinyl CoA) thiokinase
(E) inhibit the malate shuttle, which transports electrons from the cytosol into the mitochondrion

69. Which one of the following individuals has the highest risk of developing schizophrenia?

(A) The brother of a schizophrenic patient
(B) The child of two schizophrenic parents
(C) The monozygotic twin of a schizophrenic patient
(D) The child of one schizophrenic parent
(E) A child raised in an institutional setting

70. The plasma half-life of diazepam is often prolonged in elderly patients because of

(A) decreased hepatic clearance
(B) increased lean body mass
(C) increased volume of distribution
(D) decreased hepatic clearance and increased volume of distribution
(E) decreased hepatic clearance and increased lean body mass

71. A young child moves away from his mother, but constantly returns to her for comfort and reassurance. This behavior is most common in children of what age?

(A) 8–11 months
(B) 12–15 months
(C) 16–24 months
(D) 30–36 months
(E) 36–48 months

72. Patients receiving both cimetidine and sucralfate for peptic ulcer disease should separate the administration of these drugs by 2 hours because

(A) cimetidine inhibits the metabolism of sucralfate, increasing its toxicity
(B) the combination may cause acid rebound
(C) sucralfate displaces cimetidine from plasma-protein binding sites
(D) sucralfate inhibits the absorption of cimetidine
(E) cimetidine counteracts the pharmacodynamic action of sucralfate

73. Histologic examination of a muscle biopsy specimen from a 2-month-old boy with pronounced muscular flabbiness reveals that the fibers are abnormal. Many relatives on the mother's side of the family complain of chronic fatigue and weakness, and muscle biopsy samples from these relatives show a variable histologic pattern with abnormalities similar to those that predominate in the affected child. On the other hand, the father and all of his relatives have normal muscular and fatigue patterns as well as normal biopsies. Assuming that the infant suffers from a hereditary mitochondrial myopathy with maternal transmission of the abnormal gene, an abnormality of which enzymes would be expected?

(A) Those of the tricarboxylic acid (TCA) cycle
(B) Those involved with oxidative phosphorylation
(C) Those involved with fatty acid degradation
(D) Those involved with mitochondrial membrane structure
(E) Those involved with fatty acid elongation

74. Following the administration of probenecid to a patient who is receiving penicillin V orally, which penicillin pharmacokinetic parameter will be increased?

(A) Oral bioavailability
(B) Renal clearance
(C) Hepatic clearance
(D) Volume of distribution
(E) Plasma half-life

75. The "Band-Aid" phase occurs most commonly at what age?

(A) 6–12 months
(B) 12–18 months
(C) 18–24 months
(D) 24–30 months
(E) 30–60 months

76. A patient who is receiving cimetidine for peptic ulcer disease is admitted to the hospital with an acute myocardial infarction and receives intravenous lidocaine to treat acute ventricular arrhythmias. The patient exhibits signs of lidocaine toxicity. What is the most likely cause of the toxicity?

(A) Decreased hepatic clearance of lidocaine
(B) Decreased renal clearance of lidocaine
(C) A direct effect of cimetidine on cardiac automaticity
(D) A direct effect of cimetidine on central nervous system (CNS) excitability
(E) Displacement of lidocaine from plasma proteins

77. How does insulin promote the growth and differentiation of hepatocytes?

(A) It increases adenylate cyclase activity
(B) It binds to a nuclear receptor
(C) It activates protein kinase C
(D) It activates a tyrosine kinase
(E) It activates protein kinase A

78. Patients should not receive concomitant terfenadine and ketoconazole because

(A) ketoconazole increases terfenadine inactivation
(B) terfenadine antagonizes the antifungal effect of ketoconazole
(C) ketoconazole inhibits terfenadine metabolism
(D) terfenadine potentiates ketoconazole toxicity
(E) terfenadine bioavailability is decreased by ketoconazole

79. Differences between the means of two samples are tested using which one of the following methods?

(A) *t*-Test
(B) Analysis of variance
(C) Chi-square test
(D) Correlation analysis
(E) Regression analysis

80. Which one of the following psychiatric diagnoses is associated with the lowest risk for suicide?

(A) Unipolar depression
(B) Schizophrenia
(C) Alcoholism
(D) Obsessive–compulsive personality disorder
(E) Barbiturate abuse

81. What is the average life expectancy for a black woman in the United States?

(A) 65 years
(B) 72 years
(C) 74 years
(D) 78 years
(E) 80 years

82. A patient describes his relatives and associates as either all good or all bad. Which one of the following best describes the defense mechanism he is using?

(A) Sublimation
(B) Rationalization
(C) Regression
(D) Splitting
(E) Identification

83. The relative risk of developing lung cancer for smokers versus non-smokers is 24. This implies that

(A) 24% of all lung cancer patients smoke cigarettes
(B) the incidence of lung cancer among smokers is 24 times that among non-smokers
(C) the prevalence of lung cancer among smokers is 24 times that among non-smokers
(D) 24% of all smokers develop lung cancer
(E) 24 out of 100 people develop lung cancer

84. A patient has ingested mushrooms containing a toxin that has been found to specifically inhibit messenger RNA (mRNA) production. The toxin is most likely to directly inhibit

(A) RNA polymerase I
(B) RNA polymerase II
(C) RNA polymerase III
(D) DNA polymerase
(E) reverse transcriptase

85. After starting a continuous intravenous infusion of a drug whose elimination half-life is 2 hours, what percentage of the steady-state plasma drug concentration will be achieved in 6.6 hours?

(A) 75%
(B) 87%
(C) 90%
(D) 94%
(E) 97%

86. A 53-year-old man with pancreatic cancer tells his physician that he is calm and prepared to die. This patient is in the stage of dying known as

(A) acceptance
(B) denial
(C) reaction formation
(D) positive regard
(E) displacement

87. Which one of the following reactions is the committed step in *de novo* purine biosynthesis?

(A) Ribose 5-phosphate → 5-phosphoribosyl-1-pyrophosphate (PRPP)
(B) PRPP → 5-phosphoribosylamine
(C) Hypoxanthine → inosine monophosphate (IMP)
(D) Carbamoyl phosphate → carbamoyl aspartate
(E) Xanthine → uric acid

88. The Fuelgen reaction is employed in static cytometry to study ploidy in various cancers. What portion of the cell stains?

(A) RNA
(B) DNA
(C) Nucleolus
(D) Barr bodies
(E) Microtubules

89. *Bacteroides fragilis* and *Clostridium perfringens* are similar in that they both

(A) cause food poisoning
(B) produce potent endotoxins
(C) lack superoxide dismutase
(D) are spore-forming bacteria found in the colon
(E) are transmitted from poultry and domestic animals to humans

90. Which of the following statements is true about both hexokinase and glucokinase?

(A) They are expressed in liver cells
(B) They are inhibited by glucose 6-phosphate
(C) They operate at maximum velocity rates at normal fasting blood glucose concentrations
(D) They are expressed in muscle cells
(E) They are involved in the normal phosphorylation of fructose

91. In descending order, what are the leading causes of death in the United States across all age groups?

(A) Cancer, heart disease, stroke
(B) Heart disease, cancer, stroke
(C) AIDS, heart disease, cancer
(D) Heart disease, AIDS, cancer
(E) Cancer, stroke, heart disease

92. Which one of the following statements is true concerning nitric oxide?

(A) Nitric oxide raises the blood pressure by contracting smooth muscle
(B) The anesthetic effect of "laughing gas" (nitrous oxide) is caused by its oxidation to nitric oxide by nitric oxide synthetase
(C) Nitric oxide activates guanylate cyclase, which increases cyclic guanosine monophosphate (cGMP) levels
(D) Nitric oxide causes vasodilation, which enhances bacterial invasion of tissues
(E) Nitric oxide enhances blood clotting by activating calcium calmodulin

93. Which one of the following statements regarding Na^+ transport is correct?

(A) Active transport of Na^+ across all cells consumes most of the energy derived from cellular metabolism
(B) The Na^+ concentration is highest in the intracellular fluid (ICF)
(C) Na^+ reabsorption across proximal tubular cells is mainly active and transcellular
(D) The Na^+ concentration gradient provides energy for the cotransport of H^+
(E) The transport of Na^+ across the apical membrane of the nephron is an active transport process

94. Three patients received an intravenous infusion of the same drug and the resultant plasma drug concentration curves are shown below.

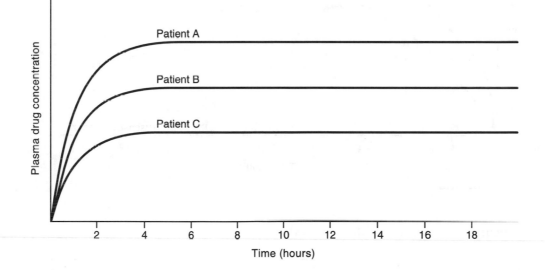

Which one of the following factors is most likely responsible for the differences in the curves?

(A) Duration of drug infusion F
(B) Serum half-life F
(C) Dosage
(D) Route of elimination
(E) Renal clearance

95. What is the most rapid means of identifying the etiologic agent of acute meningitis?

(A) Culture of cerebrospinal fluid (CSF) on a blood agar plate
(B) Culture of CSF in thioglycollate broth
(C) Counterimmunoelectrophoresis
(D) An agglutination test for the detection of soluble antigen in CSF
(E) Acute and convalescent serum antibody titers

96. Which sacroplasmic inclusion serves as an energy depot?

(A) Actin
(B) Myosin
(C) Glycogen
(D) Ribosomes
(E) Mitochondria

97. Three patients (A, B, and C) receive a continuous intravenous infusion of the same drug, and the consequent plasma drug concentrations are shown below.

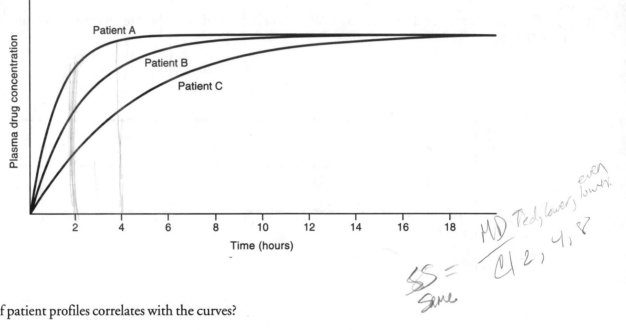

Which set of patient profiles correlates with the curves?

	Patient A		Patient B		Patient C	
	Half-life	Dose	Half-life	Dose	Half-life	Dose
(A)	2 hours	20 μg/kg/min	2 hours	10 μg/kg/min	2 hours	5 μg/kg/min
(B)	2 hours	20 μg/kg/min	4 hours	20 μg/kg/min	8 hours	20 μg/kg/min
(C)	2 hours	5 μg/kg/min	2 hours	10 μg/kg/min	2 hours	20 μg/kg/min
(D)	2 hours	20 μg/kg/min	4 hours	10 μg/kg/min	8 hours	5 μg/kg/min
(E)	8 hours	5 μg/kg/min	4 hours	10 μg/kg/min	2 hours	20 μg/kg/min

Questions 98-99

98. Test X for rheumatoid arthritis is positive in 150 out of 200 patients with rheumatoid arthritis and is negative in 180 out of 200 people without rheumatoid arthritis. In the population of people under study, what is the chance that a positive test result in a randomly selected individual indicates that the person has rheumatoid arthritis?

(A) 70%
(B) 75%
(C) 88%
(D) 90%
(E) 95%

99. If the prevalence of rheumatoid arthritis in the previous question is changed to 10%, what is the chance that a positive test result indicates that the person has rheumatoid arthritis?

(A) 45%
(B) 50%
(C) 55%
(D) 60%
(E) 65%

100. A physically normal 7-year-old boy insists on wearing girls' clothing and often expresses displeasure with the fact that he has a penis. The most correct diagnosis for this child is

(A) normal
(B) homosexual
(C) transvestic fetishism
(D) gender identity disorder
(E) intersex condition

101. What is the source of prothymocytes?

(A) Liver
(B) Spleen
(C) Thymus
(D) Bone marrow
(E) Lymph nodes

102. The exotoxin of which one of the following organisms is comprised of protective antigen, edema factor, and lethal factor?

(A) *Clostridium difficile*
(B) *Bacillus cereus*
(C) *Clostridium tetani*
(D) *Bacillus anthracis*
(E) *Haemophilus influenzae*

103. During her pediatric clerkship, a student observes a case involving a newborn infant suffering from transient bouts of hyperammonemia. The attending physician asks each student to make a list of enzyme deficiencies that could be responsible for this condition. The resident castigates the student for including which one of the following?

(A) Glutamate dehydrogenase
(B) Carbamoyl synthetase I
(C) Branched amino acid aminotransferase
(D) Glutamine synthetase
(E) Arginase

104. What is the primary site of B-cell maturation?

(A) Spleen
(B) Lymph nodes
(C) Bone marrow
(D) Thymus
(E) Tonsils

105. What are the unique immunogenic properties of the variable region of an antibody molecule collectively known as?

(A) Allotype
(B) Isotype
(C) Idiotope
(D) Idiotype
(E) Hinge

106. The incidence of which one of the following cancers has increased the most in the United States in the past 5 years?

(A) Breast cancer
(B) Pancreatic cancer
(C) Stomach cancer
(D) Malignant melanoma
(E) Malignant lymphoma

107. Arrange the following cancers in men and women, first in order of decreasing incidence and then in order of decreasing mortality.

Men		Women
Colon	(1)	Colon
Prostate	(2)	Breast
Lung	(3)	Lung

	Men		Women	
	Incidence	Mortality	Incidence	Mortality
(A)	3-2-1	2-3-1	3-1-2	3-2-1
(B)	2-1-3	3-2-1	2-1-3	2-3-1
(C)	2-3-1	3-2-1	2-3-1	3-2-1
(D)	3-2-1	2-3-1	3-2-1	2-1-3
(E)	2-3-1	3-1-2	3-1-2	3-2-1

108. Levels of α-fetoprotein (AFP), β-human chorionic gonadotropin (β-hCG), or both are likely to be elevated in the presence of which type of cancer?

(A) Lung cancer
(B) Testicular cancer
(C) Liver cancer
(D) Colon cancer
(E) Ovarian cancer

109. Pitting edema would be expected in a patient with

(A) syndrome of inappropriate antidiuretic hormone (SIADH)
(B) primary aldosteronism
(C) nephrotic syndrome
(D) diabetic ketoacidosis
(E) diabetes insipidus

110. A 72-year-old man with urinary retention from benign prostatic hyperplasia suddenly develops fever and chills. His skin feels warm and his pulse is hyperdynamic. Within 24 hours, he develops tachypnea and dyspnea. The chest radiograph reveals bilateral, diffuse infiltrates in his lungs. The arterial blood gas report indicates that the patient is experiencing hypoxemia. On the second hospital day, blood begins to seep from all of the patient's venipuncture sites. The event that occurred on the second day most closely relates to

(A) disseminated intravascular coagulation (DIC)
(B) adult respiratory distress syndrome (ARDS)
(C) endotoxemia
(D) hypovolemic shock
(E) renal failure

111. What are the most common causes of death in 15-year-old boys and 30-year-old men, respectively?

(A) Motor vehicle accidents/acquired immunodeficiency syndrome (AIDS)
(B) Drowning/motor vehicle accidents
(C) Motor vehicle accidents/suicide
(D) Suicide/cancer
(E) Motor vehicle accidents/motor vehicle accidents

112. Which one of the following would most likely result in an elevated α-fetoprotein (AFP) level in a pregnant woman?

(A) Thalidomide
(B) Valproate
(C) Phenytoin
(D) Systemic lupus erythematosus (SLE)
(E) Heroin addiction

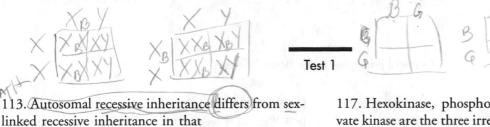

113. Autosomal recessive inheritance differs from sex-linked recessive inheritance in that

(A) children of two asymptomatic carrier parents would have symptomatic disease

(B) males are more commonly affected than females

(C) females are more commonly affected than males

(D) children of an asymptomatic carrier woman and a normal man would have symptomatic disease

(E) the children of a symptomatic man and a normal woman would have symptomatic disease

114. Which one of the following is an age-related, rather than an age-dependent, finding?

(A) Decreased skin turgor

(B) Coronary artery disease

(C) Prostate hyperplasia

(D) Osteoarthritis

(E) Cataracts

115. Which one of the following represents a deformation rather than a malformation?

(A) Hypospadias

(B) Ventricular septal defect

(C) Club foot

(D) Open neural tube defect

(E) Potter's syndrome

116. An endocrinologist prescribes a drug. The patient is told that the drug will have no effect for several days, and that it will take at least 1 week before the drug is operating at its maximal effect. Which one of the following drugs was most likely prescribed?

(A) Epinephrine

(B) Glucagon

(C) Insulin

(D) Thyroxine

(E) Antidiuretic hormone (ADH)

117. Hexokinase, phosphofructokinase-1, and pyruvate kinase are the three irreversible enzymes of glycolysis. All three are subject to metabolic regulation in

(A) skeletal muscle

(B) brain tissue

(C) adipocytes

(D) hepatocytes

(E) cardiac muscle

118. Why are all newborns administered an intramuscular injection of vitamin K?

(A) Newborns are deficient in bile salts

(B) Vitamin K is absent in breast milk

(C) Newborns lack bacterial colonization of the bowel

(D) The liver does not synthesize adequate amounts of vitamin K–dependent coagulation factors in newborns

(E) The small intestine of newborns cannot adequately reabsorb fat-soluble vitamins

119. Which one of the following biochemical processes occurs partly in the mitochondria and partly in the cytosol?

(A) β-Oxidation of fatty acids

(B) Heme synthesis

(C) Glycogen synthesis

(D) Oxidative phosphorylation

(E) Collagen synthesis

120. In what way does carboxyhemoglobin differ from methemoglobin?

(A) Carboxyhemoglobin causes a left shift in the oxygen dissociation curve

(B) Carboxyhemoglobin produces tissue hypoxia

(C) Carboxyhemoglobin blocks cytochrome oxidase

(D) Carboxyhemoglobin decreases the oxygen saturation

(E) Carboxyhemoglobin decreases the oxygen content

121. Proteins that have been chemically altered by the addition of ubiquitin are most likely to be

(A) degraded
(B) secreted from the cell
(C) incorporated into the lysosomes
(D) transported into the nucleus
(E) transported out of the mitochondria

122. Which type of bacteria derives energy from the oxidation of organic molecules?

(A) Prototrophs
(B) Heterotrophs
(C) Autotrophs
(D) Chemoautotrophs
(E) Auxotrophs

Questions 123-125

In 1992, there were 900 deaths in a midwestern city with a population of 1,000,000. At the beginning of that year, 900 cases of AIDS existed in this population. During the year, 300 new cases of AIDS were diagnosed, and 60 people died of the disease during 1992.

123. What is the incidence rate of AIDS (per 100,000 population) in this city in 1992?

(A) 6
(B) 12
(C) 30
(D) 90
(E) 120

124. What was the crude mortality rate (per 100,000 population) in 1992 for the data given?

(A) 6
(B) 12
(C) 30
(D) 90
(E) 120

125. Using the data given above, what was the prevalence rate per 100,000 at the end of 1992 for AIDS?

(A) 6
(B) 12
(C) 30
(D) 90
(E) 120

DIRECTIONS:

Each of the numbered items or incomplete statements in this section is negatively phrased, as indicated by a capitalized word such as NOT, LEAST, or EXCEPT. Select the ONE lettered answer or completion that is BEST in each case.

126. Studies by Harlowe involving infant monkeys reared in relative social isolation demonstrated that all of the following are true about these monkeys EXCEPT that

(A) they do not develop normal mating behavior as adults

(B) they do not develop normal maternal behavior as adults

(C) they do not develop normal social behavior as adults

(D) females are more likely to be affected than males

(E) they cannot recover if they have been isolated from other monkeys for more than 6 months

127. Which one of the following is LEAST likely to be associated with bile salt deficiency?

(A) Chronic pancreatitis

(B) Cholestyramine therapy

(C) Crohn's disease

(D) Cirrhosis

(E) Bacterial overgrowth in the small bowel

128. Which one of the following clinical situations would be LEAST likely to result in a newborn who is small for gestational age?

(A) Premature rupture of the membranes

(B) Abruptio placentae

(C) Congenital cytomegalovirus infection

(D) Gestational diabetes mellitus

(E) Pre-eclampsia

129. Which of the following processes does NOT require reduced nicotinamide adenine dinucleotide phosphate (NADPH)?

(A) Formation of reduced glutathione (GSH)

(B) Cytochrome P-450 metabolism

(C) Alcohol metabolism

(D) Cholesterol and fatty acid metabolism

(E) Ketogenesis

130. All of the following statements regarding B lymphocytes are true EXCEPT

(A) they secrete antibody only when helped by T cells

(B) they differentiate into plasmacytes

(C) their antigen receptor is monomeric immunoglobulin M (IgM)

(D) they function as antigen-presenting cells

(E) they mature in the bone marrow

131. Which one of the following statements concerning fatty acid synthesis is NOT correct?

(A) Generation of malonyl coenzyme A (malonyl CoA) inhibits the β-oxidation of fatty acids in the mitochondria

(B) Acetyl coenzyme A (acetyl CoA) carboxylase is the rate-limiting reaction in fatty acid synthesis

(C) Linoleic and linolenic acids provide the reducing equivalent for fatty acid synthesis and reduced nicotinamide adenine dinucleotide (NADPH) supplies the double bonds

(D) Fatty acids form complexes with albumin

(E) Palmitate, a 16-carbon fatty acid, is the end-product of the fatty acid synthase complex

132. Which one of the following statements regarding normal resident flora of the human body is NOT correct?

(A) The microorganisms that are constantly present on body surfaces are commensals

(B) Strepococci of the viridans group are the most common resident organisms of the upper respiratory tract

(C) If large numbers of viridans streptococci are introduced into the bloodstream, they may cause infective endocarditis

(D) *Bacteroides* species are the most common resident bacteria in the peritoneal cavity and pelvic tissues

(E) The normal flora of the body may be aerobic or anaerobic

133. Which of the following does NOT occur in a state of prolonged fasting (i.e., starvation)?

(A) Muscle use of ketones for fuel decreases

(B) Brain use of ketones for fuel increases

(C) Red blood cell use of glucose for fuel remains the same

(D) Urea excretion is lower than during the early fasting state

(E) Glycogenolysis takes place in the liver

134. All of the following statements regarding secondary follicles within peripheral lymphoid tissues are true EXCEPT

(A) they are normally present at birth

(B) they contain germinal centers

(C) they consist primarily of B cells and plasma cells

(D) they enlarge during infection

(E) they are found in the lymph nodes and spleen

135. All of the following attributes of neonates typically alter drug pharmacokinetics EXCEPT

(A) less cytochrome P-450–dependent drug metabolism

(B) less glucuronyl transferase activity

(C) a decreased glomerular filtration rate

(D) a lower percentage of body weight in the form of body water

(E) less plasma-protein binding of drugs

136. Mature B lymphocytes have all of the following markers EXCEPT

(A) FcγR protein

(B) major histocompatibility complex (MHC) class II molecules

(C) intracellular adhesion molecule (ICAM)

(D) terminal deoxynucleotidyl transferase (TdT)

(E) immunoglobulin M (IgM), with or without immunoglobulin D (IgD)

137. Which one of the following diseases is caused by an organism that is LEAST likely to be found in the normal human microbial flora?

(A) Subacute bacterial endocarditis

(B) Uncomplicated urinary cystitis

(C) Bacillary dysentery

(D) Actinomycosis

(E) Brain abscess

138. All of the following statements regarding immunoglobulins are correct EXCEPT

(A) they are glycosylated proteins

(B) treatment with pepsin produces two Fc fragments and one Fab fragment

(C) they consist of four globular chains

(D) each chain has only one variable region

(E) each antibody is specific for one epitope

139. A 54-year-old man, terminally ill with cancer, has feelings of helplessness, extreme guilt, and suicidal ideation. He wakes up at 3 A.M. each morning and cannot fall back asleep. All of the following statements are likely to be true about this patient EXCEPT

(A) the patient's emotional symptoms are more severe than would be expected
(B) the patient probably has a history of similar episodes
(C) the patient's emotional symptoms may be related to the cancer
(D) antidepressant medications will not help this patient
(E) the patient is suffering from a major depressive episode

140. All of the following virulence factors allow a bacterium to resist phagocytosis EXCEPT the

(A) M protein
(B) protein A
(C) peptidoglycan cell wall
(D) opacity (Opa) proteins
(E) polysaccharide capsule

141. All of the following statements about suicide are correct EXCEPT

(A) women are more likely than men to attempt suicide, but men are more likely to kill themselves
(B) middle-aged African-Americans are more likely to commit suicide than middle-aged whites
(C) suicide tends to run in families
(D) suicide is rare in children younger than 12 years of age
(E) suicide is more common in adolescents from broken homes

142. Which molecule is NOT found in the Entner-Doudoroff pathway for the fermentation of glucose?

(A) Glucose-6-phosphate
(B) 6-Phosphogluconate
(C) Xylulose-5-phosphate
(D) Glyceraldehyde-3-phosphate
(E) Pyruvate

143. Changes associated with normal aging include all of the following EXCEPT

(A) decreased intelligence
(B) decreased rapid eye movement (REM) sleep
(C) diminished sense of taste and smell
(D) increased sleep latency
(E) thinning of the vaginal mucosa

144. The process of phagocytosis involves all of the following EXCEPT

(A) phagolysosome formation
(B) a respiratory burst
(C) hypochlorite ion formation
(D) creation of memory cells
(E) proteolytic enzyme activation

145. All of the following are true about health care in the United States EXCEPT

(A) approximately 80% of physicians are specialists
(B) prior to 1900, people generally died of infections
(C) there are more than 25,000 nursing homes
(D) men are hospitalized more often than women
(E) the largest cost associated with running a hospital is staff salaries and benefits

146. All of the following statements are correct for natural killer (NK) cells EXCEPT

(A) they are a subset of T lymphocytes
(B) they do not express CD3 on their surfaces
(C) they are capable of killing via antibody-dependent cell-mediated cytotoxicity (ADCC)
(D) they can kill more than one type of target cell
(E) they are activated by interleukin-2

147. All of the following are true about health care expenses EXCEPT

(A) the percentage of the gross domestic product spent on health care in 1992 was approximately 1.3%
(B) federal and state governments pay approximately 41% of personal health care expenses
(C) private insurance pays approximately 32% of personal health care expenses
(D) hospital costs represent 41% of health care expenditures
(E) physician fees represent 20% of health care expenditures

148. All of the following statements regarding induction of the cytochrome P-450 enzyme system are true EXCEPT

(A) induction requires DNA transcription
(B) induction may occur after phenobarbital administration
(C) induction may increase the elimination half-life of other drugs
(D) induction increases the maximum rate of drug metabolism
(E) induction increases the hepatic concentration of cytochrome P-450 enzymes

149. All of the following are true about hospice care EXCEPT that it is

(A) becoming more common in the United States
(B) family-oriented
(C) paid for under Medicare
(D) autonomy-oriented
(E) cure-oriented

150. The Gram stain is useful in the diagnosis of all of the following diseases EXCEPT

(A) syphilis
(B) acute gonococcal urethritis
(C) candida vaginitis
(D) chancroid
(E) bacterial meningitis

151. Hospice care is characterized by all of the following EXCEPT

(A) grief counseling
(B) support groups
(C) inpatient supportive care
(D) outpatient supportive care
(E) restricted use of pain medication

152. Prokaryotes include all of the following EXCEPT

(A) *Giardia lamblia*
(B) *Ureaplasma urealyticum*
(C) L-form bacteria
(D) *Rickettsia*
(E) *Listeria monocytogenes*

153. Cells of the monocyte-macrophage lineage include all of the following EXCEPT

(A) microglia
(B) osteoclasts
(C) Langerhans' cells
(D) Kupffer's cells
(E) killer cells

154. All of the following statements are correct regarding macrophages EXCEPT

(A) they lack an oxygen-dependent myeloperoxidase system
(B) they express antigen-specific receptors
(C) they secrete interleukin-1
(D) they secrete growth factors
(E) they function as antigen-presenting cells

155. All of the following are true about the thymus EXCEPT

(A) the majority of lymphocytes eventually leave the thymus
(B) the thymus begins to atrophy after puberty
(C) the thymus is most active in fetal life
(D) the cortex of the thymus contains densely packed, immature, dividing cells
(E) the thymus is the major site of T-cell maturation

156. All of the following statements regarding T lymphocytes in the thymus are true EXCEPT

(A) CD4$^+$CD8$^+$ T lymphocytes are killed
(B) lymphocytes respond to thymic hormones
(C) lymphocytes express receptors for autoantigens
(D) CD4$^-$CD8$^-$ leave the thymus in the highest numbers
(E) negative selection is mediated by at least two cell types

157. Cells that assist in generating specific immune responses include all of the following EXCEPT

(A) CD4$^+$ T lymphocytes
(B) T$_H$0 lymphocytes
(C) T$_H$1 lymphocytes
(D) T$_H$2 lymphocytes
(E) CD8$^+$ T lymphocytes

158. All of the following statements are correct regarding the T-cell antigen receptor EXCEPT

(A) it consists partly of the CD3 molecule
(B) its ligand binding site is a dimer of α and β chains
(C) it binds free-floating soluble antigens
(D) its binding site is highly polymorphic
(E) each cell has receptors of a single specificity

159. Which one of the following relationships is NOT correct?

(A) Caisson's disease/divers
(B) Air embolism/head and neck surgery
(C) Paradoxical embolus/patent foramen ovale
(D) Amniotic fluid embolism/disseminated intravascular coagulation (DIC)
(E) Pulmonary embolus/superficial saphenous vein

160. All of the following laboratory abnormalities are directly associated with an increase in reduced nicotinamide adenine dinucleotide (NADH) from the metabolism of alcohol EXCEPT

(A) hypoglycemia
(B) lactic acidosis
(C) β-hydroxybutyric acid ketoacidosis
(D) hypertriglyceridemia
(E) increased serum aspartate aminotransferase (AST)

DIRECTIONS:

Each set of matching questions in this section consists of a list of four to twenty-six lettered options (some of which may be in figures) followed by several numbered items. For each numbered item, select the ONE lettered option that is most closely associated with it. To avoid spending too much time on matching sets with a large number of options, it is generally advisable to begin each set by reading the list of options. Then for each item in the set, try to generate the correct answer and locate it in the option list, rather than evaluating each option individually. Each lettered option may be selected once, more than once, or not at all.

Questions 161-162

For each type of mutation, select the agent that causes it.

(A) Bromodeoxyuridine

(B) Nitrous acid

(C) Ultraviolet light

(D) 2-Aminopurine

(E) Acridine orange

161. Frameshift mutations   E

162. Helix distortion mutations   B

Questions 163-166

For each pharmacokinetic profile, select the representative set of plasma drug concentration curves. The same dose of all drugs was injected intravenously at time zero.

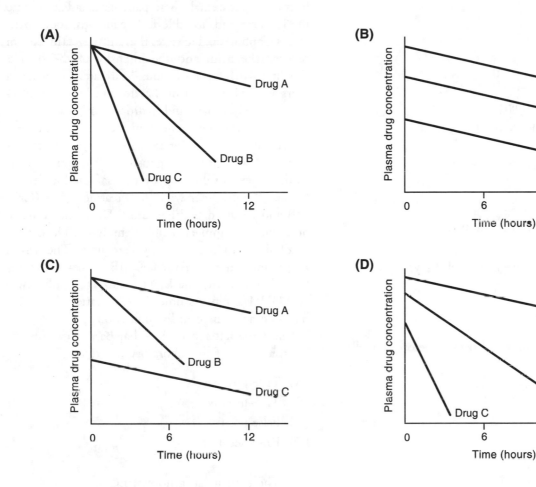

163. Drugs A, B, and C have the same half-life but different volumes of distribution

164. Drugs A, B, and C have different half-lives and different volumes of distribution

165. Drugs A, B, and C have different half-lives but the same volume of distribution

166. Drugs A and C have the same half-life; drugs A and B have the same volume of distribution

Questions 167-171

For each of the numbered phrases, choose the lettered interviewing technique with which it is most closely associated.

(A) Facilitation
(B) Confrontation
(C) Reflection
(D) Direct questioning
(E) Open-ended questioning
(F) Support
(G) Recapitulation
(H) Validation

167. "What brings you to see me?"

168. "When did you begin to feel dizzy?"

169. "And then?"

170. "You say that you felt dizzy just before you fell?"

171. "You seem to be very sad."

Questions 172-173

A 60-year-old African-American man with a long history of coronary artery disease presents with a 10-hour history of substernal chest pain with radiation into the left arm and jaw. He feels nauseous, looks pale, and is diaphoretic. He states that nitroglycerin has not relieved the pain, and the intensity of the pain is similar to that in a previous heart attack he had 4 years ago. His present medications include nitroglycerin p.r.n. chest pain and hydrochlorothiazide for essential hypertension. The clinician strongly suspects an acute myocardial infarction; however, an electrocardiogram (ECG) is not diagnostic for any acute injury. In the process of drawing a blood sample for electrolytes and serum isoenzymes for creatine kinase (CK)-MB and lactate dehydrogenase (LDH), the clinician notes that the sample is visibly hemolyzed. The patient is admitted to the coronary care unit. The serum potassium is increased, the CK-MB isoenzyme is positive (elevated), and the LDH isoenzyme results show an LDH 1/2 flip. Assume that the patient has a 10-hour-old acute myocardial infarction.

Select the lettered option that best represents the interpretation of the laboratory test result.

(A) True-positive
(B) True-negative
(C) False-positive
(D) False-negative

172. The patient has a normal ECG.

173. The patient has a positive CK-MG.

Questions 174-175

Match the following lettered areas representing portions of the nephron with the appropriate descriptions.

(A) Proximal tubule
(B) Descending limb
(C) Loop of Henle
(D) Thin ascending limb
(E) Medullary segment of the thick ascending limb
(F) Cortical segment of the thick ascending limb
(G) Macula densa
(H) Distal convoluted tubule
(I) Collecting duct

174. Location of the sodium/potassium-2 chloride co-transport pump is blocked by a loop diuretic, hence interfering with the generation of free water.

175. Peritubular capillary hydrostatic and oncotic pressure are important in the reabsorption or excretion of sodium, urea, and other solutes at this location.

Questions 176-180

Match each of the following functions or descriptions with the appropriate organelle/inclusion.

(A) Microfilaments
(B) Intermediate filaments
(C) Microtubules
(D) Microtubule-associated proteins
(E) Peroxisomes
(F) Rough endoplasmic reticulum
(G) Smooth endoplasmic reticulum
(H) Golgi complex
(I) Mitochondria
(J) Ribosomes
(K) Primary lysosomes
(L) Glycogen

176. Alzheimer's disease neurofibrillary tangles

177. Cell-surface receptor movement

178. Breakdown of hydrogen peroxide

179. Detoxification of drugs, carcinogens, pesticides

180. Most prominent organelle of the proximal convoluted tubule

ANSWER KEY

1. B	31. A	61. C	91. B	121. A	151. E
2. D	32. B	62. E	92. C	122. B	152. A
3. E	33. D	63. A	93. B	123. C	153. E
4. A	34. B	64. D	94. C	124. D	154. B
5. A	35. C	65. A	95. D	125. E	155. A
6. E	36. B	66. C	96. C	126. D	156. D
7. C	37. A	67. D	97. D	127. A	157. E
8. C	38. C	68. C	98. C	128. D	158. C
9. C	39. C	69. C	99. A	129. E	159. E
10. A	40. D	70. D	100. D	130. A	160. E
11. E	41. D	71. C	101. D	131. C	161. E
12. B	42. B	72. D	102. D	132. D	162. C
13. A	43. E	73. B	103. C	133. E	163. B
14. C	44. A	74. E	104. C	134. A	164. D
15. C	45. C	75. E	105. D	135. D	165. A
16. B	46. C	76. A	106. D	136. D	166. C
17. E	47. C	77. D	107. C	137. C	167. E
18. C	48. A	78. C	108. B	138. B	168. D
19. C	49. B	79. A	109. C	139. D	169. A
20. D	50. E	80. D	110. A	140. C	170. C
21. C	51. A	81. C	111. A	141. B	171. B
22. C	52. B	82. D	112. B	142. C	172. D
23. D	53. B	83. B	113. A	143. A	173. A
24. C	54. D	84. B	114. B	144. D	174. E
25. A	55. B	85. C	115. E	145. D	175. A
26. B	56. C	86. A	116. D	146. A	176. D
27. A	57. D	87. B	117. D	147. A	177. A
28. D	58. B	88. B	118. C	148. C	178. E
29. C	59. C	89. C	119. B	149. E	179. G
30. D	60. C	90. A	120. C	150. A	180. I

ANSWERS AND EXPLANATIONS

1. The answer is B. *(Behavioral science)*
Smiling in response to a human face, the social smile, develops at 1–2 months of age. The social smile is one of the first markers of the infant's responsiveness and attachment to another individual.

2. The answer is D. *(Microbiology)*
If histidine is added to the growth medium, the first enzyme in the biosynthetic pathway will be inhibited. Control over enzymatic activity seems to be responsible for the moment-to-moment control of intermediary metabolism. During this regulatory process, known as feedback inhibition, a metabolite binds to an allosteric enzyme causing it to gain or lose catalytic activity (i.e., activating or inhibiting catalytic activity, respectively). These activators and inhibitors are intermediates of metabolism and act as effectors. The concentrations of end products of various pathways allow the cell to monitor and regulate the flow of materials, providing the most efficient use of resources. This control serves to maintain a relatively constant internal concentration of metabolites in the face of changing demands for them and their availability in the medium. Usually only the first enzyme of a biosynthetic pathway is regulated. Inhibition of later enzymes causes wasteful accumulations of intermediates in that pathway. The rate of synthesis is not directly increased by the added nutrient, nor is the rate of synthesis slowed down because of the direct inhibition of the enzymes required by the pathway. Only the specific biochemical pathway (histidine in this example) is affected by this control process. No specific end product (one amino acid, for example) is able to affect all other amino acid pathways.

3. The answer is E. *(Biochemistry)*
Pyruvate is an important crossroad in metabolism. It can be transaminated to form alanine, carboxylated to form oxaloacetate, oxidatively decarboxylated to form acetyl coenzyme A (acetyl CoA), or reduced to form lactate. However, it cannot be phosphorylated to form phosphoenolpyruvate. The pyruvate kinase reaction is irreversible.

4. The answer is A. *(Microbiology)*
Lysogenic conversion is the change from nonpathogenicity to pathogenicity following the incorporation of a prophage from a temperate bacteriophage into the chromosome of a bacterial host. The acquisition of the beta phage by *Corynebacterium diphtheriae* induces the production of the diphtheria toxin by this organism. Diphtheria toxin halts all protein metabolism in a cell by inhibiting cellular elongation factor-2. A similar situation allows *Streptococcus pyogenes* to produce erythrogenic toxins involved in scarlet fever. Another example of lysogenic conversion is the ability of *Staphylococcus aureus* to make enterotoxins (responsible for staphylococcal food poisoning). Endotoxin, on the other hand, is part of any gram-negative cell wall. M proteins (seen in group A streptococci) and protein A (seen in *S. aureus*) are fimbriae. The ability to produce these proteins does not appear to be related to bacteriophage involvement. The ability to produce polysaccharide capsules, the tetanus toxin, or the botulism toxin is under bacterial chromosomal control, with no evidence of any bacteriophage involvement.

5. The answer is A. *(Pathology)*
Disease onset is likely to be early in patients with autosomal recessive disease, and late in patients with autosomal dominant disease. Autosomal dominant disorders usually involve abnormalities in the synthesis of structural proteins, membrane receptors, or transport proteins.

6. The answer is E. *(Microbiology)*
Almost all surfaces of the human body are colonized by a mixed group of bacteria that are referred to as normal, or usual, flora. These bacteria do not normally cause disease and are considered to be commensal (i.e., they offer no advantage or disadvantage). If these organisms escape from their normal ecological niche, however, they may cause opportunistic infections. Normal flora may be facultative or anaerobic in their metabolic processes. Body areas where microorganisms actively grow and colonize include the skin and contiguous mucous surfaces, the nose, throat, mouth, intestine, vagina, and outer portion of the urethra. The trachea, bronchi, esophagus, stomach, and upper urinary tract are normally sterile. Both gram-negative and gram-positive cocci and rods make up this flora. The colon contains the largest concentration of bacteria of any region of the body. Healthy individuals

contain bacterial populations exceeding 10^{11} organisms per gram of colonic content and consisting of more than 400 species. Up to 99% of these organisms are anaerobic because of the biochemical conditions found in the area. The anaerobic bacteria that colonize the skin (e.g., *Proprionibacterium* and *Brevibacterium*) are usually found in the sebaceous gland area. The mouth represents a complex system of ecological niches. Anaerobes and spirochetes are found in the gingival crevices. Vaginal anaerobic flora includes at least six genera. The lungs are normally sterile and contain no anaerobes. This location is at great risk of infection (aspiration pneumonia) if anaerobes are accidentally introduced.

7. The answer is C.   *(Biochemistry)*
Insulin and nitric oxide receptors are similar in that both have a short, rod-like transmembranal domain. Agonists binding to nitric oxide receptors increase guanylate cyclase activity; agonists binding to insulin receptors increase tyrosine kinase activity. Neither receptor is coupled to adenylate kinase. The nitric oxide receptor is monomeric; the insulin receptor is a dimer of dimers (i.e., a tetramer).

8. The answer is C.   *(Pathology)*
The edema associated with both the swelling of tissue following a bee sting and adult respiratory distress syndrome (ARDS) is the result of increased vessel permeability. Bee stings involve a type I hypersensitivity reaction that results in the local release of histamine from mast cells, leading to increased vessel permeability and tissue swelling. In ARDS, neutrophils in the pulmonary capillaries emigrate into the alveoli, damaging the capillaries and contributing to increased vessel permeability and the presence of an exudate in the alveoli. Edema may be transudative or exudative in nature. Transudates relate to an alteration in Starling's forces such that the oncotic pressure (serum albumin) is decreased, the intravascular hydrostatic pressure is increased, or both. Exudates imply an increase in vessel permeability, most commonly associated with an inflammatory condition. Right-sided heart failure and minimal change disease both produce transudative edema, as do left-sided heart failure and celiac disease; therefore, these conditions are not associated with increased vascular permeability. The cerebral edema of encephalitis is caused by increased vessel permeability, but the cerebral edema in hyponatremia is an intracellular edema related to osmotic forces that favor the movement of water into the intracellular fluid (ICF) compartment from the extracellular fluid (ECF) compartment. The pleural effusion seen in pneumonia results from increased vessel permeability, but the ascites seen in cirrhosis results from alterations in Starling's forces and an inability to degrade aldosterone.

9. The answer is C.   *(Biochemistry)*
Muscle maintains a large store of phosphocreatine as a reserve energy supply. As soon as adenosine triphosphate (ATP) is degraded to adenosine diphosphate (ADP) by muscle contraction, creatine kinase rephosphorylates the ADP by transferring a phosphate group from phosphocreatine. Glycerol kinase, aldolase B, an allosterically regulated pyruvate kinase isozyme, and glucokinase are generally liver-specific and not found in muscle.

10. The answer is A.   *(Pathology)*
Primary cancers of the ovary (most commonly serous cystadenocarcinoma) are more common than metastasis to the ovary. It is more likely to find metastatic, rather than primary, cancer in the lymph nodes (the most common site for metastasis), brain, bone, lungs, liver, and adrenals. Breast, prostate, and thyroid cancers commonly metastasize to bone. Lung cancers, especially small cell carcinomas, commonly metastasize to the brain. Gastrointestinal cancers commonly metastasize to the liver. Metastasis is defined as the discontinuous spread of malignant cells from one organ to another. It is the single best criterion for malignancy. The majority of patients already have metastasis when the tumor is first discovered, and most patients die from the metastases, rather than the primary tumor. For metastasis to occur, malignant cells must have the capacity to invade tissue. Dissemination of tumor occurs by seeding within body cavities, lymphatic spread, or hematogenous spread. Seeding is commonly seen with colorectal cancers and ovarian cancers. Lymphatic invasion is more common in carcinomas than sarcomas. Hematogenous spread is favored by sarcomas (but not exclusively); spread to the lungs and liver is a common finding.

11. The answer is E. *(Biochemistry)*
Acetyl coenzyme A (acetyl CoA) carboxylase adds a carbon to acetyl CoA to form malonyl CoA. This is the rate-determining step in fatty acid synthesis. This step, like all carboxylation reactions, requires biotin pyrophosphate as an essential cofactor. Although acetyl CoA carboxylase is activated by citrate, no fatty acid synthesis occurs in muscle. Insulin (the hormone of the fed state) activates fatty acid synthesis and glucagon (the enzyme of the fasted state) inhibits fatty acid synthesis; acetyl CoA carboxylase activity would be activated or inhibited accordingly. Malonyl CoA inhibits acetyl CoA in a negative feedback loop. Fatty acid degradation, not synthesis, takes place in the mitochondrial matrix; synthesis occurs in the cytosol.

12. The answer is B. *(Microbiology)*
Body secretions (e.g., saliva, tears, mucus secretions of the respiratory and intestinal tracts, prostatic fluid, milk) contain large amounts of immunoglobulin A (IgA). This class of immunoglobulin is known as the "secretory antibody." IgA in secretions is present primarily as a dimeric molecule held together by a joining (J) chain, a small protein synthesized by the plasmacytes that produce polymeric IgA. The J chain is attached to the antibody by disulfide bonds and bears no structural relationship to the heavy or light chains. IgA in secretions also has a secretory component that is produced by submucosal epithelial cells close to lymphoid tissues (e.g., Peyer's patches). The secretory component facilitates transport of the antibody to the outside of the body and may also stabilize polymeric IgA so that it is less apt to be degraded by enzymes and acids that may be present in secretions. Immunoglobulin G (IgG) represents approximately 80% of the antibody found in blood. Approximately 10% of the antibody in the blood is immunoglobulin M (IgM), the first antibody to appear in primary immune responses against most antigens. Only a small amount of immunoglobulin D (IgD) is ever secreted. The exact function of IgD is unknown. Immunoglobulin E (IgE) accounts for approximately 0.004% of the antibody in the serum. However, during infections with helminths and other multicellular parasites, high levels of IgE are pro-

duced. IgE is also very important in allergic disorders (e.g., type I hypersensitivity).

13. The answer is A. *(Biochemistry)*
The glycosaminoglycans are large polysaccharides attached to relatively smaller protein structures. They are usually negatively charged. The negative charges are provided by sulfate groups and the carboxyl groups of uronic acid moieties. The negative charges on the glycosaminoglycans repel each other, forcing the molecule to fan out, forming a gel-like viscous solution. Glycosaminoglycans are found in synovial fluid, vitreous humour, and the ground substance of connective tissues. Glycogen, proteins, phosphosphingolipids, and lysosomal membranes are generally not sulfonated.

14. The answer is C. *(Pathology)*
Fat embolization follows fractures of the shafts of long bones (most commonly the femurs) or severe soft tissue trauma and is the most likely mechanism behind this patient's clinical condition. One theory is that microglobules of fat from the marrow enter the circulation and damage tissue. The fatty acids damage vessel endothelium, resulting in thrombosis. A more recent theory is that swelling of adipose tissue in the area of injury pushes fat into the circulation. Symptoms and signs of fat embolism are usually delayed 24–72 hours. Neurologic findings are the most common cause of death and result from vessel occlusion by fat globules. Acute dyspnea is caused by plugging of the pulmonary capillaries with fat. Laboratory findings include thrombocytopenia (because platelets adhere to fat), severe hypoxemia (fat in the pulmonary capillaries interferes with gas exchange), and fat in the urine or sputum. Death occurs in 10%–15% of cases. Although disseminated intravascular coagulation (DIC) can complicate fat embolism, there is no evidence of bleeding related to the consumption of coagulation factors or prolongation of the prothrombin and partial thromboplastin times (PT and PTT). Pneumonia would not cause the neurologic abnormalities seen in this patient and would be associated with a productive cough. Atelectasis (alveolar collapse) commonly occurs in postoperative patients, and pulmonary embolism is a common complication in hospitalized patients, but neither condition would be associated with neurologic abnormalities, thrombocytopenia or petechial lesions.

15-16. The answers are: 15-C, 16-B. (*Biochemistry*)

The symptoms are consistent with those of gout. The meal the man ate is extraordinarily rich in foods that would be expected to precipitate an attack of gout in a susceptible patient. Attacks of gout have long been associated with alcohol consumption, in particular red wines. In addition, sweetbreads and pâté are foods derived from organs that actively synthesize proteins and as a consequence are a rich source of RNA, while caviar (sturgeon roe) is a rich source of DNA. Assuming monosodium urate crystals are observed in the synovial fluid, the diagnosis is confirmed and there would be no need to conduct any of the other tests listed in the question.

Some patients suffering from gout have been found to have a mutant form of phosphoribosyl-ribose-pyrophosphate (PRPP) synthetase that is less susceptible to allosteric inhibition by inorganic phosphate or to feedback inhibition by guanosine diphosphate (GDP), adenosine diphosphate (ADP), or both. Failure to inhibit PRPP activity leads to overproduction of purines and excessive uric acid (following degradation of the purines). Xanthine oxidase converts hypoxanthine and xanthine to uric acid. The objective of allopurinol therapy in the treatment of gout is to inhibit this enzyme; therefore, it is illogical to expect a deficiency of the enzyme to cause gout. Adenosine deaminase is another enzyme involved in the degradation of a purine. Therefore, a deficiency of this enzyme does not cause gout. Glucose-6-phosphatase deficiency (Von Gierke's glycogenosis) can lead to gout. Because hepatocytes cannot convert glucose-6-phosphate to glucose, they divert more carbon into the transketolase and transaldolase reactions of the pentose phosphate shunt. This increases ribose 5-phosphate levels and consequently increases PRPP levels and purine synthesis. However, a 55-year-old man with a glycogen storage disease would be a real rarity. Complete hypoxanthine-guanine phosphoribosyltransferase (HGPRTase) deficiency, a sex-linked recessive disorder, leads to the Lesch-Nyhan syndrome. This disease is associated with mental retardation and self mutilation, traits that do not apply to this patient. However, a partial HGPRTase deficiency does lead to gout in some patients who have an aberrant enzyme with some, but not full, activity.

17. The answer is E. (*Pathology*)

Venous clots primarily consist of coagulated blood (i.e., coagulation factors, erythrocytes and platelets), while arterial clots are primarily composed of aggregated platelets. Venous clots most frequently develop in the setting of stasis, while arterial clots develop over atherosclerotic plaques or in areas of turbulence (injury to the vessel endothelium predisposes to platelet adhesion). Arterial clots are paler than venous thrombi because they are primarily composed of platelets. Aspirin inhibits platelet aggregation and is the primary agent used to prevent arterial clots. Because venous clots are primarily composed of clotted blood, heparin and warfarin derivatives are usually used to prevent venous thrombosis.

18. The answer is C. (*Biochemistry*)

Pepsin begins the process of protein digestion, which continues in the small intestine by the action of a group of pancreatic proteases. Enteropeptidase from intestinal mucosal cells activates trypsinogen to form active trypsin. Trypsin then autocatalytically activates additional trypsinogen molecules as well as the precursors of other pancreatic proteases. Chymotrypsinogen, for example, is converted to chymotrypsin. Trypsin, chymotrypsin, and other pancreatic proteases then degrade the protein molecules to oligopeptides. Digestion is completed by aminopeptidase in the small intestine.

19. The answer is C. (*Microbiology*)

After 120 minutes, there would be 6.4×10^4 bacteria. Bacteria divide by binary fission. Increases in numbers are logarithmic, not merely additive. The increase in number is calculated as follows:

Time	Bacterial Concentration
0	4×10^3
40 (lag phase)	4×10^3
60 (1 generation time)	8×10^3
80 (2 generation times)	16×10^3 or 1.6×10^4
100 (3 generation times)	32×10^3 or 3.2×10^4
120 (4 generation times)	64×10^3 or 6.4×10^4

20. The answer is D. *(Biochemistry)*
By convention, oligopeptides are written with the amino terminus on the left and the carboxy terminus on the right. Because trypsin cleaves on the carboxy side of arginine and lysine residues, it would cleave the peptide in question at point D. Chymotrypsin preferentially cleaves on the carboxy side of the aromatic amino acids phenylalanine, tyrosine, and tryptophan. Elastase cleaves on the carboxy side of alanine, glycine, and serine. Carboxypeptidase cleaves one amino acid at a time from the carboxy terminus, while aminopeptidase cleaves one amino acid at a time from the amino terminus.

21. The answer is C. *(Pathology)*
Antithrombin III deficiency and oral contraceptives are both associated with venous thrombosis. Antithrombin III normally inactivates coagulation factors that are serine proteases (e.g., thrombin, factors XII, XI, and X), while the estrogen in oral contraceptives increases the levels of coagulation factors and decreases the concentration of antithrombin III. The postoperative state leaves a patient susceptible to venous stasis and venous thrombosis, while aspirin inhibits platelet aggregation (and, therefore, arterial thrombi) by blocking cyclooxygenase. Disseminated malignancy is frequently accompanied by thrombocytosis and elevated coagulation factors, thus predisposing to venous thrombosis, while heparin, an anticoagulant, enhances antithrombin III activity. Tissue plasminogen activator therapy causes activation of plasminogen leading to the formation of plasmin, which dissolves clots, while polycythemia rubra vera increases blood viscosity, predisposing to clots. Protein C deficiency predisposes to venous thrombosis because protein C normally inactivates factors V and VIII, while coumarin inhibits epoxide reductase, which decreases vitamin K_1 levels, leaving the patient anticoagulated. Vitamin K_1 is necessary for the carboxylation of the vitamin K–dependent factors (i.e., II, VII, IX, and X), protein C, and protein S.

22. The answer is C. *(Biochemistry)*
Prior to exercising, the patient was in negative nitrogen balance and his body fat content was increasing. Since beginning the diet and exercise regimen, the patient is in positive nitrogen balance and his body fat content is decreasing. Wasting of muscle due to any cause, including lack of exercise, is generally associated with a negative nitrogen balance (excretion of more nitrogen than is ingested), as a result of the net loss of muscle protein and a concomitant increase in nitrogen excretion. While losing muscle, the patient gained weight. Therefore, his body fat content was increasing. Exercise increased his muscle mass, putting him into positive nitrogen balance (i.e., excreting less nitrogen than he ingested). Because the patient is gaining muscle mass without gaining weight, his body fat content is decreasing.

23. The answer is D. *(Behavioral science)*
The diagnosis for the 9-year-old boy who tricks fellow students into giving him their lunch money, rarely follows the school rules, and shows little interest in the feelings of others is conduct disorder. Conduct disorder involves failure to follow social norms and would be considered criminal behavior in an adult. Although conduct disorder in childhood has many of the characteristics of antisocial personality disorder and is associated with antisocial personality disorder in adulthood, personality disorder is generally not diagnosed before age 16. Children with attention deficit/hyperactivity disorder show increased activity and failure to pay attention and children with oppositional defiant disorder may challenge authority; neither group shows behavior that would be considered criminal in an adult.

24. The answer is C. *(Biochemistry)*
Insulin levels are very low or nonexistent in untreated type I diabetes, which permits blood glucose levels to increase. The inhibitory effect of glucose on glucagon excretion also requires insulin. Thus, at least initially, the glucagon levels increase despite the high glucose levels, which further increases glucose levels, activates hepatic adenyl cyclase, and increases fatty acid mobilization from the adipocytes. These actions increase circulating fatty acid levels, and provide more substrate for hepatic ketone body formation, resulting in a ketoacidosis that is more severe than that observed during fasting. In the normal physiologic response to fasting, the regulatory mechanisms are intact. The stimulus for increased glucagon levels and lower insulin concentrations is low blood glucose. Although the glucagon—

insulin ratio is markedly increased, insulin is never completely absent. In addition, blood glucose levels are, by definition, never increased during fasting. In both diabetic and physiologic ketoacidosis, the increase in glucagon increases hepatic cyclic adenosine monophosphate (cAMP) levels. In diabetes, blood fatty acid levels are elevated, whereas in fasting they are lowered. This difference may result from the fact that the increase in the glucagon–insulin ratio is more exaggerated in diabetes than in fasting, or that in fasting the driving force is a need for fuel and the mechanisms for its utilization remain intact.

25. The answer is A.   *(Microbiology)*
The presence of catalase (or peroxidase in lactobacilli) and superoxide dismutase indicates that the bacterium is able to grow under aerobic conditions because it is capable of degrading the potentially harmful byproducts of aerobic respiration (i.e., hydrogen peroxide and oxygen radicals). Superoxide dismutase converts superoxide (the most toxic metabolite) to hydrogen peroxide and oxygen. Catalase degrades hydrogen peroxide to water and oxygen. Hydrogen peroxide and oxygen radicals would be injurious to the bacteria and would prevent normal metabolism and growth unless destroyed by the enzymes. Anaerobic bacteria are anaerobic because they do not contain sufficient amounts of catalase and superoxide dismutase to destroy the toxic byproducts of aerobic respiration. Some anaerobes do contain flavoproteins, indicating that some oxygen radicals, hydrogen peroxide, or both may be produced. Growth of these bacteria would not be affected by a lowered oxygen concentration. Spore germination into vegetative bacteria would not be directly affected by the presence of these enzymes.

26. The answer is B.   *(Biochemistry)*
The toxin that causes the diarrhea of cholera acts by inducing adenosine diphosphate (ADP) ribosylation of a G_s protein. *Vibrio cholerae*, *Escherichia coli*, and *Bacillus cereus* produce heat-labile enterotoxins that consist of an active subunit and a cell surface binding subunit. The active subunit of the toxin is an enzyme that catalyzes a reaction between the α subunit of the cellular G_s protein and oxidized nicotinamide adenine dinucleotide (NAD^+), forming an ADP ribosyl–$G_{\alpha s}$

protein complex. This complex results in the irreversible activation of the G_s protein, which, in turn, activates adenylate cyclase and increases cyclic adenosine monophosphate (cAMP) levels. Consequently, protein kinase A (cAMP-activated protein kinase) activity increases and water and electrolytes are excreted from the cell, causing a voluminous "rice-water" diarrhea. Because the fluid is isotonic, the diarrhea is referred to as "secretory." Exotoxins produced by *Corynebacterium diphtheriae* and *Pseudomonas aeruginosa* catalyze the ADP ribosylation of elongation factor-2 (EF-2), terminating protein synthesis in the affected cells and killing them. Pertussis toxin induces an ADP ribosylation of a G_i protein. In this case, the G_i protein is inactivated, resulting, once again, in overproduction of cAMP.

27. The answer is A.   *(Pharmacology)*
Drug C is a weak base because it is more ionized and rapidly excreted in urine of an acidic pH. The pH of the urine determines the proportion of ionized and unionized forms of weak acids and bases. Because ionized drugs are less lipid-soluble than unionized drugs, they are not reabsorbed as well as unionized drugs. Therefore, the urine pH influences the renal clearance of acidic or basic drugs. Weak acids are more ionized at an alkaline pH and weak bases are more ionized at an acidic pH. Drug A is not a weak acid or base because its renal clearance is the same in acidic and basic urine. Drug B is a weak acid, not a weak base, because it is more ionized and rapidly excreted in urine with an alkaline pH.

28. The answer is D.   *(Biochemistry)*
Glutamate serves as the central "way station" through which most of the ammonia in urea passes, because most of the amino acids transaminate with α-ketoglutarate. The newly formed glutamate either presents the ammonia to carbamoylphosphate synthetase I (the first enzyme of the urea cycle) via the action of glutamate dehydrogenase, or passes it, via transamination, to oxaloacetic acid to form aspartate, the source of the second nitrogen in urea. The rate-limiting step of the urea cycle is catalyzed by carbamoylphosphate synthetase I. Arginase is the last reaction in the sequence. Rarely, if ever, will the last reaction in a sequence be rate-limiting, because metabolites would

pile up behind this step. The normal dietary requirement for protein is a little less in grams than a person's weight in kilograms, or roughly 40–50 grams per day. However, the daily turnover is an order of magnitude greater. Normally, 400–500 grams of protein are broken down and resynthesized per day. In other words, approximately 90% of the amino acids liberated by the daily hydrolysis of protein are salvaged and reincorporated into protein. Amino acids are not stored. Those lost every day must be replaced the same day or negative nitrogen balance will occur. Whereas alanine is the primary transport form of carbon from muscle to liver during gluconeogenesis, it is not particularly abundant in muscle.

29. The answer is C.   (*Microbiology*)
Selective toxicity refers to the fact that antibacterial agents are useful for combating infections caused by microbes because the microbes will be adversely affected, while the host will not be adversely affected (or, at least, only minimally affected) by the antimicrobial. For example, many antibacterial agents target a bacterial component (e.g., the cell wall) that is not possessed by the host cell. The relatively high amounts of antimicrobials needed to kill some microorganisms (e.g., *Pseudomonas* species) is not a situation where the term selective toxicity would be meaningful. Similarly, differences in the responses of gram-positive and gram-negative bacteria to antibiotics is not described by selective toxicity. Here, the term "range of activity" (i.e., broad or narrow) is usually used. A broad-spectrum antimicrobial will kill both gram-positive and gram-negative bacteria. Finally, isolating a pathogenic strain of a microorganism from a disease process gives no indication as to whether or not that organism will respond to a specific antimicrobial. A sensitivity test would need to be performed in the laboratory on the purified organism.

30. The answer is D.   (*Biochemistry*)
Most of the nitrogens in urea existed, if only briefly, as the α-amino group of glutamate; therefore, glutamate dehydrogenase and arginosuccinate synthetase account for the majority of the nitrogen excreted as urea. With the exception of lysine, all of the amino acids transaminate, directly or indirectly, with α-ketoglutarate to form glutamate. Glutamate transaminates with oxaloacetic acid to form aspartic acid or is deaminated by

glutamate dehydrogenase to form ammonia, which is used by carbamoyl synthetase I to form carbamoylphosphate. Carbamoylphosphate condenses with ornithine to form citrulline. Arginosuccinate synthetase combines aspartate to the citrulline forming arginine, which is then cleaved by arginase to produce urea. Carbamoyl synthetase I, the initiating enzyme of the urea cycle, should not be confused with carbamoyl synthetase II, which catalyzes the first step in pyrimidine synthesis. D-Amino acid oxidase liberates free ammonia from glycine. This ammonia can also be converted to carbamoyl phosphate, but produces only a small fraction of the ammonia in urea relative to that produced by the glutamic acid dehydrogenase, which produces ammonia from all of the amino acids that transaminate with α-ketoglutaric acid. Glutamine synthetase uses ammonia to form the amide of glutamic acid, glutamine. Glutaminase is induced by lower-than-normal plasma pH and plays an important role in protecting the body against acidosis, because ammonia binds with hydrogen ion an is excreted in the urine. Urease is an enzyme used to break down urea and is not found in mammals.

31. The answer is A.   (*Physiology*)
Phospholipase C is activated by hormones whose receptors are coupled to a Gp protein. It cleaves the phosphoester bond between carbon 3 of glycerol and inositol 4,5 bisphosphate on phosphatidylinositol diphosphate (PIP_2), producing diacylglycerol (DAG) and inositol triphosphate (IP_3). DAG and IP_3 are second messengers. IP_3 raises the free intracellular calcium ion levels. Calcium ion and DAG act synergistically to activate protein kinase C. Phospholipase C does not directly stimulate reactions that affect the activity of protein kinase A, tyrosine kinase, or guanylate kinase. Phospholipase A_2 cleaves ester bonds at carbon 2.

32. The answer is B.   (*Biochemistry*)
Cystinuria, one of the most common inherited diseases, is caused by a deficiency of the transport system that is responsible for the reabsorption of the amino acids cysteine, ornithine, arginine, and lysine in kidney tubules. In patients with this disease, the levels of these four amino acids in the urine is increased. Cysteine becomes oxidized to form cystine, which precipitates to form kidney stones.

33. The answer is D. *(Microbiology)*
The gram-positive bacteria are capable of surviving in the patient, despite antimicrobial treatment. The reappearance of disease (relapse) indicates that the microorganism has not been totally eradicated by the antibiotics that have been used. Penicillin, bacitracin, cephalosporin, and vancomycin all affect the development of the gram-positive cell wall. However, it is known that protoplasts (gram-positive bacteria that lack a cell wall) and L-form bacteria may survive if an osmotically-protected environment can be found. Therefore, most of the bacteria involved in an acute infection episode would probably be killed by penicillin, bacitracin, cephalosporin, or vancomycin, but use of these agents may lead to protoplast or L-form bacteria formation. Once the host's system eliminates the antibiotic, these organisms could again develop the ability to produce cell walls, grow in the host, and cause disease. In this patient, choosing tetracycline as an alternative antibiotic would be an excellent decision because another bacterial metabolic target (protein synthesis) would be affected. Tetracycline is a broad-spectrum agent that affects gram-positive and gram-negative organisms. Use of this antimicrobial would not lead to protoplast or L-form formation.

34. The answer is B. *(Pharmacology)*
Drug B has the highest bioavailability. The oral bioavailability (F_o) is the fraction of drug reaching the systemic circulation after oral administration. It depends on the fraction absorbed (f) and the degree of "first-pass" elimination by the liver, as expressed by the ratio of hepatic clearance to hepatic blood flow [i.e., the extraction ratio (ER)]: $F_o = f \times (1-ER)$. According to the data in the table, drug E is the best absorbed, but has a high ER and a bioavailability of 0.200. Drug B is less well absorbed but has a low ER, resulting in the highest bioavailability (0.300). Drugs C and D are better absorbed than drug B, but they have higher ERs, resulting in bioavailabilities of 0.250 and 0.125, respectively. Drug A has a bioavailability of 0.225.

35. The answer is C. *(Microbiology)*
Innate, or natural, immunity consists of a broad range of factors that are protective to the host. All of these factors are relatively nonspecific (i.e., specific antigenic

stimulation is not required). Neutrophils, along with macrophages and natural killer (NK) cells, are among the most important cells in innate immunity. Neutrophils, which survive for only a few days, are phagocytes. They are sometimes referred to as granulocytes (because of the numerous granules in the cytoplasm) or polymorphonuclear cells (because of their lobulated, pinched-off nuclear configuration). Neutrophils are the most abundant leukocytes present in the circulation—50% are circulating and 50% are members of the marginating pool (i.e., they are adherent to the endothelium). Neutrophils can migrate into tissues in response to chemical mediators (e.g., C5a and leukotriene B_4). T and B lymphocytes are important cells of acquired immunity, which involves highly specific interactions between antigen and receptor molecules on the lymphocyte surface. Plasmacytes are activated antibody-producing B lymphocytes. Mast cells are scattered throughout tissues and are important in type I hypersensitivity reactions.

36. The answer is B. *(Biochemistry)*
Calcium and magnesium ions act antagonistically: calcium stimulates, magnesium relaxes. Calcium and sodium are mainly extracellular ions, whereas magnesium and potassium are primarily intracellular ions. Because the serum water compartment contains only approximately 9% of the water in the body, and because magnesium and potassium are primarily intracellular ions, the amount of magnesium and potassium in serum represents only a small fraction of the total body content. Therefore, measurement of serum concentration of these ions is an unreliable measure of the total body stores. A small but significant fraction of the total body magnesium is found in association with bone. It is believed to be chemi-absorbed on the surface of the hydroxyapatite crystals and is, for the most part, readily available to the fluids of the body. The adenosine triphosphate (ATP)-dependent sodium–potassium pump accounts for more than half of the basal metabolic energy expended. Cells are constantly working against a large gradient to exclude sodium and retain potassium.

37. The answer is A. *(Microbiology)*
Neutrophils appear at the site of tissue injury within approximately 30 minutes. The injury may be the

—Eliminat'n was Not proportional to plasma ccn t½ is

result of microbial, physical, chemical, or immunologic damage to tissues. Neutrophils are attracted to the injury site by chemical mediators (e.g., chemotactic agents such as C5a and leukotriene B_4). Some chemical mediators (e.g., histamine) increase vascular permeability, facilitating neutrophil migration from the blood into the damaged tissues. The initial increase in blood flow accounts for the redness (rubor) and heat (calor) at the injured site. These early events, which increase in intensity over a period of hours, are known as acute inflammation. Neutrophils are phagocytic and begin engulfing cell debris and foreign materials immediately upon arrival. Phagocytosis is enhanced by a variety of proteins known as opsonins. The most important ones are complement derivatives and immunoglobulins (e.g., C3b and IgG, respectively). Opsonins increase phagocytic ability because neutrophils, monocytes, and macrophages have receptors for them. The mechanisms by which neutrophils accomplish phagocytosis are nonspecific and are believed to be very similar to those of macrophages. Neutrophils have a short life span and do not replicate. As more and more of them are released from the bone marrow following interleukin-1 stimulation, neutrophilic leukocytosis occurs. If the reaction is prolonged, mononuclear cells begin to accumulate, especially macrophages. In addition to being phagocytic, macrophages act as accessory cells in generating humoral and cell-mediated responses from B and T lymphocytes, which eventually also accumulate in the area of injury. Activation of lymphocytes results in specific acquired immunity (as opposed to innate or natural immunity). If the cause of the problem is not removed or destroyed, chronic inflammation may occur. In these cases, the inflammatory response may be only temporarily alleviated with the use of anti-inflammatory agents like aspirin or nonsteroidals.

38. The answer is C. *(Pharmacology)*
When the drug elimination mechanism is saturated, such as is observed with high doses of phenytoin, the plasma drug concentration declines at a constant rate. In such cases, the plasma half-life is proportional to the plasma drug concentration and slowly declines until the elimination mechanism is no longer saturated. First-order kinetics are observed when the elimination mechanism is no longer saturated. In this case, phenytoin was eliminated at a constant rate that was not proportional to plasma drug concentration. Phenytoin is almost entirely eliminated by hepatic metabolism and very little is excreted unchanged. Hence, acidification of the urine would not accelerate phenytoin elimination.

39. The answer is C. *(Microbiology)*
Neutrophils are most important in mediating the acute inflammatory reaction seen in immune complex glomerulonephritis. Immune complex glomerulonephritis occurs when a circulating antibody binds to an antigen and activates the complement cascade, resulting in the generation of C5a, a potent inflammatory factor that is chemotactic for neutrophils. The infiltrating neutrophils attempt to phagocytose immune complexes lodged in the glomeruli. Abortively released lysosomal enzymes and free oxygen radicals damage the glomerular capillaries. The endothelial cells that line the blood vessel walls swell and proliferate, platelets aggregate on top of injured endothelial cells, and fibrin deposition occurs. This type of inflammation is called fibrinoid necrosis and accompanies all immune complex–mediated disease (e.g., poststreptococcal glomerulonephritis). Eosinophils are primarily associated with allergic reactions and infections with parasitic helminths. Cytotoxic (and helper) T lymphocytes and macrophages are also considered to be major inflammatory cells, but appear later during the reaction. Natural killer (NK) cells are non-T cells that are important in innate (natural) immunity. They are best known for their ability to kill virally-infected cells and tumor cells.

40. The answer is D. *(Behavioral science)*
AIDS is the leading cause of death in people 25–44 years old in the United States. Accidents, cancer and heart disease, homicide, and suicide are the second, third, fourth, and fifth leading causes of death in this age group.

41. The answer is D. *(Microbiology)*
Ureaplasma urealyticum is one of several causes of nongonococcal urethritis in men. Ureaplasma can be distinguished from mycoplasma by its ability to produce the enzyme urease. The only other organism that could cause this man's symptoms is *Neisseria*

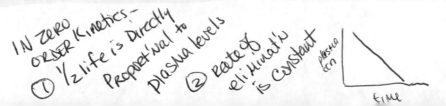

IN ZERO ORDER Kinetics – (1) ½ life is Directly Proport'nal to plasma levels (2) Rate of eliminat'n is constant

gonorrhoeae; however, if *N. gonorrhoeae* were the causative agent, a Gram stain of the urethral discharge would demonstrate gram-negative diplococci, often within white blood cells. *Treponema pallidum, Candida albicans,* and *Staphylococcus aureus* would be unlikely to cause nongonococcal urethritis.

42. The answer is B.   *(Behavioral science)*
The percentage of all health care costs incurred by the elderly in the United States is approximately 30%. This figure is expected to raise to 50% by the year 2020.

43. The answer is E.   *(Microbiology)*
Activated macrophages are the epithelioid cells of granulomas. Macrophages accumulate around foreign targets that are large and difficult to destroy (e.g., mycobacteria, fungi, mineral oil) and interdigitate to form a continuous sheet resembling an epithelium. The epithelioid-like macrophages, fused macrophages (multinucleated giant cells), lymphocytes, fibroblasts, and other cell types are found in granulomas, which are characteristic of type IV hypersensitivity reactions (cellular immunity). Activated macrophages do not specifically destroy normal or abnormal tissues. Although they bind to some particles directly, the molecular interactions are nonspecific. CD4$^+$ T lymphocytes, not activated macrophages, are the major producers of interleukin-2. Activated macrophages secrete more than 100 other substances, including interleukin-1 and tumor necrosis factor-α. Activated macrophages express many surface molecules, including receptors for complement components (C3b), immunoglobulin G (IgG), bacterial carbohydrates, cytokines (interleukin-1, interleukin-3, interferon-α, -β, and -γ, and transforming growth factor-β, but not antigen-specific receptors. The presence of receptors for IgG (Fc receptors) and C3b is important in the pathogenesis of autoimmune hemolytic anemia, thrombocytopenia, and neutropenia. Most macrophages constitutively express major histocompatibility complex (MHC) class I and class II molecules. Class II expression increases on the activated macrophage surface. B7, a costimulatory molecule for T lymphocytes, appears on the activated macrophage after a single encounter with antigen. These molecules are involved in macrophage presentation of antigenic peptides to T lymphocytes, making macrophages important accessory cells in specific immune responses. Activated macrophages are better at antigen presentation than nonactivated cells.

44. The answer is A.   *(Biochemistry)*
Fatty acids are synthesized from glucose under high energy charge (energy-rich) conditions. In order for fatty acid synthesis to occur, the glucose carbons must first traverse the glycolytic pathway. Under energy-rich conditions, the concentrations of citrate and adenosine triphosphate (ATP), negative modulators of phosphofructokinase-1, will be high, deactivating the enzyme. However, there is a simultaneous increase in fructose 2,6-bisphosphate levels, an activator that overrides the inhibition. This latter compound is synthesized by phosphofructokinase-2 when insulin levels are high and glucagon levels are low, as in the fed condition. Thus the normal response to a carbohydrate meal is an increase in fructose 2,6-bisphosphate levels; this activates phosphofructokinase-2 and stimulates the flux of glucose through the glycolytic sequence to form acetylcoenzyme A (acetyl CoA) and, eventually, fatty acids. However, in the case of the individual in this question, the increase in fructose 2,6-bisphosphate would be in vain because of the lowered affinity of phosphofructokinase-1 for this activator [i.e., the increased dissociation constant (K_d)].

45. The answer is C.   *(Microbiology)*
Natural killer (NK) cell activity is thought to provide an important early defense against viruses, and possibly other infectious agents and tumor cells. NK cells do not need to be activated or primed in order to kill cells expressing viral antigens. NK cell activity is dramatically increased (20- to 100-fold) by the production of interferon-α and -β after viral infection. Activated cytotoxic T lymphocytes are able to kill virally-infected target cells; however, because many viruses replicate rapidly and generation of cytotoxic T lymphocytes takes several days, these cells are not of major importance in early defense. The term "virgin lymphocytes" refers to lymphocytes that have not yet encountered the antigen to which they can respond, hence they would provide no defense until after activation and clonal expansion have taken place. Most virgin

lymphocytes (mature, resting B and T cells) have a short life span and die within a few days of leaving the bone marrow or thymus. Plasmacytes are antibody-secreting B lymphocytes. As with T lymphocytes, activation and clonal expansion requires several days; therefore, plasmacytes do not wage an immediate response. T and B lymphocytes proliferate extensively after they are activated by the appropriate antigen. Some of the progeny of these cells develop into memory cells. Memory cells resemble the virgin lymphocytes from which they are derived, but they are long-lived (i.e., they can survive for years, sometimes for the life of the individual). In a subsequent encounter with the same infectious agent, the memory cells provide a more rapid and more effective defense. It should be noted that memory cells are not generated in response to a T-independent antigen.

46. The answer is C. *(Behavioral science)*
Medicare was designed primarily for people eligible for Social Security (i.e., those over 65 years of age or chronically ill). Medicaid was designed primarily for economically disadvantaged people and their families. Long-term nursing home care is not covered under Medicare. People without health insurance may lose their lifetime accumulation of assets if they become seriously ill and require hospitalization.

47. The answer is C. *(Microbiology)*
Clostridium difficile causes antibiotic-associated pseudomembranous enterocolitis. *C. difficile* is a part of the normal flora of the gastrointestinal tract in approximately 3%–10% of the general population. When broad-spectrum antimicrobials (e.g., ampicillin) are used, the drug-sensitive normal flora are killed. *C. difficile* is relatively resistant to many of these antibiotics, leading to bacterial overgrowth. It produces exotoxin A (an enterotoxin), which causes a watery diarrhea, and exotoxin B, a cytotoxin that damages the gut mucosa, leading to an accumulation of inflammatory cells and fibrin (pseudomembrane). Pseudomembranous enterocolitis is not an invasive enterocolitis. Although *Staphylococcus aureus* is also relatively resistant to broad-spectrum antibiotics and can cause diarrhea and fever, there is less damage to the gut mucosa. Blood loss and leukocytosis would not usually be observed, except in neonates. *C. perfringens* and *Bacillus*

cereus can cause diarrhea, but the diarrhea is associated with food poisoning, not antibiotics. *Streptococcus pyogenes* does not cause diarrhea.

48. The answer is A. *(Behavioral science)*
The average citizen of the United States visits the doctor 5.5 times per year. In countries with systems of socialized medicine, the average number of visits made by patients to doctors per year is higher. Currently, most physicians in the United States are paid on a fee-for-service basis, a fact that probably influences patient behavior. With a system of socialized medicine or of managed care, patients pay through their taxes or pay an annual premium for health care.

49. The answer is B. *(Pharmacology)*
The elimination half-life of this drug is 4 hours. The elimination half-life depends on the volume of distribution and clearance rate and can be calculated as $t_{1/2} = 0.7 \times Vd / CL$, where $t_{1/2}$ = the elimination half-life, Vd = the volume of distribution, and CL = clearance. Therefore, the elimination half-life is directly proportional to the volume of distribution and inversely related to clearance. The hepatic extraction ratio and T_{max} are factors relating to oral bioavailability and the rate of absorption, and these do not affect elimination half-life.

50. The answer is E. *(Behavioral science)*
This widow's first few years in the nursing home will be paid for by her savings. The current cost of nursing home care in the United States is between $35,000 and $75,000 per year. After her $300,000 in savings are gone, she will become one of the elderly indigent, and her nursing home care will be paid for by Medicaid. Medicare only covers nursing home care for elderly people for a limited time following a medical hospitalization. Health maintenance organizations (HMOs) and independent practice associations (IPAs) do not generally cover nursing home care.

51. The answer is A. *(Microbiology)*
The Gram stain is a fundamental staining technique based on the properties of bacterial cell walls. Gram-positive bacteria, which have a thick peptidoglycan cell wall, stain blue and gram-negative bacteria, which have lipid-rich, thin walls, stain red. This student

probably added too much acetone, a destaining agent, which can cause gram-positive organisms to appear gram-negative. The Gram stain procedure is performed as follows:

1. The bacterial smear is heat-fixed on a glass slide.
2. Crystal violet dye is applied for 1 minute.
3. The slide is rinsed with water.
4. Iodine solution is applied for 1 minute.
5. The slide is rinsed with water.
6. The slide is briefly rinsed with an organic solvent (e.g., acetone, alcohol).
7. The slide is counterstained with safranin for 1 minute.
8. The slide is rinsed with water and examined.

The crystal violet–iodine complex is retained by the thick peptidoglycan cell wall of gram-positive organisms, causing them to appear blue. In gram-negative organisms, the organic solvent extracts the blue dye from the lipid-rich, thin-walled gram-negative bacteria. The safranin then stains the colorless bacteria red.

52. The answer is B.   *(Behavioral science)*
In Freud's topographic model of the mind, the unconscious mind contains repressed thoughts and feelings while the preconscious mind is characterized by memories that are available to both the conscious and the unconscious minds. The conscious mind operates in close relationship with the preconscious mind but does not have access to the unconscious. In Freud's structural model of the mind, the mind contains the id (sexual and aggressive drives), the ego (control of the expression of these drives), and the superego (the conscience), all of which operate on a primarily unconscious level.

53. The answer is B.   *(Microbiology)*
Chlamydia and *Rickettsia* are true obligate intracellular parasites (i.e., they require host cells to produce new progeny organisms). They cannot grow outside host cells because they cannot produce sufficient adenosine triphosphate (ATP). In other words, they are energy deficient. *Chlamydia* species cause psittacosis, trachoma, and genital and upper respiratory tract infections. Laboratory diagnosis (culture and isolation) involves the detection of inclusion bodies using immunofluoresence microscopy or the detection of antibodies using enzyme-linked immunosorbent assay

(ELISA) techniques. *Rickettsia* typically infect the vascular system, particularly the endothelial lining of the blood vessels. *Mycoplasma* (a genus of bacteria that lack cell walls) and true bacteria can be grown in the laboratory on media of various kinds. Even bacteria that prefer intracellular locations (e.g., *Mycobacterium tuberculosis, Brucella*) can be grown on media that contains the proper nutrients and growth factors.

54-55. The answers are: 54-D, 55-B.   *(Behavioral science)*
The crude birth rate is defined as the number of live births among residents in an area in a calendar year divided by the average population of the area in that same year. The number of live births was 4000 and the total population was 1,450,000; therefore, the crude birth rate was 4000/1,450,000.

The maternal mortality rate is the number of deaths from causes related to childbirth in a year divided by the number of live births in the same year. Therefore, the maternal mortality rate is 40/4000. The maternal mortality rate reflects the adequacy of prenatal care as well as the general socioeconomic status of the area.

56. The answer is C.   *(Behavioral science)*
The mortality rate for African-American infants is 2.4 times higher than that for white infants in the United States. The infant mortality rate is higher among African-Americans primarily because of decreased access to health care services as a result of low socioeconomic status.

57. The answer is D.   *(Behavioral science)*
Bipolar disorder has been linked to markers on the X chromosome. The concordance rate is the chance of a relative of an affected individual developing the illness. For bipolar illness, the concordance rate is 14%–20% for dizygotic twins or for siblings, 50%–75% for the child of two affected parents, 65%–67% for a monozygotic twin, and 27% for the child of one parent with bipolar illness. The concordance rate is higher for bipolar than for unipolar disorder. The lifetime incidence of unipolar disorder is approximately 15%–20% in women and only 10% in men. In contrast, the lifetime incidence of bipolar disorder is approximately equal in men and women.

58. The answer is B. *(Pharmacology)*
The elimination half-life is the time required to reduce the plasma drug concentration by 50%. In this example, the drug concentration was reduced by 87.5%, which would require 3 half-lives. Because 12 hours had elapsed, the half-life must be 4 hours.

59. The answer is C. *(Behavioral science)*
Latency age children (i.e., those 6–11 years of age) prefer to play with children of the same sex. Younger children do not have a preference for playing with same-sex children; adolescents often seek the company of those of the opposite sex.

60. The answer is C. *(Pharmacology)*
Hydroxylation of phenytoin is catalyzed by the cytochrome P-450 enzyme system. Cytochrome P-450 participates in a wide range of oxidative reactions, including hydroxylations, dealkylations, deaminations, and other reactions catalyzed by mixed function oxidases (MFOs). Cytochrome P-450 is also involved in some reductive reactions, but it is not involved in hydrolytic or synthetic (conjugative) reactions.

[handwritten: involved in Phase I Metab.]

61. The answer is C. *(Behavioral science)*
Following childbirth, 33%–50% of new mothers experience sadness, i.e., "baby blues." The sadness is short-lived (i.e., it usually resolves after 1 week) and results from changes in hormone levels, the stress of childbirth, fatigue, and an awareness of increased responsibility. Approximately 5%–10% of women suffer from a more severe depression after childbirth and require psychiatric treatment.

62. The answer is E. *(Behavioral science)*
In the United States, the infant mortality rate is lowest among Japanese infants (6.4 deaths per 1000 live births). The mortality rates for Anglo-American, Chinese-American, Native American, and African-American infants are 7.3, 7.6, 14.4, and 18.3 per 1000 live births, respectively.

63. The answer is A. *(Behavioral science)*
Mahler described the first month of postnatal life as the normal autistic phase because the infant has little

interaction with people or with the external environment at this age. Freud described early infant development as the oral phase because the major site of gratification is the mouth. Erikson described the first year of life as the stage of trust versus mistrust, when the child learns to rely on and trust the caregiver to provide for his needs. Piaget described the period from birth to 2 years of age as the sensorimotor stage, when the child learns to master her environment through assimilation and accomodation. Harlowe studied the role of attachment in early infant development in monkeys.

64. The answer is D. *(Pharmacology)*
Cimetidine inhibits the hepatic cytochrome P-450 enzyme system, thereby interfering with the metabolism of many drugs, including warfarin. Inhibition of the hepatic cytochrome P-450 enzyme system decreases hepatic warfarin clearance and increases its plasma concentration and anticoagulant effect. Other histamine$_2$-blockers (H$_2$-blockers), such as ranitidine, have little or no effect on the cytochrome P-450 system and are preferred when patients are receiving warfarin and other drugs metabolized by cytochrome P-450. Cimetidine has no effect on blood coagulation, renal tubular secretion, plasma-protein binding, or oral drug bioavailability.

65. The answer is A. *(Behavioral science)*
This child is demonstrating stranger anxiety (i.e., the infant's tendency to cry and cling to the mother when a stranger approaches). Stranger anxiety is normal in infants between 7 and 9 months of age. Stranger anxiety indicates that the infant has a specific attachment to his mother and is able to distinguish her from strangers. Infants exposed to multiple caregivers are less likely to show stranger anxiety than those exposed to only one caregiver.

66. The answer is C. *(Pharmacology)*
This patient should be administered 480 mg of amikacin every 8 hours to maintain an average steady-state plasma concentration of 20 mg/L. The steady-state plasma drug concentration is directly proportional to the dosage and inversely proportional to clearance. Therefore, the dosage required to obtain a desired steady-state plasma concentration can be

calculated as the desired steady-state concentration multiplied by the clearance:

Dosage = 20 mg/L × 0.05 L/min × 60 min = 60 mg/hour; 60mg/h × 8 hours = 480 mg

The volume of distribution is used in calculating a loading dose but is not used in calculating a maintenance dose required to produce a desired steady-state plasma drug concentration.

67. The answer is D.   *(Behavioral science)*
Family therapy is based on the assumption that even if only one person in the family has a psychological problem, all family members should be involved in treatment. Sessions are usually held once weekly and last approximately 2 hours. Therapy involves identification of dysfunctional behavior followed by problem solving. Uncovering repressed events and bringing the unconscious into consciousness are not strategies used in family therapy.

68. The answer is C.   *(Biochemistry)*
2,4-Dinitrophenol is an uncoupler of oxidative phosphorylation. It acts by provoking the flux of protons from the proton-rich, low pH, intermembranous space across the inner mitochondrial membrane and into the mitochondrial matrix. In the absence of an uncoupler, a proton gradient is established between the matrix and the intermembranous space of the mitochondria. The transfer of electrons to reduced nicotinamide adenine dinucleotide (NADH) or reduced flavin adenine dinucleotide (FADH$_2$), and the subsequent conveyance of these electrons to oxygen via the electron transport chain in the membrane and cristae of the mitochondria, drives the formation of this gradient. Through the action of the electron transport system, the concentration of protons becomes higher in the intermembranous space and lower in the matrix. Driven by this gradient, these protons try to return to the matrix. Normally, they pass through the adenosine triphosphate (ATP) synthetase (complex V or F$_1$) stalk, where the energy potential of the gradient is used to synthesize ATP from adenosine diphosphate (ADP) and inorganic phosphate (Pi). The complete functioning system, including the passage of electrons to oxygen to establish the gradient and flow of the protons back through the ATP synthetase stalk to phosphorylate

ADP, is called a coupled oxidative phosphorylation system. When electrons are transported but ADP is not phosphorylated, oxidation is said to be uncoupled from phosphorylation. By "poking holes" in the membrane, 2,4-dinitrophenol destroys the chemosmotic gradient and allows electrons to be transported through the electron transport system without doing the work required to generate ATP. Therefore, it functions as an uncoupler of oxidative phosphorylation. Because most of the energy produced through the oxidation of food is generated via the coupled oxidative phosphorylation system, the net result of uncoupling is that foods are oxidized without producing the energy required to synthesize fat, resulting in weight loss. Unfortunately, ATP is required for many other important functions, therefore, 2,4-dinitrophenol is not a viable option for weight loss.

2,4-Dinitrophenol does not inhibit NADH dehydrogenase, the first enzyme in the electron transport sequence, nor does it affect the malate shuttle, a series of reactions that effectively transports reducing equivalents from the cytoplasm into the mitochondrial matrix. Substrate-level phosphorylations involve the direct transfer of Pi from compound to compound and do not involve the electron transport system. Therefore, 2,4-dinitrophenol has no effect on these reactions.

69. The answer is C.   *(Behavioral science)*
The monozygotic twin of a schizophrenic patient has the highest risk of developing the disorder. The concordance rate (i.e., the chance of a relative of an individual with schizophrenia developing the illness) is 35%–58% for a monozygotic twin of a schizophrenic patient, 9%–26% for a dizygotic twin or for a sibling of a schizophrenic patient, 30%–40% for the child of two parents with schizophrenia, and 10%–13% for the child of one parent with schizophrenia. Stress, such as that engendered by being a child in an institutional setting, can interact with genetic factors and contribute to the development of psychiatric illness (the stress-diathesis mode); however, environmental factors play a much smaller role in the development of schizophrenia than genetic and other biological factors.

70. The answer is D.   *(Pharmacology)*
The plasma half-lives of most drugs are increased in elderly patients. Because the half-life is determined by

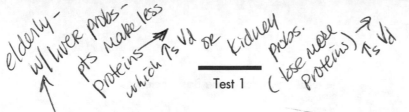

the volume of distribution and the clearance rate ($t_{1/2}$ = 0.693 × Vd/CL), an alteration in either the volume of distribution or the clearance rate will affect the half-life of a drug. In the case of many benzodiazepines (e.g., diazepam), the half-life is prolonged in elderly patients as a result of both decreased clearance and increased volume of distribution. Lorazepam, temazepam, and oxazepam are less affected by these changes than other benzodiazepines because they are metabolized by phase II reactions (conjugation), which are less affected by age.

71. The answer is C. *(Behavioral science)*
Margaret Mahler called the period when the child moves away but returns to the mother for comfort and reassurance the rapprochement phase. This behavior occurs most commonly in toddlers 16–24 months of age. This is the period when the child begins to develop physical and emotional distance from the mother.

72. The answer is D. *(Pharmacology)*
Sucralfate, which adheres to ulcer proteins, also binds to other drugs and prevents their absorption from the gut. Cimetidine, which inhibits cytochrome P-450 drug metabolism, does not affect the metabolism of sucralfate, which is minimally absorbed and acts locally in the stomach and intestine. Because it is not absorbed, sucralfate has no effect on plasma-protein binding, metabolism, or excretion of other drugs. Antacids may inhibit the binding of sucralfate to ulcer proteins; therefore, these drugs should not be administered within 30 minutes of each other.

73. The answer is B. *(Biochemistry)*
An abnormality of the enzymes involved in oxidative phosphorylation should be suspected in this infant. Maternal transmission of a trait expressed equally in males and females is characteristic of traits carried on mitochondrial DNA (mtDNA). Mitochondria carry circular molecules of DNA. Each molecule carries the genetic information that codes for 13 of the 100 or so proteins involved in oxidative phosphorylation. (The remainder of the mitochondrial proteins are coded by nuclear DNA.) mtDNA is only inherited from the mother, because sperm mitochondria do not pass into the fertilized egg. Therefore, any genetic marker or defect involving genes carried on mtDNA is passed

only from mother to child. Mothers transfer mtDNA to both sons and daughters, but only daughters can transmit their mtDNA to their children. It follows, then, that genetic defects involving oxidative phosphorylation are often inherited maternally. All of the other choices involve mitochondrial proteins, but only those involved in oxidative phosphorylation are coded by mtDNA.

The proofreading mechanism does not seem to be as efficient for mtDNA as for nuclear DNA, which accounts for a higher mutation rate in mtDNA replication. Because each cell has many mitochondria, there are multiple copies of each mtDNA. The expression of such mutations varies depending on the fraction of mtDNAs affected and their subsequent distribution. Therefore, there is variability of clinical expression among affected individuals, even within the same pedigree. However, tissues having a high energy requirement (e.g., muscle, brain, kidney, liver) are always the most susceptible to adverse effects associated with such mutations. Although phenotypic expression is rarely noted, mutations of mtDNA are responsible for clinical myopathies as well as Leber's hereditary optic neuropathy, a disease in which central vision is lost as a result of neuroretinal degeneration.

74. The answer is E. *(Pharmacology)*
Administration of probenecid to a patient receiving penicillin V orally will affect the plasma half-life of the penicillin V. Probenecid is a weak organic acid that competitively inhibits the renal tubular secretion of other organic acids (e.g., penicillin), thereby decreasing the renal clearance and increasing the plasma half-life and concentration of such drugs.

75. The answer is E. *(Behavioral science)*
The "Band-Aid" phase occurs most commonly in pre-school children between $2\frac{1}{2}$ and 5 years of age. At this age, children become overly concerned about illness and injury; they want to put a bandage on every injury.

76. The answer is A. *(Pharmacology)*
Cimetidine inhibits cytochrome P-450 metabolism of many drugs including lidocaine, resulting in decreased hepatic clearance and an increased plasma drug concentration and half-life. A direct interaction between

lidocaine and cimetidine on cardiac or central nervous system (CNS) tissue has not been demonstrated and there is no evidence that cimetidine displaces drugs from plasma proteins or affects the renal clearance of drugs.

77. The answer is D. *(Biochemistry)*
Insulin promotes the growth and differentiation of hepatocytes by activating a tyrosine kinase. Insulin has many functions, all of which are presumably mediated through interaction with receptors. The insulin receptor is a rod-like transmembrane protein with an external binding site for the hormone; a short, hydrophobic, transmembrane segment; and an internal domain (on the cytoplasmic side of the membrane) with tyrosine kinase activity. Binding of insulin to the receptor activates the internal tyrosine kinase, causing autophosphorylation of the receptor as well as phosphorylation of other targeted proteins. Such tyrosine kinase activity is always associated with hormones that influence mitosis, and thus, the growth of tissues.

78. The answer is C. *(Pharmacology)*
Ketoconazole, itraconazole, and erythromycin inhibit the cytochrome P-450–mediated inactivation of the histamine$_1$ (H$_1$)-receptor antagonists, terfenadine and astemizole. Elevated levels of these antihistamines as a result of drug interactions or overdose may prolong the QT inverval, leading to torsade de pointes and, possibly, sudden death. Terfenadine has no significant effect on the pharmacokinetics or pharmacologic activity of ketoconzole.

79. The answer is A. *(Behavioral science)*
Differences between the means of two samples are tested using a *t*-test. An analysis of variance is used to test for differences between the means of more than two samples. A chi-square test examines the differences between frequencies in a sample. Regression analysis examines the relationship between many variables, while correlation analysis examines the relationship between two variables.

80. The answer is D. *(Behavioral science)*
Obsessive–compulsive personality disorder is not associated with a high suicide risk. In contrast, unipolar depression, schizophrenia, alcoholism, and barbiturate abuse are all associated with an increased risk for suicide.

81. The answer is C. *(Behavioral science)*
The average life expectancy for a black woman in the United States is 73.8 years. Black men, on the other hand, have an average life expectancy of only 64.6 years. White men and women have average life expectancies of 72.9 and 79.6 years, respectively.

82. The answer is D. *(Behavioral science)*
Splitting is the perception of individuals as either all good or all bad. Regression is the return to an earlier form of thought or behavior, often in response to a current stress or threat. Rationalization is substituting an acceptable motive for an attitude or behavior that might otherwise be self-serving or unacceptable.

83. The answer is B. *(Behavioral science)*
The relative risk of developing lung cancer for smokers versus non-smokers is 24. This implies that the incidence of lung cancer among smokers is 24 times that among non-smokers.

84. The answer is B. *(Biochemistry)*
Because messenger RNA (mRNA) production is specifically inhibited, the target of the toxin must be a cell component involved only in the synthesis of mRNA. Eukaryotes contain three RNA polymerases: RNA polymerase I synthesizes ribosomal RNA (rRNA), RNA polymerase II synthesizes mRNA, and RNA polymerase III synthesizes transfer RNA (tRNA) and 5S rRNA. An inhibitor of DNA polymerase would inhibit DNA replication.

85. The answer is C. *(Pharmacology)*
Drug accumulation is a first-order process and the plateau steady-state is achieved at the same rate as drug elimination. Ninety percent of the steady-state plasma drug concentration is achieved after 3.3 half-lives, 94% after 4 half-lives, and 97% after 5 half-lives.

86. The answer is A. *(Behavioral science)*
The final stage of the five stages of dying, as described by Dr. Elizabeth Kubler Ross, is acceptance. In acceptance, the patient is calm and accepting of his fate.

The other four stages of dying are denial, anger, bargaining, and depression. In denial, the patient refuses to believe that he or she is dying. In anger, the patient may become angry at the physician or hospital staff. In bargaining, the patient may try to make promises or strike a deal with a supreme being in an effort to be cured. In depression, the patient becomes preoccupied with death and emotionally detached.

87. The answer is B. (Biochemistry)

The formation of 5-phosphoribosylamine from 5-phosphoribosyl-1-pyrophosphate (PRPP) is the first committed step, and a major regulated step, in de novo purine biosynthesis. Although PRPP synthesis is often considered to be the first step in purine biosynthesis, this is not the committed step because PRPP is also used in de novo pyrimidine biosynthesis and in base salvage.

88. The answer is B. (Anatomy)

Static cytometry is used on Fuelgen-stained tumor sections to describe ploidy patterns. The technique is used in combination with a digitized imaging system that measures the absorption of light in the Fuelgen-stained cells. The Fuelgen reaction produces a red color in the presence of DNA that can be quantitated. This method has been useful in the studies of breast cancer, kidney cancer, endometrial cancer, and gastrointestinal cancers. RNA, which is contained in the nucleolus, does not stain in the Fuelgen reaction. Barr bodies are the interphase chromatin expression of the X chromosome, appearing adjacent to the nuclear membrane. Such chromatin would react with the Fuelgen stain, but Barr bodies are only apparent in females. Microtubules contain the protein tubulin and do not react with the Fuelgen stain.

89. The answer is C. (Microbiology)

Bacteroides fragilis and Clostridium perfringens are both obligate anaerobes that lack superoxide dismutase. In facultative and aerobic organisms, respiration produces two toxic molecules: hydrogen peroxide (H_2O_2) and the free radical superoxide (O_2^-). Superoxide dismutase and catalase, two enzymes found in facultative and aerobic organisms, neutralize the adverse effects of these chemicals. Superoxide dismutase catalyzes the reaction: $2O_2^- + 2H^+ \rightarrow H_2O_2 + O_2$ and catalase catalyzes the reaction: $2H_2O_2 \rightarrow 2H_2O + O_2$. Small amounts of these enzymes in some anaerobic organisms may allow the bacterium to survive in the presence of oxygen for short periods of time; however, the levels are insufficient to allow growth and metabolism to occur in an oxygen-containing atmosphere.

Although both organisms are routinely found in the intestinal tract, only Clostridium produces endospores. B. fragilis does not commonly cause any form of food poisoning, but C. perfringens may cause food poisoning following the ingestion of improperly stored cooked foods containing C. perfringens spores. Only B. fragilis is gram-negative and can be a source of endotoxin, a cell wall component. Poultry and domestic animals serve as reservoirs for Salmonella species; the bacteria can be transmitted to humans and cause disease.

90. The answer is A. (Biochemistry)

Liver cells express both hexokinase and glucokinase. Hexokinase has a low Michaelis constant (K_m) value (i.e., a high affinity) for glucose and is saturated at normal glucose blood levels. Glucokinase has a high K_m value (i.e., a low affinity) for glucose and has very little activity at normal blood glucose levels. Glucokinase becomes more active as the glucose concentration increases; its primary function is to remove glucose from the portal blood after a meal. Hexokinase, not glucokinase, is inhibited by glucose 6-phosphate. This mechanism prevents cells from taking in more glucose than they can metabolize. Inhibition of glucokinase by glucose 6-phosphate would be counterproductive and does not occur. Most cells, including muscle cells, only express hexokinase, not glucokinase. Normally, fructose is primarily phosphorylated by fructokinase, a liver enzyme.

91. The answer is B. (Behavioral science)

Heart disease is the leading cause of death in the United States, followed by cancer and stroke.

92. The answer is C. (Biochemistry)

Nitric oxide is a potent vasodilator, normally formed from arginine by the action of nitric oxide synthetase. It binds to a rod-like receptor with a short transmembrane domain (similar to the tyrosine kinase activating receptors). Binding of nitric oxide to its receptor activates guanyl kinase and elevates cyclic guanosine monophosphate (cGMP) levels. cGMP is the second messenger in this system. Although it induces vasodilation, vasodilation does not normally enhance bacterial invasion. The conversion of nitroglycerin and amyl nitrate to nitric oxide is what gives these agents their vasodilator properties, but nitrous oxide, or "laughing gas," is not converted to nitric oxide. Nitric oxide does not enhance blood clotting and calcium calmodulin is not a factor that promotes blood clotting. Rather, calmodulin is an intracellular protein that binds calcium and modulates many of its effects.

93. The answer is C.

Most of the proximal reabsorption of Na^+ occurs by active transport and is transcellular. The transcellular pathway consists of the apical and basolateral membranes. The Na^+-K^+-ATPase pump in all cell membranes is responsible for active Na^+ transport (efflux) and active K^+ transport (influx). This enzyme maintains the low intracellular Na^+ concentration and the high extracellular Na^+ concentration. Active Na^+ transport consumes 30%–50% of the energy derived from metabolism in most cells. Although the influx of Na^+ from the tubular lumen to the proximal tubular cell is in the direction favored by the electrochemical potential, this transport is mediated by specific membrane carrier proteins and not by simple diffusion. These membrane proteins couple the active movement of other solutes to the passive moment of Na^+. Examples include Na^+-glucose and Na^+-amino acid symporters and a Na^+ antiporter. In each case, the potential energy released by the downhill transport of Na^+ is used to power the uphill transport of the other substance. These transport systems are referred to as Na^+-coupled, secondary active transport processes. It is essential to understand that reabsorption includes not only Na^+ influx from the tubular lumen but also active transport of Na^+ out of the cell into the bloodstream.

94. The answer is C. *(Pharmacology)*

The differences in the plasma drug concentration curves among the three patients are attributable to the dosage administered to each. The plateau (steady-state) drug concentration is directly proportional to the dosage (dose/time) and inversely proportional to the clearance. A change in drug clearance or half-life would change the time required to reach steady-state, because the time to reach steady-state is approximately four to five half-lives. Because the time to reach steady-state is the same in all three patients, the drug half-life and clearance must be about the same in all three patients. The duration of drug infusion is the same for all three patients. If it were not, the plasma drug concentrations would begin to decline as soon as the infusion was stopped. The plasma drug concentration curve does not provide information about the route of elimination.

95. The answer is D. *(Microbiology)*

Detection of soluble antigen in cerebral spinal fluid (CSF) using a latex particle agglutination assay has been proven to be an accurate and quick method of identifying the causative agent of acute meningitis. Latex agglutination tests can identify all of the most probable causative organisms, are accurate, and are easy to perform. It has been shown that culture and isolation of agents causing central nervous system (CNS) infections can be time-consuming. Many organisms (e.g., *Neisseria meningitis*) may be difficult to grow routinely in the laboratory and require special media or procedures to obtain an accurate diagnosis. Because decisions, such as which antibiotic is most appropriate, depend on an accurate and timely laboratory result, other methods may be better. Counterimmunoelectrophoresis and antibody titers are time-consuming and difficult to perform. The time required to collect both the acute and convalescent sera samples would delay an accurate diagnosis.

96. The answer is C. *(Physiology)*

Glycogen is considered an inclusion because it is a transitory, "nonliving," component of the muscle cytoplasm (sarcoplasm). Skeletal muscle rapidly metabolizes glucose from glycogen during exercise. Glycogen is also found in clusters in hepatocytes. Actin and myosin are the proteins of the thin and thick filaments, respectively. Ribosomes are involved in protein synthesis; they are not numerous in muscle cells. Mitochondria produce energy that is easily accessible by the cell; therefore, they are not considered energy depots. In addition, they are organelles, not inclusions.

97. The answer is D. *(Pharmacology)*

The set of patient profiles in choice D correlates with the plasma drug concentration curves shown in the figure. The time required to achieve the plateau steady-state is approximately four to five times the plasma drug elimination half-life. Because the time to reach plateau increased from patient A to C, the half-life must also increase from patient A to C. On the basis of this information, all of the choices can be eliminated but choices B and D. The plasma plateau drug concentration is directly proportional to dosage (dose/time) and half-life. Because the steady-state plasma drug concentrations were the same in all three patients and the serum half-lives increased from patient A to patient C, then the dosage must have decreased from patient A to patient C. In choice B, the dosage remained the same (20μ/kg/min); therefore, only choice D is viable.

98-99. The answers are: 98-C, 99-A. *(Behavioral science)*

Test results return either positive or negative (normal). Patients with disease either have a true-positive (TP) or false-negative (FN) test result, whereas those without disease either have a true-negative (TN) or false-positive (FP) test result. The **sensitivity** of a test refers to how often the test returns positive in disease. Sensitivity = TP/ (TP + FN) × 100. A test with 100% sensitivity has no FNs; therefore, when a test result returns negative, it must be a TN rather than a FN. Tests with high sensitivity are used to screen for asymptomatic disease (e.g., phenylketonuria) and to retain or exclude diseases on a list of differential diagnoses. In a test with 100% sensitivity, a negative test result excludes disease, but a positive test result may be either a TP or a FP—the sensitivity of a test does not distinguish between the two.

The **specificity** of a test refers to how often a test is negative in a patient without the disease. Specificity = TN/ (TN + FP) × 100. A test with 100% specificity has no FPs; therefore, a positive test result must be a TP. Tests with high specificity are used to differentiate a TP from an FP test result, thus serving a primary role in confirming disease.

Sensitivity and specificity describe how the test performs in patients with and without disease, respectively. A positive test result is either a TP or FP, whereas a negative test result is either a TN or FN. In the former situation, the clinician must determine what the chance is that the positive test result indicates that the patient has the disease. This is called the predictive value of a positive test result (PV+): PV+ = TP/ (TP + FP) × 100. Similarly, when a test result returns negative, the clinician must determine what the chance is that the negative test result indicates that the patient does not have the disease. This is designated the predictive value of a negative test result (PV-): PV- = TN/ (TN + FN) × 100.

The following chart is useful for calculating sensitivity, specificity, and the predictive value of positive and negative test results:

	Disease	
Test Result	**Present**	**Absent**
Positive	TP	FP → PV+ = TP/(TP + FP) × 100
Negative	FN	TN → PV- = TN/(TN + FN) × 100
	↓	↓
	Sensitivity	Specificity
	TP/(TP + FN) × 100	TN/(TN + FP) × 100

It is necessary to calculate the PV+ to answer the first portion of the question ("In the population of people under study, what is the percent chance that a positive test result in a randomly selected individual indicates that the person has rheumatoid arthritis?"). The PV+ can be calculated as follows:

Test Result	Disease	
	Present	Absent
Positive test	140	20 → PV+ = 140/(140 + 20) × 100 = 88%
Negative test	60	180

Other calculations are as follows:
sensitivity = 140/140 + 60 × 100 = 70%
specificity = 180/180 + 20 × 100 = 90%

That is, there is an 88% chance that the test result is a TP and a 12% chance it is an FP.

Prevalence of disease refers to the actual number of patients with the disease in the population under study. The prevalence of a disease affects how the clinician interprets the test result. The formula is:

$$\text{Prevalence} = \frac{\text{Patients with disease}}{\text{Total population studied}} \times 100$$

In the first part of the question, the prevalence of rheumatoid arthritis in the total population studied is 50% (200/400 100 = 50%). In order to calculate the effect of prevalence on the predictive value of positive and negative test results, an arbitrary number, such as 1000, is used from which the total number of people with and without disease is calculated. For example, in the second part of the question, the prevalence of rheumatoid arthritis is 10%; therefore, 900 out of 1000 people are normal and 100 people have rheumatoid arthritis. Out of the 900 normal people, the specificity of the test (90%) indicates that 810 are TNs and 90 are FPs. Similarly, out of the 100 people who have rheumatoid arthritis, the sensitivity of the test (75%), indicates that 75 are TPs and 25 are FNs:

Test Result	Disease	
	Present	Absent
Positive test	75	90 → PV+ = 75/(75 + 90) × 100 = 45%
Negative test	25	810

That is, there is a 45% chance that the test result is a TP and a 55% chance it is a FP.

100. The answer is D.   *(Behavioral science)*
Gender identity disorder is a sense of being born into the body of the wrong sex; therefore, this is the most correct diagnosis for the 7-year-old boy in the question. Gender identity is an individual's sense of being male or female. Gender identity is normal in homosexual and transvestic individuals—homosexual individuals have sexual and love interest in people of the same sex but are content with their physical sex, and transvestites are heterosexual men who dress in women's clothing for sexual pleasure. In an intersex condition, the individual has biological characteristics of both sexes and is not physically normal.

101. The answer is D. *(Anatomy)*

The adult bone marrow contains pluripotent stem cells that differentiate along erythroid, myeloid, and lymphoid pathways. The lymphoid pathway is responsible for producing B cells and prothymocytes. In the diagram below, several intermediate differentiation stages have been omitted.

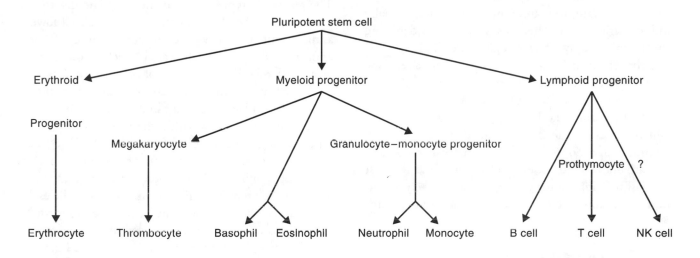

The liver and spleen exhibit hematopoietic activity in the fetus until about the fourth or fifth month of gestation. In adults, the liver and spleen resume this function in a process known as extramedullary hematopoiesis if the marrow is incapable of meeting the demand for hematopoietic elements. The thymus is a primary lymphoid organ that is important in lymphopoiesis.

102. The answer is D. *(Microbiology)*

Bacillus anthracis causes anthrax. A toxic factor demonstrated in the plasma of animals dying from anthrax has been partially characterized into three components: protective antigen, edema factor, and lethal factor. At the portal of entry, bacterial growth produces a gelatinous edema and congestion. Bacteria enter the bloodstream via the lymphatics, where they multiply. At one time, death was thought to be caused by massive septicemia leading to capillary blockage and organ dysfunction, but exact mechanisms remain unclear as far as the pathogenicity of *B. anthracis* is concerned. Toxin A (an enterotoxin) and toxin B (a cytotoxin) are produced by *Clostridium difficile*. *Bacillus cereus* can cause two forms of food poisoning. The emetic form is caused by a heat-labile enterotoxin, while the diarrheal form is caused by a heat-stable toxin. *Clostridium tetani* produces tetanospasmin, a neurotoxin. *Haemophilus influenzae* derives its pathogenicity from polysaccharide capules (designated a through f). *H. influenzae* does not produce an exotoxin, but the gram-negative cell wall does contain endotoxin.

103. The answer is C. *(Biochemistry)*

A deficiency of a branched amino acid aminotransferase will not directly lead to hyperammonemia because deficiency of this enzyme will not accelerate the release of free ammonia or inhibit its uptake.

Glutamate dehydrogenase plays a central role in amino acid and ammonia metabolism. Most amino acids transaminate with α-ketoglutarate, forming glutamate plus the conjugate α-keto acid (e.g., pyruvic acid from alanine). The α-keto acid carbon skeleton is then available to be catabolized. The amino group passed onto the α-ketoglutarate is transferred to another α-keto acid, using a second aminotransferase, thereby synthesizing an amino acid in short supply. Alternatively, the amino group can be liberated as free ammonia by glutamate dehydrogenase. The ammonia is then passed into the urea cycle via carbamoyl phosphate. Glutamate dehydrogenase is a reversible enzyme and, in times of ammonia excess, will transfer free ammonia to α-ketoglutarate to form glutamic acid. Therefore, a deficiency of glutamate dehyrdogenase, while not creating ammonia itself, could lead to transient bouts of hyperammonemia. In fact, it is believed that overstimulation of this enzyme, in an attempt to protect the brain from ammonia intoxication, actually induces serious central nervous symptoms by depleting the brain's supply of α-ketoglutarate. This inhibits tricarboxylic acid (TCA) cycle activity and adenosine triphosphate (ATP) production.

Glutamine synthetase plays a prominent role in regulating ammonia levels by forming glutamine, which serves as the major vehicle for transporting ammonia in a nontoxic form through the blood.

Carbamoyl synthetase I and arginase are the first and last reactions in the urea cycle, respectively. Obviously, an inability to form urea will lead to a hyperammonemia.

104. The answer is C.　(Anatomy)
The bone marrow is the major site of B cell maturation. In the adult bone marrow, the lymphoid stem cell proceeds through several stages of maturation as identified by the expression (or lack of expression) of certain markers. The lymphoid stem cell differentiates into the pro-B cell (the earliest B cell progenitor), which becomes the pre-B cell (defined as a cell that does not yet express light chains of antibody, but has heavy chains in the cytoplasm). Cell mitosis stops, proliferation resumes in response to stimulation by antigen, and rearrangements of light chain V (variable) and J (joining) gene segments occurs. The pre-B cell differentiates into the early B cell. Surface immunoglobulin M (IgM), with or without immunoglobulin D (IgD), is expressed; all immunoglobulin gene segment rearrangements cease and the cell becomes a mature B lymphocyte. The bone marrow is equivalent to the bursa of Fabricius in birds, the first animal species in which a specific site of B cell maturation was discovered. Therefore, the bone marrow is sometimes referred to as "bursa-equivalent" tissue. The spleen filters blood and removes dying and dead erythrocytes from the circulation. The lymph nodes, which consist of lymphocytes and macrophages associated with reticulin fibers, filter foreign materials. The thymus is the site of T lymphocyte maturation. The tonsils, nodular aggregates of lymphocytes and macrophages directly underneath the epithelium that lines the nasopharynx

and soft palate, may participate as a secondary B cell maturation site.

105. The answer is D.　(Microbiology)
The term "idiotype" refers to the antigenic determinants found in the hypervariable portion [also known as the complementarity-determining region (CDR) or antigen-binding site] of the variable (V) region of any given antibody. Immunization of one individual with antibody from another individual can induce the production of anti-idiotypic antibodies, which bind to these specific sequences within the V region. An idiotope is a single antigenic epitope within the V region of an antibody. The sum total of idiotopes in an immunoglobulin molecule is known as the idiotype. The term "allotype" is derived from the word "alleles;" alleles are variants of the same gene. The heavy and light chains of antibody are encoded in separate gene loci that exist in more than one form in the human population (i.e., they are polymorphic). The different forms (alleles) result in immunoglobulins that differ from each other in only one or a few amino acids. These alternative forms are known as allotypes. Allotypes found on human heavy$_\gamma$ chains are referred to as Gm; those on light$_\kappa$ chains are referred to as Inv. The term "isotype" is used to refer to antigenic differences in the constant (C) regions of the heavy and light chains of an antibody. These differences are used to distinguish among the classes and subclasses of immunoglobulins. Thus, IgG, IgA, IgM, IgD, and IgE are different isotypes because the C regions of their heavy chains are different; IgG1, IgG2, IgG3, and IgG4, as well as IgA1 and IgA2, are different isotypes because of differences in the C region of their heavy chains. The κ and λ light chains are different isotypes because of antigenic differences in their C regions. The hinge, a part of the C region of the heavy chains, is located at the base of each Fab arm. It allows the two arms to swing freely and gives the antibody molecule flexibility.

106. The answer is D.　(Pathology)
Malignant melanoma has increased in incidence more than any other cancer in recent years. Both sexes are affected equally, but fair-skinned, blue- or green-eyed people with red or blond hair are most at risk. Malignant melanoma is on the rise as more people experience

the repercussions of excessive exposure to ultraviolet light. A history of severe sunburn is a major risk factor for malignant melanoma.

107. The answer is C. *(Pathology)*
Estimated cancer incidence and mortality in both men and women for 1994 in order of decreasing incidence and mortality are:

Men		Women	
Incidence	**Mortality**	**Incidence**	**Mortality**
(2) Prostate	(3) Lung	(2) Breast	(3) Lung
(3) Lung	(2) Prostate	(3) Lung	(2) Breast
(1) Colon	(1) Colon	(1) Colon	(1) Colon

Lung cancer is the most common cause of cancer-related death in both men and women. Breast cancer is the most common cancer in women. The incidence of breast cancer is steadily increasing as a result of advances in technology (e.g., mammography) that allow detection of masses that previously went undetected. Approximately 1 in 8 women will develop breast cancer. Prostate cancer is the most common cancer in men. Approximately 1 in 10 men will develop prostate cancer. Prostate cancer is more common in blacks than in whites and is age-dependent.

108. The answer is B. *(Pathology)*
α-Fetoprotein (AFP) and β-human chorionic gonadotropin (β-hCG) levels are likely to be elevated in patients with testicular cancer. Seminomas, as a rule, are not associated with an increase in either tumor marker. In embryonal carcinoma, both markers are usually elevated. In choriocarcinomas β-hCG levels are usually elevated, and in endodermal sinus (yolk sac) tumors AFP levels are usually elevated.

109. The answer is C. *(Physiology)*
Pitting edema is most commonly the result of increased total body sodium. Because sodium is primarily located in the extracellular fluid (ECF) compartment and the interstitial space is larger than the vascular space, an increase in total body sodium results in excess salt and water in the interstitial space. The physical manifestation of this shift is pitting edema. An increase in hydrostatic pressure, a decrease in oncotic pressure (hypoalbuminemia, as occurs in nephrotic syndrome), or both predisposes to leakage of transudate out of the vascular compartment and into the interstitial space. The syndrome of inappropriate antidiuretic syndrome (SIADH) results in an excess of free water, which lowers the serum sodium. The resultant hyposmolarity in the ECF leads to a movement of water into the intracellular fluid compartment. Eventually, there is an excess in the interstitium and vascular compartment as well, but an excess of water in the interstitium without an excess of salt does not result in pitting edema. In primary aldosteronism, the excess reabsorption of sodium in the distal and early collecting ducts causes an increase in plasma volume, which increases the arterial blood volume. The increase in arterial blood volume increases the peritubular capillary hydrostatic pressure, resulting in a loss of salt in the proximal tubule that offsets the gain of salt in the distal tubule. Therefore, pitting edema does not occur. In diabetic ketoacidosis, there is a hypotonic loss of fluid in the kidneys as a result of osmotic diuresis from glucosuria. More water is lost than salt, resulting in a decrease in total body sodium and clinical evidence of dehydration, because the tissue turgor related to salt and water in the interstitial space is decreased. In diabetes insipidus, the loss or lack of activity of antidiuretic hormone (ADH) results in a loss of free water without affecting the total body sodium. Because total body sodium is normal, there is no evidence of either pitting edema or dehydration.

110. The answer is A. *(Pathology)*
The patient has endotoxic shock from septicemia related to urinary obstruction. The endotoxic shock caused widespread tissue damage, resulting in disseminated intravascular coagulation (DIC), the most likely mechanism behind the seepage of blood from the venipuncture sites on the second hospital day. Endotoxins damage endothelial cells and activate macrophages, causing the release of nitric oxide, a potent vasodilator that contributes to the pathophysiology of shock. The release of other mediators ultimately results in vessel dilatation (which would explain the patient's warm skin), high cardiac output failure, and sinus tachycardia. DIC is characterized by the intravascular consumption of clotting factors, which would result in blood oozing from puncture sites and eventual hypovolemia and shock. The patient probably also has

adult respiratory distress syndrome (ARDS) as a result of endotoxic shock, which would account for the bilateral diffuse infiltrates seen on the chest x-ray and the hypoxemia. Hypovolemic shock is likely present as well in this patient, but it is not responsible for the oozing of blood on the second hospital day. Renal failure is likely to develop in this patient, but none of the data supplied in the question would indicate that uremia is present at this time.

111. The answer is A. *(Behavioral science)*
In the 1- to 24-year-old age bracket, motor vehicle accidents are the number one cause of accidental death, followed closely by burns and drowning. Alcohol plays a significant role in adolescent vehicle-related deaths. Acquired immunodeficiency syndrome (AIDS) has replaced injury as the most common cause of death in the 25- to 44-year-old age bracket.

112. The answer is B. *(Anatomy)*
Valproate, an anti-epileptic drug, is associated with open neural tube defects, which lead to increased maternal serum and amniotic fluid α-fetoprotein (AFP) levels. Amniotic fluid AFP levels are more sensitive than maternal serum AFP levels for diagnosing open neural tube defects, which is why serum levels are used as a screen and amniotic fluid levels are used to confirm the diagnosis (along with the finding of increased acetylcholinesterase activity). AFP, which is synthesized by fetal hepatocytes and yolk sac cells, is thought to represent fetal albumin. AFP levels may also be increased by exposure of fetal abdominal viscera (i.e., omphalocele), which allows fetal serum to leak into the amniotic fluid, and esophageal or duodenal atresia, which interferes with fetal swallowing and uptake of AFP out of the amniotic fluid. Normal levels of AFP in both amniotic fluid and maternal serum are gestationally dependent, so proper interpretation depends on an accurate gestational age—diagnostic testing is best performed during the 16th to 18th week of gestation. Low levels of AFP in maternal serum or amniotic fluid are seen in fetuses with Down's syndrome. Maternal ingestion of thalidomide to control nausea causes limb abnormalities such as amelia (absent limbs) and phocomelia (seal-like limbs). Maternal ingestion of phenytoin (dilantin) may result in fetal growth disturbances, hypoplasia of the distal phalanges, central nervous system (CNS) abnormalities, and congenital heart disease. Systemic lupus erythematosus (SLE) can lead to complete heart block. Heroin or methadone addiction can produce irritability, hyperactivity, tremors, excessive hunger and salivation, temperature instability, seizures, and low birth weight in neonates. Neonates born to mothers who are heroin addicts are also at greater risk for infections [e.g., hepatitis B, human immunodeficiency virus (HIV)].

113. The answer is A. *(Pathology)*
In autosomal recessive disease, both parents must have the abnormal gene to transmit the disease to their children, whereas in sex-linked recessive disease, the asymptomatic carrier (heterozygote) mother transmits the disease to her sons. In autosomal recessive disease, siblings have a 25% chance of being affected if both parents are heterozygotes (asymptomatic carriers), a 50% chance of being affected if one of the parents is symptomatic and the other is a carrier, and a 100% chance of being affected if both parents are symptomatic (homozygous).

114. The answer is B. *(Pathology)*
Coronary artery disease is not inevitable as one gets older but the greatest risk factor for coronary artery disease is age; therefore, it is an age-related disorder. Age-dependent changes are an inevitable aspect of aging; examples include decreased skin turgor, prostate hyperplasia or cancer, osteoarthritis, and cataracts. Examples of age-related disorders include atherosclerosis, ischemic heart disease, and type II diabetes.

115. The answer is E. *(Anatomy)*
A deformation is an anatomical defect resulting from mechanical factors. Deformation tends to occur during the last two trimesters of pregnancy, after the organs have developed. Potter's syndrome, characterized by floppy ears, flexion contractures, and pulmonary hypoplasia, is caused by oligohydramnios as a result of renal cystic disease. Maternal factors that can result in deformations include leiomyomas (the most common cause of an obstructive delivery) and multiple gestations. Fetal factors that can lead to deformations include abnormal position and poor fetal movement. Malformations occur during the first trimester; they result from problems in the morphogenesis of organs. The cause of 40%–60% of malformations is unknown.

Genetic disorders are the next most common cause of malformations, with multifactorial inheritance (genetic disease plus environmental factors) leading the list. Teratogenic agents, such as drugs and viruses, have also been implicated. Hypospadias is the most common congenital malformation, followed by club foot and ventricular septal defects. Open neural tube defects associated with folate deficiency are another example.

116. The answer is D. *(Biochemistry)*
Thyroxine binds to a nuclear receptor and influences the rate of transcription of specific proteins, usually enzymes. Therefore, the response time is relatively slow because the drug will have no visible effect until sufficient protein has been synthesized. Maximal effect occurs after the steady-state level has been achieved, usually 7–10 days after initiating therapy. Epinephrine, glucagon, insulin, and antidiuretic hormone (ADH) bind to surface receptors that influence the concentration of second messengers. The second messengers induce post-transcriptional phosphorylation of preexisting proteins. The effects of these agents are manifested in a matter of minutes.

117. The answer is D. *(Biochemistry)*
Hepatocytes have more control over glycolysis than most other cell types because they synthesize fatty acids and carry out gluconeogenesis. Under fasting conditions, liver pyruvate kinase is inactivated by a glucagon-induced phosphorylation, allowing gluconeogenesis to occur without establishing a futile energy consuming cycle at this site. Phosphofructokinase-1 is regulated in all tissues by metabolites, but the liver enzyme is also hormonally regulated. Low insulin and high glucagon levels increase the concentration of fructose 2,6-bisphosphate, a potent activator of phosphofructokinase-1. Hexokinase is also subject to metabolic regulation in the liver.

118. The answer is C. *(Pathology)*
Bacterial colonization of the bowel is not present in neonates, so vitamins that are normally synthesized by gut bacteria (e.g., vitamin K) are dangerously lacking 2–5 days after birth. (Although vitamin K is not present in high quantities in breast milk, this is not the primary reason for the deficiency in newborns.) A deficiency of vitamin K results in an anticoagulated state that predisposes the newborn to a condition called "hemorrhagic disease of the newborn." Intracerebral hemorrhage is one of the serious complications associated with this condition. Adequate amounts of vitamin K–dependent coagulation factors are synthesized by the liver in newborns, but the precursors cannot be γ-carboxylated into an active form in the absence of vitamin K. Newborns are not deficient in bile salts. The small bowel of newborns can reabsorb fat-soluble vitamins.

119. The answer is B. *(Biochemistry)*
Heme, a component of hemoglobin, is partially synthesized in the cytosol and partially in the mitochondria:

	Succinyl CoA + Glycine + Vitamin B_6 (pyridoxine)
	↓
Mitochondria	δ-aminolevulinic acid
	↓
	Porphobilinogen
	↓
Cytosol	Uroporphyrinogen
	↓
	Coproporphyrinogen
	↓
Mitochondria	Protoporphyrin + Iron = Heme

β-Oxidation of fatty acids and oxidative phosphorylation occur in the mitochondria. Glycogen synthesis occurs in the cytoplasm. Collagen synthesis occurs in the cytosol and the extracellular space.

120. The answer is C.   *(Physiology)*
Both methemoglobinemia and carboxyhemoglobin-emia produce tissue hypoxia. Methemoglobin, which is hemoglobin with iron in the ferric (+3) state rather than the oxygen-binding ferrous (+2) state, is similar to carboxyhemoglobin, except it does not block cytochrome oxidase. Carbon monoxide has a 240 times greater affinity for hemoglobin than oxygen, which means that it decreases the oxygen saturation of hemoglobin (i.e., the total number of binding sites occupied by oxygen). Decreased oxygen saturation decreases the total amount of oxygen carried by blood, or the oxygen content. In addition, carbon monoxide shifts the oxygen dissociation curve to the left, so the little oxygen that the hemoglobin is carrying is not released to the tissue. Methemoglobin also decreases the oxygen content by decreasing the oxygen saturation, because oxygen can only combine with heme in the ferrous state. In addition, methemoglobin causes a left shift in the oxygen dissociation curve.

121. The answer is A.   *(Biochemistry)*
Ubiquitin is a small, heat-stable protein that is attached to another protein as a posttranslational modification to signal that the latter protein is to be degraded. Mannose-6-phosphate is a posttranslational modification that occurs on proteins that are destined to be incorporated into lysosomes. Precursors of proteins that are secreted from the cell contain a hydrophobic signal sequence at their amino termini. Proteins that contain nuclear or mitochondrial entry sequences are transported into their appropriate organelles.

122. The answer is B.   *(Microbiology)*
Bacteria that derive their energy and carbon from organic molecules are called heterotrophs. All medically significant bacteria are heterotrophs. Chemoautotrophs derive their energy from the oxidation of inorganic compounds and their carbon by metabolizing carbon dioxide. Autotrophs, in general, are microorganisms that do not require organic nutrients for growth. Auxotrophs are genetic mutants that require essential growth factors to be included in the medium on which they are grown. A prototroph is an organism capable of growing in a minimal essential medium containing only salts and glucose.

123–125. The answers are: 123-C, 124-D, 125-E.   *(Behavioral science)*
The incidence rate is defined as the number of new cases occurring per year divided by the total population. With 300 new cases occurring per 1,000,000 population in 1992, the incidence rate for AIDS in this population is 30 per 100,000.

The crude mortality rate is defined as the total number of deaths divided by the total population. With 900 deaths per 1,000,000 population, the crude mortality rate is 90 per 100,000.

The prevalence rate is defined as the number of existing cases of a disease divided by the total population during a specific period (1992). Because the prevalence of AIDS in this population in 1992 was 900 (previous cases), plus 300 (new cases), and the population size was 1,000,000, the prevalence rate at the end of 1992 for AIDS is 1200 per 1,000,000 or 120 per 100,000.

126. The answer is D.   *(Behavioral science)*
Infant monkeys reared in relative social isolation are more likely to be adversely affected if they are male. Monkeys reared in social isolation do not develop normal mating, maternal, or social behavior as adults and, if isolated for more than 6 months, do not recover.

127. The answer is A.   *(Pathology)*
Chronic pancreatitis and the resulting deficiency of pancreatic enzymes produces steatorrhea (fat in the stool as a result of maldigestion of fats), but the deficiency of pancreatic enzymes does not directly affect the production or reabsorption of bile salts. Because cholesterol cannot be degraded by the liver, it is either solubilized in bile and excreted or converted into the primary bile acids (cholic acid and chenodeoxycholic acid). Primary bile acids are further conjugated to glycine and taurine to form the primary bile salts (glycholic acid, glycochenodeoxycholic acid, taurocholic acid, taurochenodeoxycholic acid). Acting as detergents, the primary bile salts form 1-μm micelles in the small intestine with fatty acids and 2-monoglycerides. These micelles enhance absorption of bile salts by the small intestinal villi. In the intestine, some of the primary bile salts, bile acids, and secondary bile salts are deconjugated by bacteria into the secondary bile acids (deoxycholic acid and lithocholic acid). Deoxycholic acid and approximately 95% of the primary

(conjugated) bile salts are reabsorbed in the terminal ileum and recycled back to the liver. Lithocholic acid, a carcinogen that predisposes to colorectal cancer, is not reabsorbed. Potential causes of bile salt deficiency include:

- Cirrhosis, which decreases bile salt synthesis
- Bacterial overgrowth in the small bowel, which increases degradation
- Terminal ileal disease (e.g., Crohn's disease) which decreases reabsorption
- Binding agents (e.g., cholestyramine), which decrease reabsorption
- Obstruction of the common bile duct (e.g., as the result of gallstones), which decreases delivery to the small intestine

128. The answer is D.　(Pathology)

Pregnancies associated with gestational diabetes mellitus usually produce newborns who are large for gestational age (macrosomia). Hyperglycemia in the mother causes fetal release of insulin, which increases the synthesis of fat and muscle. Fetal, placental, and maternal causes can result in a newborn who is small for gestational age. Fetal abnormalities include chromosome disorders, congenital anomalies, and infection. Placental abnormalities (uteroplacental insufficiency) can result from infection, infarction, abruptio placentae, and premature rupture of the membranes. Maternal factors are most common and include pregnancy-induced hypertension (pre-eclampsia), malnutrition, smoking, alcohol consumption, and drug addiction.

129. The answer is E.　(Biochemistry)

Reduced nicotinamide adenine dinucleotide phosphate (NADPH) is extremely important in providing reducing equivalents (reductive biosynthesis) for many biochemical reactions in the body. However, reduced nicotinamide adenine dinucleotide (NADH), not NADPH, is primarily used in ketogenesis. NADPH is involved in the formation of reduced glutathione (GSH), in cytochrome P-450 metabolism, in fatty acid and cholesterol synthesis, and in the metabolism of alcohol into acetaldehyde via the P-450 route.

130. The answer is A.　(Microbiology)

B lymphocytes do not always require help from T cells in order to produce antibody. T-independent antigens, such as the polysaccharides that comprise bacterial capsules, are not readily processed and presented to the T helpers. However, these types of antigens can directly activate B cells by crosslinking B-cell antigen receptors. The crosslinked receptors become aggregated at one pole of the cell by a process known as "capping," resulting in the transmission of a signal sufficient for B-cell activation. Nearly all of the antibody produced is immunoglobulin M (IgM) and the kinetics of production resemble a primary response. B cell differentiation occurs in two phases, an antigen-independent phase and an antigen-dependent phase, during which B cells become activated and differentiate into antibody-secreting plasmacytes. Monomeric IgM is embedded in the cytoplasmic membrane of each immunocompetent B cell and acts as a highly specific B-cell antigen receptor. In addition to the secretion of antibody, B cells can present antigen to $CD4^+$ T cells. The surface IgM efficiently traps the antigen, which is then engulfed by the B cells via endocytosis (B cells are not capable of phagocytosis). The engulfed antigen is processed and the critical peptides are presented on the B-cell surface in the context of major histocompatibility complex (MHC) class II molecules. The bone marrow, a central lymphoid organ, is the major site of B cell maturation. The maturation process involves assistance from bone marrow stromal cells.

131. The answer is C.　(Biochemistry)

Linoleic and linolenic acids are unsaturated fatty acids and do not provide the double bonds for fatty acid synthesis. Reduced nicotinamide adenine dinucleotide phosphate (NADPH) provides the reducing equivalents. Acetyl coenzyme A (acetyl CoA) cannot diffuse out of the mitochondria into the cytosol for fatty acid synthesis, so it is first converted into citrate, which, when it reaches a high enough concentration in the mitochondria, is translocated into the cytosol. In the cytosol, citrate is converted back into oxaloacetic acid and acetyl CoA by citrate lyases. Oxaloacetic acid is further converted into malate and malate back to pyruvate by a nicotinamide adenine dinucleotide phosphate (NADP)–dependent malate dehydrogenase reaction, resulting in the generation of NADPH. This NADPH, in combination with the NADPH from the pentose phosphate shunt, provides the reducing equivalents for fatty acid synthesis. Acetyl CoA is converted into malonyl coenzyme A (malonyl CoA) by acetyl CoA carboxylase. This is the rate-limiting step of fatty acid synthesis. Malonyl CoA, in addition to playing a role in fatty acid synthesis, prevents carnitine acyltransferase in the mitochondrial membrane from accepting fatty acids for β-oxidation. The remaining series of reactions in fatty acid synthesis is catalyzed by the fatty acid synthase complex, which utilizes pantothenic acid as a cofactor. Palmitate, a 16-carbon fatty acid, is the end-product of this complex. It is the precursor for the longer-chained fatty acids or can be desaturated by separate enzyme reactions. Fatty acids form a complex with albumin in the peripheral blood and are used as a source of energy in the fasting state and for triacylglycerol synthesis in the fed state.

132. The answer is D.   *(Microbiology)*
Bacteroides organisms are the largest component of the intestinal flora, not the flora of the peritoneal cavity or pelvic tissues. They grow well in the anaerobic atmosphere of the intestines. These organisms are opportunistic and will cause abscesses if they escape their normal ecological niche; infections of the peritoneal cavity and pelvic tissues by *Bacteroides* is common. The microorganisms that are constantly present on body surfaces are commensals. Streptococci of the viridans group are the most common resident organisms of the upper respiratory tract. If large numbers of viridans streptococci are introduced into the bloodstream, infective endocarditis may result. The normal flora of the body may be aerobic or anaerobic.

133. The answer is E.   *(Biochemistry)*
A starvation state exists after 4–5 days of prolonged fasting. Because red blood cells can only use glucose for fuel and glycogen stores are depleted 10–18 hours after fasting, gluconeogenesis, not glycogenolysis, occurs to maintain blood glucose levels during prolonged fasting. Lipolysis occurs, generating fatty acids, which the muscles use for fuel. In the starvation state, ketone body synthesis is markedly increased, because ketone bodies are the byproduct of increased β-oxidation of fatty acids. Muscle use of ketones for fuel is decreased to make more ketones available for the brain tissue to use as fuel. In the early fasting state, urea excretion is greatly increased over normal because of the catabolism of muscle for the release of amino acids as a

substrate for gluconeogenesis. However, as fasting becomes prolonged, urea excretion decreases because less muscle breakdown of protein occurs.

134. The answer is A.   *(Microbiology)*
Secondary follicles are not normally present at birth; their presence signals an ongoing immune response by B cells that is predominantly humoral. They are formed from primary follicles in peripheral lymphoid tissues after antigenic stimulation. Primary follicles are spherical or ovoid collections of lymphoid tissue in the cortex of the lymph nodes and the white pulp of the spleen. They consist of mature resting B cells, relatively few T lymphocytes, and follicular dendritic cells with long appendages that surround the lymphocytes. Upon exposure to antigen, which is processed by the follicular dendritic cells and presented to T helper lymphocytes, secondary follicles develop. Secondary follicles have a pale germinal center containing activated lymphocytes in various stages of maturation. A mantle of mature B lymphocytes surrounds the germinal center. Many macrophages and some plasma cells can be identified. The antibody that is secreted by the plasma cells enters the lymphatic and blood circulatory systems to seek out the inducing antigen.

135. The answer is D.   *(Pharmacology)*
The volume of distribution of drugs is affected by the percentage of body water and fat, as well as muscle mass and protein concentrations in the plasma and tissues. Neonates have a higher, rather than lower, percentage of body weight in the form of water (75% versus 60% in adults), which tends to increase the volume of distribution of water-soluble drugs and decrease the volume of distribution of fat-soluble drugs. Neonates also have lower cytochrome P-450–dependent and conjugative (glucuronyl transferase) drug metabolism activity than adults. The glomerular filtration rate is also lower in neonates as compared with older children and adults.

136. The answer is D.   *(Anatomy)*
Terminal deoxynucleotidyl transferase is a nuclear enzyme expressed in immature B (and T) lymphocytes. It appears early in the pro-B cell and disappears when the early B cell expresses surface immunoglobulin. Some B cells express both immunoglobulin M (IgM) and immunoglobulin D (IgD). The FcγR protein, a

receptor for the Fc region of immunoglobulin G (IgG), is expressed during the early and mature stages of B cell development, as are major histocompatibility complex (MHC) class II molecules. Intracellular adhesion molecule (ICAM), leukocyte function-associated antigen (LFA), and L-selectin are homing and adhesion proteins that facilitate the movement of mature B cells from the bone marrow to the lymph nodes and other peripheral sites. The following table summarizes the order of appearance of the various markers:

	Pro-B cell	Pre-B cell	Early B cell	Mature B cell
TdT	+	–	–	–
CD10	+	+	–	–
RAG-1 and RAG-2	+	+	–	–
Cytoplasmic IgM	–	+	–	–
Surface IgM, IgD	–	–	+	+
MHC class II molecules	–	–	+	+
FcγR protein	–	–	+	+
Complement receptor	–	–	+	l
L-selectin	–	–	–	+
LFA	–	–	–	+
ICAM	–	–	–	+

FcγR = receptor for the Fc region of immunoglobulin G (IgG); ICAM = intercellular adhesion molecule; IgD = immunoglobulin D; IgM = immunoglobulin M; LFA = leukocyte function-associated antigen; MHC = major histocompatibility complex; RAG-1 and RAG-2 = recombinase components; TdT = terminal deoxynucleotidyl transferase.

137. The answer is C. *(Microbiology)*
Bacillary dysentery (enterocolitis) is caused by *Shigella* species; these organisms are not part of the normal human flora. Of the enteric bacteria, *Shigella* are among the most virulent; as few as 100 organisms can cause disease, whereas at least 10^5 *Vibrio* or *Salmonella* organisms must be present to cause infection. Shigellosis is only a human disease and is passed by the fecal-oral route. Subacute bacterial endocarditis is routinely caused by α-hemolytic oral streptococci. *Escherichia coli* is often the cause of uncomplicated urinary tract infections. *Actinomycosis* is caused by endogenous oral bacteria. Brain abscesses are frequently caused by intestinal obligate anaerobes, with dental extractions being the most common predisposing factor.

138. The answer is B. *(Biochemistry)*
Pepsin cleaves antibody on the carboxyl side of the disulfide bonds that hold the heavy chains together (i.e., closer to the Fab regions). This enzymatic action yields one large fragment called $F(ab')_2$, which has two antigen-binding sites and an extensively degraded Fc portion. In contrast, papain cleaves antibody on the N-terminal side of the disulfide bonds that hold the heavy chains together, thereby yielding two separate Fab fragments and an intact Fc fragment.

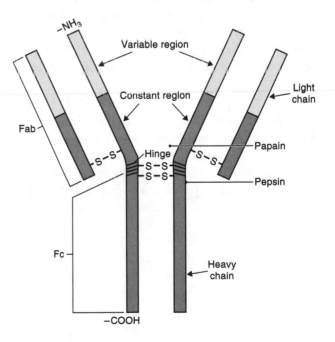

Historically, pepsin and papain have been important in elucidating the structure and function of antibodies. They are still used today for diagnostic and research purposes. Immunoglobulins are protein molecules secreted by activated B lymphocytes (plasma cells) and, as such, they consist of amino acids. All proteins have a carboxyl (-COOH) group at one end and an amino group ($-NH_3$) at the other end. Carbohydrate moieties (sugars) are added to the Fc portion of the heavy chains during their transport through the cytoplasm of the plasma cell. All antibodies consist of four protein chains. Two are relatively large and heavy chains and two are small and light chains. Each individual is capable of producing five different heavy chains of antibody (γ, α, μ, δ, and ϵ, each one representing a different immunoglobulin class or isotype) and two different light chains (κ and λ). Each antibody molecule has identical heavy chains and identical light chains. Relatively minor variations in the structure and function of the constant (C) region of the heavy chains of immunoglobulin G (IgG) are used to identify the 4 subclasses: IgG1, IgG2, IgG3, and IgG4 (γ1, γ2, γ3, and γ4 heavy chains). Similarly, there are two subclasses of IgA, IgA1 and IgA2 (α1 and α2 heavy chains). IgM, IgD, and IgE do not have subclasses. The chains are folded into globular domains (one domain per light chain; four or five domains per heavy chain). Each chain has one variable (V) region at the N-terminus (VH and VL) and one or more constant (C) regions at the carboxyl terminus (CH and CL). The specificity of an antibody is determined by the structure within paired VH and VL regions. Each antibody molecule is designed to bind to a single type of epitope.

139. The answer is D.   *(Behavioral science)*
While dying is commonly associated with sadness, this patient is demonstrating depression that is a more severe reaction. Antidepressants are often helpful in the treatment of depression associated with dying. A previous history of depression is a risk factor for depression during the dying process. Illness, including cancer, endocrine dysfunction, pneumonia, mononucleosis, AIDS, systemic lupus erythematosus, rheumatoid arthritis, multiple sclerosis, and Parkinson disease can produce depressive symptoms.

140. The answer is C.   *(Microbiology)*
The peptidoglycan cell wall of both gram-positive and gram-negative organisms provides structure and rigidity to the cell, but it cannot prevent phagocytosis from occurring. M protein, the major virulence factor of group A, β-hemolytic streptococci, has antiphagocytic properties. Opacity (Opa) proteins, found on *Neisseria gonorrhoeae*, mediate bacterial attachment to mucosal cells and have antiphagocytic properties. Protein A is a fimbrae-like series of molecules on the cell wall of *Staphylococcus aureus* that is able to bind to the Fc portion of immunoglobulin G (IgG), preventing complement binding and interfering with phagocytosis by white blood cells. Polysaccharide capsules are probably the most common antiphagocytic mechanism possessed by bacteria. *Streptococcus pneumoniae*, for example, can produce 85 different types of polysaccharide capsule.

141. The answer is B.   *(Behavioral science)*
Middle-aged whites are more likely to commit suicide than middle-aged African-Americans. Women are more likely than men to attempt suicide, but men are more likely to kill themselves. Suicide is rare in children, tends to run in families, and is more common in adolescents from broken homes.

142. The answer is C.   *(Microbiology)*
Xylulose-5-phosphate does not participate in the Entner-Doudoroff pathway, an alternate pathway for carbohydrate metabolism. 6-Phosphogluconate is dehydrated by dehydratase, and then an aldolase reaction produces pyruvate and triose phosphate (glyceraldehyde-3-phosphate):

Glucose → Glucose-6-phosphate → 6-Phosphogluconate

Pyruvate   Glyceraldehyde-3-phosphate

↓

Lactate

143. The answer is A. *(Behavioral science)*
Normal aging is not associated with decreased intelligence. Decreased rapid eye movement (REM) sleep, a diminished sense of taste and smell, increased sleep latency, and thinning of the vaginal mucosa are associated with normal aging.

144. The answer is D. *(Microbiology)*
Memory cells, long-lived B and T lymphocytes that have been primed by prior exposure to antigen, are not created during phagocytosis. The presence of memory cells results in a rapid and prolonged secondary (anamnestic) response against a specific antigen on subsequent encounter. During phagocytosis, bacteria, other microorganisms, and particulate inanimate materials are engulfed within vacuoles known as phagosomes, which fuse with the enzyme-containing lysosomes (granules) to form phagolysosomes. Shortly after ingestion, the phagocytes undergo an oxygen-dependent respiratory burst. Highly reactive oxygen radicals, such as superoxide (O_2^-) and hydrogen peroxide (H_2O_2), are generated. Hydrogen peroxide is generally more bactericidal than superoxide, but organisms that produce catalase (e.g., staphylococci) may escape its effects. The interaction of chloride (CI^-) and hydrogen peroxide is catalyzed by myeloperoxidase (present in neutrophils, but not in macrophages), resulting in the formation of hypochlorite ions (CIO^-). The green myeloperoxidase imparts a greenish appearance to pus. Hypochlorite ions are considered to be the most important agents in the killing of microorganisms. They can damage cells directly and indirectly (by reacting with hydrogen peroxide to produce singlet oxygen, which breaks down lipids). Degradation of ingested material involves proteolytic enzymes, as well as lipases and nucleases.

145. The answer is D. *(Behavioral science)*
Women are hospitalized more often than men. Prior to 1900, Americans generally died of infections, but chronic diseases are currently the most common cause of death. In the United States, there are more than 25,000 nursing homes, with a total capacity for 1.5 million beds. The largest portion of a hospital's budget goes toward salaries and benefits for health care staff.

146. The answer is A. *(Microbiology)*
Natural killer (NK) cells are not a subset of T lymphocytes. Like cytotoxic T cells, however, they are capable of killing target cells directly. NK cells do not express CD3 molecules on their surfaces; however, they are positive for CD16, which is not found on T cells. CD16 functions as a low-affinity receptor for the Fc portion of IgG. NK cells can also kill target cells by a mechanism known as antibody-dependent cell-mediated cytotoxicity (ADCC). The cytotoxic machinery of the NK cell becomes activated when the cell binds (via its CD16 protein) to the Fc region of IgG antibody coating a target cell. Unlike cytotoxic T lymphocytes, which are highly specific, a single NK cell can kill several types of target cells. Incubation of NK cells with interleukin-2 leads to activation of the NK cells. Peripheral blood mononuclear cells incubated in the presence of high-dose interleukin-2 become lymphokine-activated killer (LAK) cells (granular lymphocytes). The majority of LAK cells are thought to be activated NK cells.

147. The answer is A. *(Behavioral science)*
The percentage of the gross domestic product spent on health care in 1992 was approximately 13%, not 1.3%. The costs for personal health care are divided approximately as follows: 41%, the federal government; 32%, private insurance; 24%, the individual; and charity, 3%. Hospital costs represent approximately 41% of health care expenditures; physician costs comprise approximately 20% of these expenditures.

148. The answer is C. *(Biochemistry)*
Induction of the cytochrome P-450 enzymes increases the rate of drug metabolism, resulting in shorter elimination half-lives and increased drug clearance. Enzyme induction refers to the increased synthesis of enzyme protein and requires DNA transcription and the translation of messenger RNA (mRNA). Certain drugs (e.g., phenobarbital, rifampin) are particularly effective inducers of the hepatic cytochrome P-450 drug metabolizing enzymes.

149. The answer is E. *(Behavioral science)*
Rather than being cure-oriented, hospices provide supportive care to terminally ill patients (i.e., those expected to live less than 6 months). The hospice concept

originated in England, but hospices are becoming more common in the United States. In the United States, most hospice care is provided in the patient's home and involves the family, with the aim of providing as much autonomy for the dying patient as possible. There are currently at least 1800 hospice programs in the United States, supported since 1983 by the federal government under Medicare.

150. The answer is A.   *(Microbiology)*
Treponema pallidum, a spirochete, causes syphilis and cannot be grown on laboratory medium. Spirochetes are so thin that they can be observed only by using darkfield microscopy, silver impregnation, or immunofluorescence techniques. The spirochete does not stain well with aniline dyes, and the Gram stain would not be used to diagnose syphilis. *Neisseria gonorrhoeae*, *Candida albicans*, *Haemophilus ducreyi* (the etiologic agent of chancroid), and meningitis-causing bacteria would all stain well using a gram stain.

151. The answer is E.   *(Behavioral science)*
Primary features of hospice care include administration of pain medication as needed, grief counseling, and support groups. Supportive care is provided in both inpatient and outpatient settings.

152. The answer is A.   *(Microbiology)*
Protozoa, such as *Giardia lamblia*, belong to the protist kingdom. As such, they are eukaryotic (i.e., they have a true nucleus bounded by a membrane, mitochondria, and a flexible outer membrane). Bacteria belong to the prokaryote kingdom. Prokaryotes lack a nuclear membrane and mitochondria and have a fairly rigid cell wall. *Ureaplasma urealyticum*, L-form bacteria, *Rickettsia*, and *Listeria monocytogenes* all have a genome not bounded by a nuclear membrane.

153. The answer is E.   *(Anatomy)*
The term "killer cells" was originally given to cells capable of mediating antibody-dependent cell-mediated cytotoxicity (ADCC). However, it is now known that a number of different cell types can mediate ADCC: cytotoxic T lymphocytes, natural killer (NK) cells, lymphokine-activated killer cells, monocytes, and macrophages. Thus, although in the broadest sense

"killer cells" could include monocytes and macrophages, "E" is the best answer to this question. Monocytes migrate from the bone marrow into the blood, where they account for approximately 1%–6% of the leukocytes in the blood circulation. After approximately 1 day, the monocytes move into tissues and differentiate into macrophages (histiocytes). Nearly all parts of the body have some resident phagocytic cells. They are relatively few in number and sparsely scattered. However, some tissues have large numbers of these cells that are densely arranged. They have characteristic morphologies and have been given different names. Microglia, osteoclasts, Langerhans' cells, and Kupffer's cells (found in the brain, bone, skin, and liver sinusoids, respectively) are all derived from cells of the monocyte-macrophage series.

154. The answer is B.   *(Microbiology)*
Macrophages do not possess antigen-specific receptors. Only T and B lymphocytes express molecules specific for antigen. In contrast to neutrophils, macrophages do not contain myeloperoxidase. More than 100 different products are secreted by macrophages. Interleukin-1 is among the most important of the "monokines." Other products secreted by macrophages include platelet-derived growth factor (PDGF), transforming growth factor-β, and interferon. Macrophages play a critical role in specific immune responses in that they function as antigen-presenting cells. Ingested material is broken down into small fragments ("processed") and then expressed on the surface of the macrophage together with major histocompatibility complex (MHC) class II proteins for presentation to helper T cells. Activation of the lymphocyte involves binding of its T-cell antigen receptor to the presented antigenic peptide–class II protein complex.

155. The answer is A.   *(Anatomy)*
The thymus is a two-lobed structure with a cortex and a medulla. The cortex consists of a large number of rapidly proliferating T cell precursors. Greatest activity in the thymus occurs during fetal life; it is during this time that most of the T cell maturation occurs. Virtually all T lymphocyte maturation occurs in the thymus. However, only mature, single-positive (CD4$^+$ or CD8$^+$) cells leave the thymus and seed other parts of the body; more than 95% of the lymphocytes die in the thymus. The

thymus reaches its peak weight (approximately 35 g) at puberty, after which the lymphoid cells decline and are replaced by fatty connective tissue. In the adult, the thymus weighs only approximately 6 g and consists mostly of epithelial elements.

156. The answer is D.   *(Anatomy)*

Most of the T lymphocytes that leave the thymus are single-positive (either CD4$^+$ or CD8$^+$). CD4$^-$CD8$^-$ (double-negative) cells comprise only about 10% of the thymocytes. Approximately 75% of T cells in the thymus are double-positive (i.e., CD4$^+$CD8$^+$). These cells die during a complex and not entirely understood selection process. T lymphocyte maturation is mediated by thymic hormones (small peptides) secreted by epithelial cells within the thymus. Thymic hormones include thymosins, thymulin, thymopentin, thymostimulin, and thymic humoral factor. These hormones have been used experimentally to augment immune responses in certain viral infections and immunodeficiency diseases such as DiGeorge syndrome and ataxia-telangiectasia. Deletion of potentially self-reactive T lymphocytes occurs, at least partly, in the thymus. When a developing thymocyte binds to a self antigen, it undergoes apoptosis (programmed cell death). This process is known as negative selection. However, T cells with receptors for autoantigens found exclusively in parts of the body other than the thymus, or which appear later in life, may not be eliminated by this process. Negative selection of T lymphocytes is mediated primarily by macrophages and dendritic cells within the thymus. These cells present autoantigen to the T cells.

157. The answer is E.   *(Microbiology)*

CD8$^+$ T lymphocytes are cytotoxic cells that kill antigen-bearing targets. CD4$^+$ T lymphocytes act as helper cells, which, when activated, secrete soluble proteins called lymphokines. Lymphokines interact with many cell types (e.g., B lymphocytes, monocytes, macrophages, T cells) and regulate their activities. Most of the time, the cells with receptors for the lymphokines respond with increased growth and differentiation, as well as increased functional capacity. There are a few CD8$^+$ T lymphocytes with helper activity and a few CD4$^+$ T lymphocytes with cytotoxic activity; however, most of the time, the CD8 and CD4 designations refer to cytotoxic and helper T cells, respectively. T$_H$0, T$_H$1, and T$_H$2 lymphocytes are CD4$^+$ subsets of T helper cells. They are differentiated on the basis of the lymphokines that they secrete. The T$_H$1 subset helps in generating cell-mediated (T cell) responses. The T$_H$2 subset helps in generating humoral (B cell, antibody) responses. The T$_H$0 subset helps in generating both.

158. The answer is C.   *(Microbiology)*

The T-cell antigen receptor does not bind free-floating soluble antigens. Instead, it recognizes peptide fragments that are bound in a groove of the major histocompatibility complex (MHC) class I or class II molecule. The T-cell antigen receptor consists of eight polypeptide chains, six of which (three sets of dimers) are the same among all mature T cells and make up the structure of the CD3 molecule. The CD3 protein is noncovalently associated with the remaining two chains, the α and β chains. CD3 is involved in signal transduction. Thus, when the α,β dimer binds to the peptide–MHC complex on an antigen-presenting cell, it is CD3 that sends the message for activation. The α,β dimer is highly polymorphic and is generated through mechanisms similar to those for the light and heavy chains of antibody. Rearrangement of V (variable), D (diversity), and J (joining) gene segments, all of which act together to code for the variable portion of the α and β chains, occurs early during T cell development. Each T lymphocyte produces an α,β dimer of only one type; therefore, each T cell can bind only a certain specific antigenic peptide–MHC complex.

159. The answer is E.   *(Pathology)*

Pulmonary emboli most commonly derive from the deep saphenous, not the superficial saphenous, veins of the calf. The superficial saphenous system drains into the deep saphenous system via small penetrating branches; therefore, a thrombus in the superficial system would not be able to pass through these small vessels. Caisson's disease is associated with divers who ascend rapidly to the surface. It occurs when nitrogen dissolves in the blood, creating bubbles that lodge in the vessels of the muscles and joints. Mountaineers who ascend heights too quickly are also subject to Caisson's disease. Air embolism is a potential complication of head and neck surgery. The negative intrathoracic pressure in the pleural cavity predisposes to the suctioning of air into the venous system. The air mixes with blood in the right side of the heart; the resultant froth blocks pulmonary blood flow. Approximately 100 cc of air in the circulation can be fatal. Paradoxical emboli arise in the venous system and pass through a patent foramen ovale into the systemic circulation. They are rare and occur when an atrial septal defect, which starts as a left-to-right shunt, becomes a right-to-left shunt as a result of pulmonary hypertension, thus allowing a venous thromboembolus access to the systemic circulation. Amniotic fluid embolization may occur during a difficult labor and delivery and may be complicated by disseminated intravascular coagulation (DIC). At autopsy, lanugo and

fetal skin are often found in the mother's pulmonary capillaries. DIC occurs if the presence of tissue thromboplastin in the amniotic fluid activates the extrinsic coagulation system. The mortality rate is 80%.

160. The answer is E.   *(Biochemistry)*
Aspartate aminotransferase (AST) is located in the mitochondria and cytosol of hepatocytes. When hepatocytes are damaged by alcohol, AST is released and serum AST levels increase. This increase is not related to an increase in reduced nicotinamide adenine dinucleotide (NADH); rather, it results from physical damage to the hepatocyte. In the liver, alcohol metabolism takes place in the cytosol of hepatocytes:

$$\text{Alcohol} \xrightarrow{\text{Alcohol dehydrogenase}} \text{Acetaldehyde} + \text{NADH} \xrightarrow{\text{Aldehyde dehydrogenase}} \text{Acetate} + \text{NADH} \rightarrow \text{Acetyl (coenzyme A = CoA)}$$

and via the mircrosomal ethanol oxidizing system:

$$\text{Alcohol} + \text{NADPH} \xrightarrow[]{O_2 \quad H_2O} \text{NADP}^+ + \text{Acetaldehyde}$$

The increases in NADH, acetate (simple fatty acid), and acetyl coenzyme A (acetyl CoA) are responsible for many of the metabolic and histologic changes associated with alcoholism. Increased NADH alters the redox potential in favor of NADH over nicotinamide adenine dinucleotide (NAD), resulting in increased production of lactic acid. The increased lactic acid produces a metabolic acidosis. Because pyruvate is changed into lactate, there is less pyruvate available for gluconeogenesis, so patients experience a fasting hypoglycemia. Increased NADH increases the production of triglyceride [very low-density lipoprotein (VLDL)] in the liver by reversing one of the reactions in glycolysis. The excess build-up of VLDL in the hepatocyte results in hypertriglyceridemia (fatty liver). Increased production of the ketoacid β-hydroxybutyrate results from the increase in NADH and acetyl CoA. Ketoacids and lactic acid compete with uric acid for excretory sites in the kidney, thus leading to hyperuricemia, and possibly gout.

161-162. The answers are: 161-E, 162-C. *(Microbiology)*
Frameshift mutations are caused by intercalating agents, such as acridine orange. Intercalating agents

insert themselves between the stacked base pairs in DNA, leading to the accidental insertion or deletion of one or more base pairs during DNA replication. Messenger RNA (mRNA) produced from this region would then contain the insertion or deletion. Because the ribosome translates the mRNA molecule by reading series of three-base codons, its reading frame will become misaligned upon encountering insertions or deletions of any number of bases not divisible by three. Frameshift mutations usually seriously impact protein structure and function because the entire amino acid sequence is altered after the point of the mutation. Proflavine and other acridine dyes are also intercalating agents.

Helix distortion mutations are commonly caused by ultraviolet light. Ultraviolet light causes the formation of thymine dimers, produced when two neighboring thymine residues on the same DNA strand become covalently linked together. Thymine dimers can be repaired by photoreactivation or by excision repair mechanisms. However, if they are not repaired before the DNA undergoes replication, mutations can be permanently introduced into the molecule.

Bromodeoxyuridine and 2-aminopurine are base analogs that can cause point mutations in DNA by base pairing with the incorrect partner. Nitrous acid is a deaminating agent that chemically alters bases in DNA, causing them to form improper base pairs. These types of mutagens all cause transition mutations,

does also transversions

transition

in which a purine is substituted for another purine and a pyrimidine is substituted for another pyrimidine.

163-166. The answers are: 163-B, 164-D, 165-A, 166-C. *(Pharmacology)*

The drugs in graph B have the same half-life (evidenced by the parallel slopes of the elimination curves), but different volumes of distribution (evidenced by the fact that back-extrapolation of the curves would cause them to intersect the concentration scale at different points).

The drugs in graph D have different elimination slopes and different intercepts on the plasma concentration scale, indicating that drugs A, B, and C have different half-lives and different volumes of distribution.

The drugs in graph A have the same volume of distribution (back-extrapolation of the elimination curves will cause them to intercept the same point on the concentration scale) but different half-lives.

In graph C, drugs A and C have parallel elimination slopes and drugs A and B back-extrapolate to the same point on the concentration scale; therefore, drugs A and C have the same half-life while drugs A and B have the same volume of distribution.

167-171. The answers are: 167-E, 168-D, 169-A, 170-C, 171-B. *(Behavioral science)*

"What brings you to see me?" is an example of an open-ended question. Using the open-ended question, the interviewer encourages the patient to speak freely and elicits a great deal of information.

"When did you begin to feel dizzy?" is an example of the interviewing technique known as direct questioning. Direct questions are used to elicit specific information when time is limited (e.g., in an emergency situation).

"And then?" is an example of facilitation. In facilitation, the interviewer encourages the patient to elaborate on an answer.

"You say that you felt dizzy just before you fell?" is an example of the interviewing technique known as reflection. In reflection, the interviewer repeats the response of the patient in a questioning way to encourage the patient to elaborate on the answer.

"You seem to be very sad" is an example of the interviewing technique known as confrontation. In confrontation, the interviewer calls the patient's attention to inconsistencies in his responses or body language in order to encourage the patient to express his feelings. In this example, the patient may not have told the interviewer that he was sad, but he appears to be sad.

172-173. The answers are: 172-D, 173-A. *(Pathology)*

An electrocardiogram (ECG) has a sensitivity of $\approx 70\%$ and specificity of $\approx 100\%$ for diagnosing the changes associated with an acute myocardial infarction. In this patient, the ECG was normal in the presence of an infarct; hence, it represents a false-negative test result (patient with disease who is misclassified as normal). The CK-MB isoenzyme has a sensitivity and specificity approaching 100% and is normally increased 8 hours after an infarct and disappears by 3 days. Hence, the positive CK-MB is an expected finding after 10 hours and is therefore a true-positive. The visibly hemolyzed specimen would falsely elevate potassium (false-positive) and would also produce an $LDH^{1/2}$ flip (LDH1 is present in red blood cells), hence simulating a myocardial infarction (false-positive).

174-175. The answers are: 174-E, 175-A. *(Physiology)*

The medullary segment of the thick ascending limb has the sodium/potassium-2 chloride cotransport pump, which is important in the generation of free water. Free water is water that has been separated from sodium, chloride, and potassium via the pump. In the absence of antidiuretic hormone (ADH), the loss of free water leads to normal dilution (positive free-water clearance), and the presence of ADH results in the reabsorption of free water, hence concentrating the urine (negative free-water clearance). The pump is blocked by loop diuretics, which interfere with the generation of free water and the ability to dilute urine.

The peritubular capillary hydrostatic and oncotic pressure are important in the reabsorption of sodium, urea, and other solutes in the portion of the proximal tubule located in the cortex. An increase in peritubular capillary hydrostatic pressure (e.g., an increase in arterial blood volume) opposes the reabsorption of solute, which results in the loss of solutes in the urine. A reduction in peritubular hydrostatic pressure (e.g., decrease in glomerular filtration rate in volume depletion) results in an increase in capillary oncotic pressure, which favors the reabsorption of solute to counteract volume depletion.

176-180. The answers are: 176-D, 177-A, 178-E, 179-G, 180-I. *(Anatomy)*

Neuronal loss and disorganization of layers of the cerebral cortex are microscopic features of Alzheimer's disease. The neurofibrillary tangles of the affected neurons consist of tangled masses of paired helical filaments (PHFs). These PHFs consist of the microtubule-associated protein, tau. The tau protein becomes highly phosphorylated in Alzheimer's disease and the following entanglement leads to disruption of the microtubule network and thus impairment of axonal transport, leading to neuron death. The tangles stain well with silver stains. The other major abnormality in patients with Alzheimer's disease is the extracellular deposit of beta-amyloid, known as senile plaques.

Microfilaments, because of their short and flexible nature, can move receptors on the cell membrane. A linking protein appears to be necessary for attaching the actin filament to the receptor. An example is the linker protein talin, which connects the actin filament to the fibronectin receptor (integrin). Therefore, the arrangement of fibronectin on the cell surface can be determined by the intracellular arrangement of actin microfilaments.

Spectrin is an intermediate filament protein that is closely related to the red blood cell membrane. However, this protein adds structural rigidity to the red blood cell membrane so that it can withstand the stress of shape change.

Microtubules may play a role in cell-surface receptor movement, but this role has not been demonstrated in a conclusive manner.

Peroxisomes are membrane-bound organelles about the size of lysosomes; they contain the enzyme catalase, which controls the intracellular level of hydrogen peroxide. Peroxisomes also contain oxidases and are thereby able to oxidize various substrates, such as fatty acids and the purine bases. Ironically, H_2O_2 is formed by the oxidation process of peroxisomes and controlled by the enzyme catalase. Peroxisomes also contain alcohol dehydrogenase and are able to degrade alcohol. These organelles are present in large numbers in hepatocytes and in the apex of proximal convoluted tubule cells.

Lysosomes are membrane-bound organelles that may contain 50 or more hydrolytic enzymes. They are usually identified by a positive reaction for acid phosphatase.

The smooth endoplasmic reticulum is the site of inactivation of various drugs and substances, which occurs by means of various enzymes distributed along the endoplasmic reticulum membrane. It has been shown that smooth endoplasmic reticulum increases throughout the hepatocyte when experimental animals are treated with phenobarbital.

The cell cytoplasm of the proximal convoluted tubule is filled with mitochondria. These mitochondria are throughout the cell as well as interdigitated between basal infoldings. Mitochondria supply the energy necessary for functioning of the Na^+K^+–ATPase pump found along the basal and lateral membranes. From 70% to 80% of the plasma filtrate is reabsorbed in the proximal convoluted tubule via this energy burning mechanism.

Peroxisomes are also present in the proximal convoluted tubule but are not nearly as plentiful as the mitochondria.

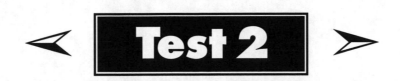

Test 2

QUESTIONS

DIRECTIONS:

Each of the numbered items or incomplete statements in this section is followed by answers or by completions of the statement. Select the ONE lettered answer or completion that is BEST in each case.

1. Compared with first marriages, second marriages are

(A) less likely to end in divorce
(B) equally likely to end in divorce
(C) more likely to end in divorce
(D) more likely to involve an older man and a younger woman
(E) more likely to result in children

2. Reverse transcriptase activity is involved in the reproduction cycles of which of the following pairs of viruses?

(A) Human immunodeficiency virus (HIV) and hepatitis A virus
(B) HIV and hepatitis B virus
(C) HIV and hepatitis C virus
(D) Hepatitis B virus and hepatitis C virus
(E) Hepatitis A virus and hepatitis D virus

Questions 3-4

Every time Katie runs out into the street she is spanked by her mother. She then begins to run into the street more often.

3. Katie's change in behavior is an example of

(A) negative reinforcement
(B) positive reinforcement
(C) punishment
(D) shaping
(E) extinction

4. The most effective and most lasting way to get Katie to stop running into the street is by using

(A) negative reinforcement
(B) positive reinforcement
(C) punishment
(D) shaping
(E) extinction

5. The first step in the catabolism of most amino acids is the transfer of the α-amino group to α-ketoglutarate to form

(A) oxaloacetate
(B) aspartate
(C) pyruvate
(D) alanine
(E) glutamate

6.   Which of the following causes of encephalitis is associated with transmission by mosquitoes?

(A) Equine encephalitis
(B) Varicella
(C) Rubeola
(D) Hantavirus
(E) Rabies

7.   Which of the following characteristics distinguishes lead poisoning from mercury and arsenic poisoning?

(A) Lead is a heavy metal
(B) Lead poisoning is associated with central nervous system signs and symptoms
(C) Lead poisoning is associated with nephrotoxic acute tubular necrosis
(D) Lead deposits are visible on x-rays of bone
(E) Lead is detectable in urine

8.   Which of the following serologic tests is positive during the serologic gap, or window, of a typical acute hepatitis B virus (HBV) infection?

(A) Anti-HBV surface antigen (anti-HBsAg)
(B) HBV core antigen (HBcAg)
(C) Anti-HBV epsilon antigen (anti-HBeAg)
(D) HBV surface antigen (HBsAg)
(E) Anti-HBV core antigen (anti-HBcAg)

9.   Aminotransferases (transaminases) require which of the following coenzymes?

(A) Biotin
(B) Pyridoxal phosphate
(C) Oxidized nicotinamide adenine dinucleotide (NAD$^+$)
(D) Oxidized nicotinamide adenine dinucleotide phosphate (NADP$^+$)
(E) Flavin adenine dinucleotide (FAD)

10. Which one of the following enzymes is in the HIV particle (virion)?

(A) DNA-dependent RNA polymerase
(B) DNA-dependent DNA polymerase
(C) Double-stranded RNA–dependent RNA polymerase
(D) RNA-dependent DNA polymerase
(E) Single-stranded RNA–dependent RNA polymerase

11. Obesity contributing to the clinical expression of type II diabetes mellitus is an example of what type of inheritance pattern?

(A) Autosomal recessive
(B) Autosomal dominant
(C) Sex-linked recessive
(D) Sex-linked dominant
(E) Multifactorial

12. Which of the following antibodies would be found in the serum of a person who received a hepatitis B virus (HBV) vaccination?

(A) Anti-HBV core antigen (anti-HBcAg)
(B) Anti-HBV surface antigen (anti-HBsAg)
(C) Anti-HBV DNA
(D) Anti-HBV DNA polymerase
(E) Anti-HBV epsilon antigen (anti-HBeAg)

13. A patient with severe viral hepatitis would primarily have elevated plasma levels of which of the following enzymes?

(A) Creatine kinase 2 (MB)
(B) Lactate dehydrogenase
(C) Aspartate aminotransferase
(D) Glutamate oxaloacetate transaminase
(E) Dihydrofolate reductase

14. Which of the following terms correctly describes the flagella of this bacterium?

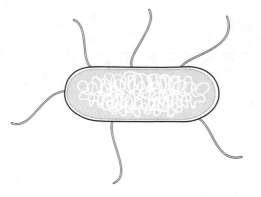

(A) Monotrichous
(B) Lophotrichous
(C) Peritrichous
(D) Polytrichous
(E) None of the above

15. A 2-year-old child has multiple nodular masses in the skin. A biopsy reveals small, basophilic-staining cells that are positive for S-100 protein. Where would this patient be expected to have a primary lesion?

(A) Cerebellum
(B) Kidney
(C) Adrenal medulla
(D) Bone
(E) Lymph nodes

16. The quellung test is a capsule-swelling test that has been used to identify strains of which of the following organisms?

(A) *Enterococcus faecalis*
(B) *Streptococcus pneumoniae*
(C) *Staphylococcus epidermidis*
(D) *Neisseria gonorrhoeae*
(E) *Gardnerella vaginalis*

17. Excess nitrogen derived from the degradation of amino acids is excreted in the urine in the form of

(A) ammonia
(B) creatinine
(C) aspartate
(D) urea
(E) uric acid

18. Which of the following statements concerning viruses is correct?

(A) All viruses, except retroviruses, have haploid genomes
(B) All viruses, except retroviruses, have diploid genomes
(C) All RNA viruses, except reoviruses, have positive-sense genomes
(D) All RNA viruses, except reoviruses, have negative-sense genomes
(E) All live, attenuated viral vaccines consist of positive-sense RNA viruses

19. The pedigree depicted below is most consistent with which one of the following inheritance patterns?

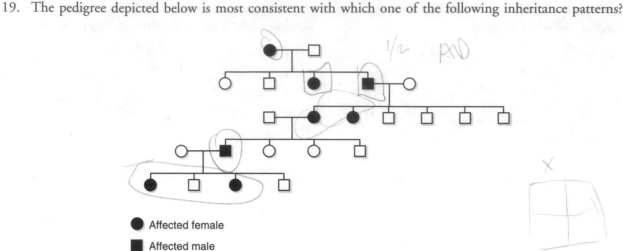

● Affected female
■ Affected male

(A) Multifactorial
(B) Autosomal recessive
(C) Autosomal dominant
(D) Sex-linked recessive
(E) Sex-linked dominant

20. Which of the following viral diseases has an approved vaccine that has been developed by recombinant DNA technology?

(A) Hepatitis A
(B) Hepatitis B
(C) Influenza A
(D) Poliomyelitis
(E) Rabies

21. Ammonia for the urea cycle is supplied by the action of which of the following enzymes?

(A) Aspartate aminotransferase
(B) Glutamate dehydrogenase
(C) Argininosuccinate synthase
(D) Argininosuccinate lyase
(E) Arginase

22. Defective viruses lack one or more functional genes required for viral replication. Which of the following viruses is a defective virus requiring helper activity from another virus for some step in replication or maturation?

(A) Hepatitis A
(B) Hepatitis B
(C) Hepatitis C
(D) Hepatitis D
(E) Hepatitis E

23. Which of the following immunoglobulins acts as the antigen receptor for B lymphocytes?

(A) IgG
(B) IgA
(C) IgM
(D) IgD
(E) IgE

24. The immediate precursor of urea in the urea cycle is

(A) arginine
(B) aspartate
(C) carbamoyl phosphate
(D) citrulline
(E) ornithine

25. Which of the following tumor–electron microscopic finding relationships is correctly matched?

(A) Squamous carcinoma—Birbeck granules
(B) Angiosarcoma—Weibel-Palade bodies
(C) Carcinoid tumor—tonofilaments
(D) Histiocytosis X—neurosecretory granules
(E) Oncocytoma—increased smooth endoplasmic reticulum

26. Which one of the following statements concerning eicosanoid metabolism is true?

(A) Cortisol and aspirin both inhibit arachidonic acid cyclooxygenase, but aspirin is an irreversible inhibitor and cortisol is a reversible inhibitor
(B) Aspirin inhibits synthesis of leukotriene A_4, thromboxane A_2, and prostaglandins PGE_2, $PGF_{2\alpha}$, and PGI_2 by irreversibly inhibiting phospholipase A_2.
(C) The prostaglandins are telecrine hormones
(D) Nonsteroidal anti-inflammatory drugs (NSAIDs) other than aspirin (e.g., indomethacin, phenylbutazone) inhibit synthesis of leukotriene A_4, thromboxane A_2, and prostaglandins PGE_2, $PGF_{2\alpha}$, and PGI_2 by reversibly inhibiting phospholipase A_2
(E) Aspirin is an irreversible inhibitor of arachidonic acid cyclooxygenase, but the action of other NSAIDs is reversible

27. The most common benign tumor in women is most commonly located in the

(A) ovary
(B) breast
(C) uterus
(D) liver
(E) stomach

28. Which of the following amino acids is ketogenic but not glucogenic?

(A) Glutamate
(B) Phenylalanine
(C) Tyrosine
(D) Valine
(E) Leucine

29. Which of the following is involved in isotype switching from immunoglobulin M (IgM) to IgG?

(A) Messenger RNA is translated in two different ways
(B) DNA for the $C\mu$ region of H chains is excised
(C) Two different immature RNA transcripts are produced
(D) There is a lack of lymphokines in the microenvironment.
(E) There is a change in the V region of the antibody

30. Albinism results from a deficiency in the metabolism of which of the following amino acids?

(A) Alanine
(B) Proline
(C) Tryptophan
(D) Tyrosine
(E) Valine

31. In which of the following combinations are gonad type, genotype, and phenotype correctly matched with the appropriate condition?

Condition	Genotype	Phenotype	Presence of Gonads Male	Presence of Gonads Female
(A) Testicular feminization	Male	Female	Yes	No
(B) 17-hydroxylase deficiency in male	Male	Male	Yes	No
(C) 17-hydroxylase deficiency in female	Female	Male	No	Yes
(D) 21-hydroxylase deficiency in female	Female	Male	Yes	No
(E) True hermaphrodite (most cases)	Predominantly male	Variable	Yes	Yes

32. *S*-adenosylmethionine (SAM) is important in metabolism because it can serve as a donor of

(A) a sulfhydryl group
(B) a methyl group
(C) an amino group
(D) ribose
(E) adenine

33. Which of the following terms correctly describes the St. Louis encephalitis virus?

(A) Enveloped helical
(B) Enveloped icosahedral
(C) Enveloped DNA
(D) Naked helical
(E) Naked icosahedral

34. An inherited deficiency of branched-chain α-keto acid dehydrogenase results in which of the following conditions?

(A) Maple syrup urine disease
(B) Phenylketonuria
(C) Homocystinuria
(D) Alcaptonuria
(E) Histidinemia

35. Which of the following disorders has a mode of inheritance that differs from the others listed?

(A) Cleft lip
(B) Essential hypertension
(C) Congenital heart disease
(D) Coronary artery disease
(E) Testicular feminization

36. Which of the following statements most accurately describes the digestion and absorption of lipids?

(A) Triacylglycerol and cholesterol esters are synthesized from smaller precursor molecules during lipid absorption
(B) Digestion and absorption of lipids does not require synthesis of specific proteins by intestinal mucosal cells
(C) Dietary triacylglycerol is digested in the intestinal lumen by pancreatic lipase, which most often liberates three molecules of free fatty acid, and one of glycerol, per molecule of triacylglycerol hydrolyzed
(D) Bile salts are required to emulsify ingested lipids into small droplets called chylomicrons
(E) Pancreatic lipase emulsifies triacylglycerol molecules before hydrolyzing them

37. Which of the following conditions is the most common manifestation of fetal alcohol syndrome?

(A) Microcephaly
(B) Atrial septal defect
(C) Maxillary hypoplasia
(D) Mental retardation
(E) Short palpebral fissures

38. The activation of a T helper lymphocyte is facilitated by interaction of the major histocompatibility complex class II molecule on an antigen-presenting cell with a coreceptor on the T helper cell surface. Which of the following is the correct designation of this coreceptor?

(A) CD2
(B) CD3
(C) CD4
(D) CD8
(E) CD10

39. A child psychiatrist was referred an overweight, but not obese, three-year-old boy by a pediatrician who was concerned by the child's weight and refusal to socialize with other children at nursery school. The child did not engage in play, particularly in games that involved exercise. The pediatrician had previously referred the child to an endocrinologist who found no abnormality.

No obvious psychological derangement was found. A muscle physiologist found that while his muscles were somewhat underdeveloped, they were not pathologically weak. There was no evidence of any dystrophy or atrophy. However, when stimulated for more than 15 minutes, they cramped, causing sufficient pain to explain his refusal to engage in strenuous play. Such stimulation also induced myoglobinuria and a marked rise in creatine kinase. On the basis of these findings, a muscle biopsy was performed.

No evidence of a glycogen storage abnormality was uncovered, and glucose could be oxidized at a normal rate. Fatty acids were oxidized very slowly in tissue slices, but at a normal rate in properly supplemental broken cell extracts. There remained sufficient material from the biopsy sample to conduct one enzymatic assay. Which of the following enzymes has the greatest possibility of having an abnormally low activity level?

(A) Acyl coenzyme A (CoA) dehydrogenase
(B) Enoyl CoA hydratase
(C) β-Hydroxyacyl CoA dehydrogenase
(D) Thiolase
(E) Carnitine acyltransferase

40. Although his alarm clock has been ringing for five minutes, a 25-year-old medical student remains asleep. Which of the following brain wave patterns is this student most likely to exhibit?

(A) Theta waves
(B) Delta waves
(C) K complexes
(D) Beta waves
(E) Alpha waves

41. Which of the following statements correctly describes the activation and role of the regulated enzyme acetyl coenzyme A (CoA) carboxylase? Acetyl CoA carboxylase is activated by

(A) acetyl CoA, in order to stimulate the rate of cholesterol synthesis
(B) acetyl CoA, in order to stimulate the rate of ketone body synthesis
(C) acetyl CoA, in order to stimulate the rate of triacylglycerol synthesis
(D) citrate, in order to stimulate the rate of ketone body synthesis
(E) citrate, in order to stimulate the rate of fatty acid synthesis

42. The designation of legal representatives to make decisions concerning one's health care in the event that one can no longer do so is most correctly known as

(A) a living will
(B) a durable power of attorney
(C) managed care
(D) involuntary treatment
(E) informed consent

43. Malonyl coenzyme A (CoA) labeled with C^{14} on the free carboxyl group is added to a cell-free system containing all the factors required for fatty acid synthesis, including unlabeled acetyl CoA. The reaction is permitted to proceed in synchrony for 32 cycles (i.e., malonyl CoA is used as a substrate 32 times). How many carbons of the resulting palmitate will be labeled?

(A) None
(B) 2
(C) 4
(D) 8
(E) 16

44. An Ouchterlony test was performed using a patient's serum (S). Antigen preparations 1, 2, 3, and 4 were dispensed into wells surrounding the S-containing center well. From the precipitin pattern shown in the figure, one can correctly conclude that

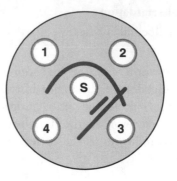

(A) antigens 1 and 2 are related, but not identical
(B) there are two totally different antigens in wells 2 and 3
(C) antigen preparation 3 contains more than two antigens
(D) the patient has antibodies against antigen 4
(E) antigens 2 and 4 are related

45. Which of the following statements concerning calcium ions is true?

(A) They circulate in the serum bound to calmodulin
(B) They bind to a calmodulin subunit, thereby activating muscle phosphorylase kinase
(C) They dampen the effect of diacylglycerol on protein kinase C
(D) Calcium ion levels increase through the action of hormones that activate membrane phospholipase A_2
(E) Calcium channels have a negligible effect in creating an action potential in heart muscle

46. A major function of interleukin-2 (IL-2) is to

(A) enhance the maturation of B lymphocyte precursors
(B) act as a chemotactic agent for macrophages
(C) induce the antiviral state in target cells
(D) promote the clonal expansion of T lymphocytes
(E) induce the acute-phase response in liver cells

47. What is the net number of ATP equivalents obtained from the complete oxidation of one molecule of palmitoleic acid (16 carbons, 1 double bond) by β-oxidation in a tightly coupled oxidative phosphorylation system?

(A) 131
(B) 129
(C) 127
(D) 125
(E) 123

48. A married 16-year-old male requires surgery. Who must give consent for the surgery?

(A) One parent
(B) The spouse
(C) Both parents
(D) A court-appointed legal guardian
(E) The 16-year-old himself

49. Which of the following correctly describes a property or function of vitamin E?

(A) It suppresses the formation of cholesterol-containing plaques on the walls of arteries by inhibiting the oxidation of unsaturated fatty acids in low-density lipoproteins
(B) Because it is stored in the liver, it is toxic when ingested chronically in higher than recommended doses
(C) It serves as an antioxidant by working together with reduced nicotinamide adenine dinucleotide phosphate (NADPH) to keep glutathione in the reduced state
(D) It is a quinone derivative with a structure similar to coenzyme Q
(E) It is an important water-soluble antioxidant

50. Part of the virion genome of which of the following viruses is synthesized by the virion polymerase?

(A) Epstein-Barr virus
(B) Hepatitis B virus
(C) Hepatitis C virus
(D) Adenovirus
(E) Parvovirus

51. Which of the following statements correctly describes ketone bodies during fasting?

(A) They provide an alternative source of fuel for the liver
(B) They are formed from fatty acids in the liver
(C) They are hydrophilic and can not pass the blood–brain barrier without the mediation of carnitine as a transporter
(D) They are used exclusively by the brain as an alternative fuel
(E) Erythrocytes use ketone bodies as a supplemental fuel during long-term fasting

52. A man's family sues a physician for malpractice after he dies while in the doctor's care. For this claim to be upheld in court the family must prove that the doctor

(A) was improperly educated
(B) intended to cause the patient harm
(C) committed a crime
(D) overcharged a patient for the care given
(E) deviated from the established standard of care in that community

53. An infant, who had been thriving well until 6 months of age, started to develop nausea with vomiting, night sweats, and lassitude. His fasting blood glucose level was 62 mg/dL. Upon taking a history, his family pediatrician determined that prior to this time, the baby's diet was limited to mother's milk and that onset of symptoms roughly coincided with intermittent addition of fruit juices to the diet. The pediatrician recommended the immediate return to mother's milk as the sole food in the baby's diet, with particular emphasis on the avoidance of fruit juices, fruits, and sweets. On this new regimen, the symptoms disappeared and the child continued to thrive. In order to obtain a *definitive* diagnosis of the infant's malady, the pediatrician would most likely recommend

(A) a fructose tolerance test
(B) isolation and culture of fibroblasts from an innocuous source with the subsequent determination of aldolase B activity
(C) determination of urinary fructose levels a week after having been placed on the restricted diet
(D) liver biopsy and determination of aldolase B activity
(E) determination of urinary reducing sugar levels immediately upon admission, while the infant is still showing symptoms.

54. Coagulase is an important virulence factor for which of the following organisms?

(A) *Streptococcus pyogenes*
(B) *Streptococcus mutans*
(C) *Streptococcus mitis*
(D) *Staphylococcus aureus*
(E) *Staphylococcus epidermidis*

55. Which of the following sets of assays involves the electrophoretic separation of proteins?

(A) Immunoelectrophoresis only
(B) Immunoelectrophoresis and zone electrophoresis
(C) Immunoelectrophoresis, zone electrophoresis, and Western blot
(D) Zone electrophoresis and Western blot
(E) Northern blot only

56. A teenager frequently shoplifted items from stores. As a young adult, he is a professional baseball player who holds the record for the most stolen bases in a season. Which one of the following best describes the defense mechanism used by this man in adulthood?

(A) Sublimation
(B) Rationalization
(C) Regression
(D) Splitting
(E) Identification

57. A patient with acute lymphocytic leukemia is treated with methotrexate. Which of the following enzymes is directly inhibited by this drug?

(A) Dihydrofolate reductase
(B) Xanthine oxidase
(C) Phosphoribosyl pyrophosphate (PRPP) synthase
(D) Thymidylate synthase
(E) Hypoxanthine-guanine phosphoribosyltransferase (HGPRT)

58. Of the following risk factors for suicide, which of the following carries the lowest risk?

(A) Unmarried status
(B) Serious medical illness
(C) Recent divorce
(D) Male gender
(E) Alcohol or drug abuse

59. Which class of nucleic acid is most likely to be chemically modified to contain a large number of unusual bases?

(A) Nuclear DNA
(B) Mitochondrial DNA
(C) Ribosomal RNA
(D) Transfer RNA
(E) Messenger RNA

60. Which of the following statements accurately describes normal development of a 3-year-old girl?

(A) She cannot engage in parallel play
(B) She may have an imaginary companion
(C) She rarely has nightmares
(D) She understands death's finality
(E) She understands the difference between right and wrong

61. Which of the following restriction endonuclease cleavages is most likely to produce fragments that could anneal and ligate to fragments generated by *Bsp*120I (G↓GGCCC)?

(A) *Stu* I (AGG↓CCT)
(B) *Hae* III (GG↓CC)
(C) *Apa* I (GGGCC↓C)
(D) *Sma* I (CCC↓GGG)
(E) *Eag* I (C↓GGCCG)

62. If a course of rifampin therapy is given to a patient who is receiving continuous warfarin (Coumadin) therapy, the patient will most likely exhibit

(A) a decreased potential for thrombus formation
(B) a decreased prothrombin time (PT)
(C) disseminated intravascular coagulation (DIC)
(D) bleeding or hemorrhage
(E) potentiation of antithrombin III

63. Which of the following parts of the mind functions to maintain a relationship to the external world?

(A) Id
(B) Ego
(C) Superego
(D) Preconscious
(E) Unconscious

64. Which of the following events occurs in the 3' → 5' direction?

(A) Synthesis of the leading strand during replication
(B) Synthesis of RNA during transcription
(C) Proofreading by DNA polymerase
(D) Synthesis of cDNA by reverse transcriptase
(E) Removal of RNA primers during replication

65. An individual with a mental age of 8 years and a chronological age of 10 years has an IQ of

(A) 40
(B) 60
(C) 80
(D) 100
(E) 180

66. Two opioid analgesics produce equivalent pain relief after intravenous doses of 60 mg for drug A and 4 mg for drug B. It can be concluded that

(A) drug A is less toxic than drug B
(B) drug A is longer acting than drug B
(C) drug A has a greater margin of safety than drug B
(D) drug B has a smaller volume of distribution than drug A
(E) drug B is 15 times more potent than drug A

67. Which one of the following is an objective test of personality?

(A) Thematic apperception test (TAT)
(B) Minnesota multiphasic personality inventory (MMPI)
(C) Sentence completion test (SCT)
(D) Rorschach test
(E) Luria Nebraska

68. A protein that regulates gene expression by binding to the operator region of a bacterial operon is called

(A) an inducer
(B) an enhancer
(C) a corepressor
(D) a promoter
(E) a repressor

69. The pattern of reinforcement least resistant to extinction is

(A) fixed ratio
(B) fixed interval
(C) variable ratio
(D) variable interval
(E) continuous

70. An 80-year-old woman is disabled and must be cared for by others. The most likely cause of her disability is

(A) musculoskeletal and joint disease
(B) depression and anxiety
(C) Alzheimer disease
(D) Parkinson disease
(E) stroke

71. The development of pharmacologic tolerance is accompanied by

(A) a shift of the log-dose response curve to the left
(B) an increase in the median effective dose
(C) an increase in the therapeutic index
(D) an increase in the number of drug receptors
(E) an increase in plasma drug half-life

72. Which of the following is the least mature defense mechanism?

(A) Altruism
(B) Suppression
(C) Sublimation
(D) Humor
(E) Denial

73. A test is performed on a population of normal people. The mean value of the test is 25 mg/dL and one standard deviation is 2.5 mg/dL. A reference interval (i.e., normal range) for this test that would encompass 95% of the normal population is

(A) 20–25 mg/dL
(B) 20–30 mg/dL
(C) 22.5–27.5 mg/dL
(D) 25–27.5 mg/dL
(E) 25–35 mg/dL

74. The percentage of children that live in the "traditional" American family, in which the father works and the mother stays at home, is approximately

(A) 5%
(B) 15%
(C) 20%
(D) 50%
(E) 80%

Questions 75-77

A man is scheduled for a physical examination. In order to obtain a fasting blood sample, his physician tells him not to eat after 8:00 P.M. the previous night. The blood is drawn at 10 A.M.

75. At the time that the blood is drawn, one would expect increased activity of

(A) pancreatic lipase
(B) acetyl coenzyme A (CoA) carboxylase
(C) propionyl CoA carboxylase
(D) hormone-sensitive lipase
(E) palmitoyl synthetase

76. In the liver, one would expect a decrease in

(A) levels of phosphorylated phosphofructokinase-2
(B) alanine transferase activity
(C) pyruvate kinase activity
(D) aldolase B activity
(E) phosphopyruvate carboxykinase activity

77. One would expect glucose transporter activity at this time to be

(A) decreased in brain cells
(B) decreased in hepatocytes
(C) enhanced in adipocytes
(D) decreased in red blood cells
(E) decreased in muscle cells

78. A medical student who wants high grades does poorly on her psychiatry examination. She explains her low grades in the following way: "the delay of 2 weeks put me out of sync, and the course isn't that important anyway." She believes this to be true, but she unconsciously hates the course. Which of the following mechanisms best describes the explanation given by the student?

(A) Sublimation
(B) Rationalization
(C) Regression
(D) Splitting
(E) Identification

79. Taxol, a drug used in the treatment of cancer, stabilizes which of the following structures in a cancer cell?

(A) Nucleoli
(B) Chromatin
(C) Microtubules
(D) Microfilaments
(E) Intermediate filaments

80. In a normal newborn infant, the palmar grasp reflex disappears at approximately what age?

(A) 2 months
(B) 4 months
(C) 6 months
(D) 9 months
(E) 12 months

81. Protection from influenza infection appears to depend primarily on

(A) passive immunity mechanisms
(B) production of interferon and secretory immunoglobulin A (IgA)
(C) macrophage activation
(D) antigenic drift
(E) stomach acids

82. A normal child shows upward extension of the large toe when the sole of the foot is stroked. This child's age is most likely to be

(A) 6 months
(B) 15 months
(C) 24 months
(D) 36 months
(E) 48 months

83. Which of the following statements concerning reducing equivalents is true?

(A) An equal number of ATPs are produced whether reducing equivalents are carried from the cytosol to the mitochondrial matrix via the α-glycerol phosphate shuttle or the malate-aspartate shuttle
(B) There is more reduced nicotinamide adenine dinucleotide phosphate (NADPH) in the mitochondria than in the cytoplasm
(C) Most catabolic processes that produce reduced nicotinamide adenine dinucleotide (NADH) are located in the cytoplasm
(D) Specific transporters carry NADH and NADPH across the inner mitochondrial membrane
(E) Biosynthetic reactions employing NADPH as the source of reducing equivalents occur primarily in the cytoplasm

84. A baseball manager unconsciously uses aggressive coaching techniques similar to the techniques used by his mother to control his behavior when he was young. Which of the following best explains the reason for the manager's aggressive coaching techniques?

(A) Sublimation
(B) Rationalization
(C) Regression
(D) Splitting
(E) Identification

85. A union trust fund contracts with physicians in private practice to provide medical care to the fund's subscribers. The entity thus created is best described as a

(A) private insurance carrier
(B) health maintenance organization
(C) preferred provider organization
(D) diagnosis-related group
(E) independent practice organization

86. Autonomy versus shame and doubt is associated with the work of

(A) Piaget
(B) Spitz
(C) Freud
(D) Chess and Thomas
(E) Erikson

87. Which one of the following is the leading cause of death among adolescents?

(A) Suicide
(B) Homicide
(C) Drug overdose
(D) Accidents
(E) Cancer

88. The sensorimotor period of development is associated with

(A) Piaget
(B) Spitz
(C) Freud
(D) Chess and Thomas
(E) Erikson

89. Lithium is used to treat bipolar disorders. Epinephrine enhances the rate of glycogenolysis in liver. Which of the following statements best describes the common mechanistic link in these two processes? Both lithium and epinephrine

(A) increase cyclic adenosine monophosphate (cAMP) levels
(B) regulate the rate of glycogenolysis
(C) affect the concentration of intracellular calcium
(D) directly affect the concentration of cyclic guanosine monophosphate (cGMP)
(E) enhance the rate of amino acid transport into the cell

90. According to Freud, when you correctly answer a question on the USMLE Step 1 exam concerning the names of the cranial nerves, that response has been retrieved from your

(A) unconscious
(B) preconscious
(C) conscious
(D) superego
(E) id

91. Which one of the following statements accurately describes a difference between fungi and bacteria?

(A) Fungi are filamentous whereas most bacteria are not
(B) Fungi have a cell wall whereas bacteria do not
(C) Fungi have a true nucleus whereas bacteria do not
(D) Fungi lack mitochondria, whereas some bacteria possess mitochondria

92. The topographic and structural theories of the mind are associated with

(A) Piaget
(B) Spitz
(C) Freud
(D) Chess and Thomas
(E) Erikson

93. Which of the following statements concerning the oxidative phosphorylation system is true?

(A) Complex V binds oxygen
(B) Complex II contains reduced nicotinamide adenine dinucleotide (NADH) dehydrogenase
(C) Coenzyme Q is an integral part of complex I
(D) Complex IV binds cyanide (CN^-)
(E) Succinate dehydrogenase is found in the mitochondrial matrix

94. Identify the organelle(s) at the asterisks in the connective tissue cell depicted in the accompanying micrograph.

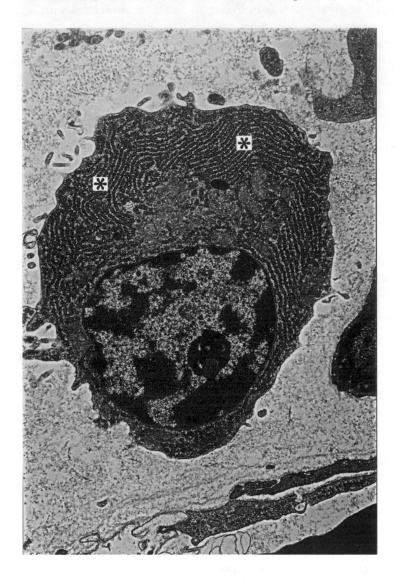

(A) Microtubules
(B) Golgi complex
(C) Collagen fibrils
(D) Rough endoplasmic reticulum
(E) Smooth endoplasmic reticulum

95. Which one of the following statements regarding the standard free energy change, ΔG^0, is correct?

(A) It is positive for a spontaneous reaction
(B) It is directly proportional to the free energy, ΔG
(C) It is algebraically additive for different reactions
(D) It varies depending upon the concentration of products and reactants
(E) It is equal to zero under standard conditions

96. Heterodimeric γ/δ receptors are found on which of the following cell types?

(A) T lymphocytes
(B) B lymphocytes
(C) Natural killer cells
(D) Neutrophils
(E) Eosinophils

97. The development of a color reaction is indicative of a positive result in which of the following assays?

(A) Immunofluorescence
(B) Flow cytometry
(C) Radioimmunoassay
(D) Enzyme-linked immunosorbent assay
(E) Neutralization test

98. Which of the following statements best applies to cytokines?

(A) They are continuously present in the peripheral blood
(B) They are very potent molecules with transient, short-range effects
(C) They are produced only by activated T lymphocytes
(D) Each cytokine mediates only one effect on a specific target cell type
(E) They are preformed mediators which are released upon cell stimulation

99. Which of the following statements regarding interferons (IFNs) is correct?

(A) IFN types I and II have equal antiviral activity
(B) Very few types of cells can synthesize type I IFN
(C) IFNs bind directly to viral genomes
(D) The antiviral activity of the IFNs is nonspecific
(E) Double-stranded RNA inhibits IFN production

100. Which one of the following cytokines suppresses cell-mediated immune responses?

(A) Interferon-γ
(B) Tumor necrosis factor-α
(C) Interleukin-1
(D) Interleukin-6
(E) Interleukin-10

101. Chronic bacterial infections, late-stage cancer, and AIDS all show a similar wasting syndrome. Which of the following factors is most likely involved in this syndrome?

(A) Interleukin-2
(B) Interleukin-4
(C) Tumor necrosis factor-α
(D) Granulocyte colony-stimulating factor
(E) Interferon-α

102. Cytotoxic T-lymphocyte activity is at least partly mediated by

(A) perforins
(B) C5b through C9
(C) class II molecules
(D) immunoglobulins
(E) oxygen radicals

103. Which of the following statements regarding memory B lymphocytes is correct?

(A) Most of them express surface immunoglobulin M (IgM)
(B) They have a low level of major histocompatibility complex class II molecules
(C) They do not interact with follicular dendritic cells
(D) They reside primarily in lymphoid follicles
(E) The affinity of their antibody is equivalent to that produced in a primary response

104. Cord red blood cells from an infant suspected of having hemolytic disease of the newborn is most likely to be tested by which of the following assays?

(A) Passive hemagglutination test
(B) Hemagglutination inhibition test
(C) Indirect Coombs test
(D) Direct Coombs test
(E) Nephelometry

105. A serum sample from a 28-year-old female bird-handler suspected of having psittacosis is evaluated by a complement fixation test. Lysis of erythrocytes in the assay indicates that the patient has

(A) no antibodies against *Chlamydia psittaci*
(B) a high level of complement activity
(C) an inadequate level of C3
(D) antibodies against *C. psittaci*
(E) a deficiency in C1 esterase inhibitor

106. A mixed lymphocyte culture (MLC) test performed prior to organ transplantation involves which of the following procedures?

(A) Incubating donor and recipient cells in the presence of tritiated thymidine
(B) Reacting donor lymphocytes with recipient serum and complement
(C) Incubating recipient lymphocytes with cells from the organ to be transplanted
(D) Mixing donor and recipient cells together with phytohemagglutinin
(E) Intradermal injection of donor lymphocytes into the recipient

107. A 45-year-old man tells you that he frequently uses his binoculars to watch an unsuspecting neighbor undressing in her apartment. Which of the following is most likely to be true about this man?

(A) He has not sought help for this problem
(B) He would like to meet the neighbor
(C) He would like to have sex with the neighbor
(D) He is unmarried
(E) He will attempt to rape the neighbor eventually

108. A 32-year-old female with a history of rheumatic heart disease was admitted to the hospital with a chief complaint of intermittent fever and headache for the past four weeks. Five weeks ago she had a root canal performed. Blood cultures taken at admission to the hospital exhibited gram-positive cocci. The most likely etiological agent in this case is

(A) *Staphylococcus aureus*
(B) *Streptococcus faecalis*
(C) *Haemophilus parainfluenzae*
(D) *Streptococcus salivarius*
(E) *Streptococcus agalactiae*

109. Which one of the following statements concerning interferon (IFN) is most accurate?

(A) The main function of IFNs is to interfere with bacterial growth
(B) IFN production is maximal after immunoglobulin-G antibodies are made
(C) IFNs are virus-specific
(D) IFNs inhibit a broad range of viruses
(E) The inhibition of animal virus growth by IFNs is caused by direct inhibition of several host enzyme functions

110. Unstimulated B lymphocytes produce membrane-bound antibody, and antigen-stimulated B lymphocytes produce secreted antibody. Which of the following statements correctly describes the mechanism that accounts for this difference? Stimulated B cells

(A) turn on a different heavy-chain gene than do unstimulated B cells
(B) selectively degrade membrane-bound antibodies
(C) splice heavy-chain messenger RNA differently from unstimulated B cells
(D) synthesize a more hydrophobic heavy chain than do unstimulated B cells
(E) synthesize a different light chain than do unstimulated B cells

111. An increase of which of the following immunoglobulins would be expected in the cord blood of a newborn with congenital toxoplasmosis?

(A) IgG
(B) IgA
(C) IgM
(D) IgD
(E) IgE

112. Which of the following descriptions most likely represents a neoplastic process?

(A) Solitary coin lesion in the lung
(B) Cold nodule in the thyroid in a woman
(C) Midline, cystic mass in the neck
(D) Mass in the right ovary of a 23-year-old woman
(E) Nontender mass in the parotid gland

113. The pedigree depicted would most likely be associated with which one of the following disorders?

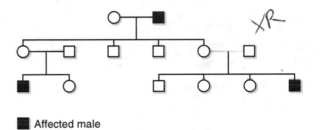

■ Affected male

(A) Lesch-Nyhan syndrome
(B) Phenylketonuria
(C) Congenital spherocytosis
(D) Gout
(E) Von Gierke's disease

114. Which of the following genetic disorders is characterized by a constellation of findings that includes cardiac defects, gastrointestinal disease, mental retardation, and a predisposition for acute leukemia?

(A) Trisomy 13
(B) Trisomy 18
(C) Trisomy 21
(D) Deletion of chromosome 5
(E) Fragile X syndrome

115. This pedigree of a proband with neurofibro-matosis exhibits the concept of

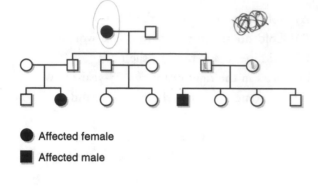

● Affected female

■ Affected male

(A) genetic heterogeneity
(B) pleiotropism
(C) variable expressivity
(D) reduced penetrance
(E) mosaicism

116. This pedigree would most likely be associated with

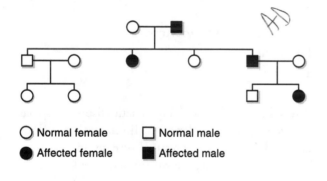

○ Normal female   □ Normal male
● Affected female   ■ Affected male

(A) Duchenne muscular dystrophy
(B) congenital spherocytosis ✓
(C) galactosemia
(D) cystic fibrosis
(E) hemophilia A

117. This pedigree would most likely be associated with which one of the following disorders?

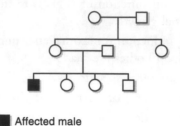

■ Affected male

(A) Huntington chorea
(B) Glucose-6-phosphate dehydrogenase deficiency
(C) Familial hypercholesterolemia
(D) Sickle cell disease
(E) Marfan syndrome

118. Which of the following concepts explains the similarity of defects associated with homocystinuria and Marfan syndrome?

(A) Genetic heterogeneity
(B) Autosomal recessive inheritance
(C) Multifactorial inheritance
(D) Reduced penetrance
(E) Pleiotropism

119. If the carrier rate for sickle cell abnormality is 1 in 12, the prevalence of sickle cell disease is approximately 1 in

(A) 144
(B) 288
(C) 576
(D) 720
(E) 1440

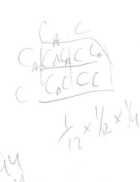

120. A 3-month-old boy is found dead in his crib. Examination of the death scene is unremarkable. The mother states that one week prior to the incident, the child had an upper respiratory infection. One of the parents is a smoker. The child is small for gestational age, and is the second of two children. A complete autopsy reveals petechia on the pleural and pericardial surfaces, pulmonary congestion, and scattered foci of lymphocytes in the interstitial tissue of the lungs. The mechanism most likely responsible for this child's death is

(A) an inborn error of metabolism
(B) abnormal temperature regulation
(C) a neural developmental delay
(D) sleeping prone on a soft mattress
(E) unknown

121. A negative Clinitest reaction would be expected in which of the following clinical specimens?

(A) Urine of a patient with fructokinase deficiency
(B) Urine of a patient with galactokinase deficiency
(C) Urine of a patient with pentosuria
(D) Urine of a patient taking ascorbic acid
(E) Filtrate of diarrhea fluid in a patient with sucrase deficiency

122. Detergents and alcohols are surface-active agents that disinfect, but should not be used together. Which of the following is the correct reason?

(A) Cationic and anionic reagents charge-neutralize each other
(B) The detergent will dissolve in an organic solvent and lose its surfactant properties
(C) Only one reagent will effectively kill bacterial spores
(D) Such a mixture will poison only selected enzyme systems
(E) Such a mixture will have less oxidizing potential than each used separately

123. The following schematic represents the development of lymphocytes.

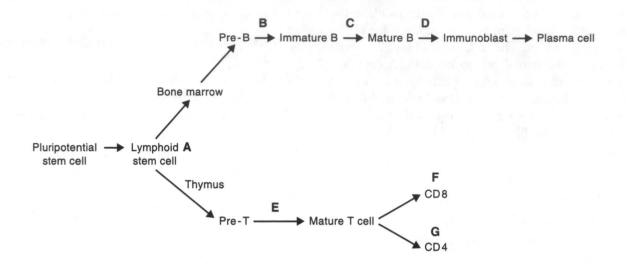

Which of the following choices lists sites that would be defective in patients with, respectively, the classic type of severe combined immunodeficiency (SCID), common variable immunodeficiency (CVID), Bruton agammaglobulinemia, and DiGeorge syndrome?

(A) A, D, B, E

(B) C, D, B, E

(C) B, D, C, E

(D) A, C, D, E

(E) E, D, B, A

124. Even after you have spoken with her extensively, a competent 26-year-old woman who is 38 weeks pregnant refuses to consent to a cesarian section that is necessary to save the baby's life. The physician should

(A) get a court order to do the procedure

(B) have the father consent to the procedure

(C) contact a law enforcement agency

(D) call a consultation liaison psychiatrist

(E) contact a social service agency

DIRECTIONS:

Each of the numbered items or incomplete statements in this section is negatively phrased, as indicated by a capitalized word such as NOT, LEAST, or EXCEPT. Select the ONE lettered answer or completion that is BEST in each case.

125. All of the following are true about rapid eye movement (REM) sleep in a patient with major depression as compared with an otherwise normal patient EXCEPT

(A) REM latency is shortened
(B) first REM period is shortened
(C) REM sleep is increased
(D) REM sleep shifts from the last half to the first half of the night
(E) REM is associated with limb movements

126. All of the following statements regarding exotoxins are true EXCEPT

(A) they are produced by gram-positive and gram-negative bacteria
(B) they are composed of polypeptides
(C) they are secreted from the cell
(D) they are part of the cell wall structure of gram-negative bacteria
(E) toxoids can be formed from them

127. Which of the following conditions is NOT associated with alcoholism?

(A) Decreased synthesis of testosterone
(B) Increased synthesis of γ-glutamyltransferase
(C) Hyperuricemia
(D) Inhibition of the cytochrome P-450 system
(E) Lactic acidosis

128. Measurements taken after an intravenous injection of inulin indicate that the substance appears to be distributed throughout 30%–35% of the total body water (TBW). This finding suggests that inulin most likely is

(A) excluded from the cells
(B) distributed uniformly throughout the TBW volume
(C) restricted to the plasma volume
(D) neither excreted nor metabolized by the body
(E) not freely diffusible through capillary membranes

129. Generation of antibody diversity includes all of the following mechanisms EXCEPT

(A) change in the specificity of antibody
(B) alternative splicing of primary RNA transcripts
(C) existence of multiple V, D, and J gene segments
(D) variation in V, D, and J gene segment joining
(E) hypermutation in the variable region

130. All of the following viruses obtain their lipid envelope from the cytoplasmic membrane of the host cell EXCEPT

(A) influenza virus
(B) measles virus
(C) mumps virus
(D) retroviruses
(E) herpesviruses

131. Inhibition of dihydrofolate reductase would be LEAST likely to inhibit the de novo biosynthesis of which of the following nucleotides?

(A) Adenosine monophosphate (AMP)
(B) Guanosine 5′-monophosphate (GMP)
(C) Thymidine monophosphate (TMP)
(D) Inosine 5′-monophosphate (IMP)
(E) Uridine 5′-monophosphate (UMP)

132. All the following statements about poliovirus infections are correct EXCEPT

(A) the virus is predominantly shed from the body and transmitted in respiratory droplets
(B) most infections are inapparent
(C) persistent viremia would favor central nervous system involvement
(D) capsid proteins are derived by post-translational cleavage from a large precursor protein
(E) both killed and live attenuated vaccines are available

133. Which of the following statements regarding monoclonal antibodies (MAbs) is LEAST accurate?

(A) MAbs are specific for a single epitope
(B) During production, activated B cells are fused with myeloma cells
(C) The term "clone" in monoclonal refers to DNA cloning
(D) All MAbs that originate from a single cell have identical light and heavy chains
(E) Chimeric MAbs are partly human and partly of another species

134. Which of the following substances is LEAST likely to be involved in the initiation of protein synthesis in bacteria?

(A) Adenosine–uracil–guanine (AUG)
(B) The 30S ribosomal subunit
(C) Formylmethionine
(D) Sigma factor
(E) Guanosine triphosphate (GTP)

135. All of the following statements regarding tolerance to self-antigens are true EXCEPT

(A) it is a highly specific state of unresponsiveness
(B) the normal individual has no potentially self-reactive lymphocytes
(C) ability to induce tolerance is partly dependent upon dose and physical characteristics of the antigen
(D) T cells are more easily made tolerant than B cells
(E) tolerance tends to break down with age

136. Each of the following statements about bacterial spores is correct EXCEPT

(A) they are formed by gram-positive rods
(B) they form under adverse environmental conditions
(C) they can be killed by heating at 121°C for 15 minutes
(D) they contain much less water than bacterial cells
(E) their survival depends on efficient aerobic metabolism

137. All of the following statements about divorce are true EXCEPT

(A) most divorced men and women remarry
(B) divorce rate is increased in offspring of divorced parents
(C) rate of divorce is higher in first marriages than in second marriages
(D) an increased rate of divorce is associated with marriage at an early age
(E) remarriage rate is higher among divorced men than among divorced women

138. A laboratory has isolated a virus from the stool of a patient with diarrhea and shown that its genome is composed of multiple pieces of double-stranded RNA. Which of the following statements about the virus is NOT correct?

(A) Each piece of RNA encodes a different protein
(B) The virus encodes an RNA-dependent RNA polymerase
(C) The virion contains an RNA polymerase
(D) The genome is incorporated into the host chromosome
(E) The virion does not contain an RNA-dependent DNA polymerase

139. A 4-year-old child screams during the night but cannot be awakened. In the morning, the child has no memory of the nighttime screams. All of the following are true about this phenomenon EXCEPT

(A) it occurs during slow-wave sleep
(B) it may develop into episodes of sleepwalking
(C) it may be an early sign of temporal lobe epilepsy
(D) careful questioning will elicit a memory of the dream that occurred at this time
(E) the child will not remember that he or she was aroused

140. Each of the following viruses is capable of establishing a chronic or latent infection EXCEPT

(A) rubeola — Measles late
(B) cytomegalovirus
(C) hepatitis A — late
(D) hepatitis B — late
(E) herpes simplex

all herpesviruses are late

141. Which of the following virus–disease relationships is NOT correctly stated?

(A) Rotaviruses—gastroenteritis in children 6 months to 2 years old
(B) Mumps virus—unilateral orchitis
(C) Measles (rubeola) virus—encephalomyelitis without sequelae
(D) Parainfluenza virus type 2—croup in children less than three years old
(E) Respiratory syncytial virus—bronchitis and pneumonitis in children under six months in age

142. Anorexia nervosa is associated with all of the following EXCEPT

(A) female gender
(B) upper socioeconomic groups
(C) mental retardation
(D) normal appetite
(E) loss of 15% or more of body weight

143. Which of the following clinical syndromes is NOT associated with adenoviruses?

(A) Keratoconjunctivitis
(B) Pharyngoconjunctival fever
(C) Acute respiratory disease
(D) Pharyngitis
(E) Heterophil-negative mononucleosis

144. Medicare part B covers all of the following EXCEPT

(A) doctors' bills
(B) home health care
(C) medical supplies
(D) long-term nursing home care
(E) ambulance service

145. All of the following illnesses are more common in African-Americans than in white individuals EXCEPT

(A) obesity
(B) hypertension
(C) bipolar illness
(D) diabetes
(E) heart disease

146. Which of the following patients is LEAST likely to be committed for involuntary treatment?

(A) A depressed man who expresses the intent to commit suicide
(B) A schizophrenic man who has threatened to kill his parents
(C) A borderline patient who has threatened to kill his psychiatrist
(D) An Alzheimer patient who regularly starts fires in his apartment
(E) A schizophrenic man who lives with other homeless people in a subway station

147. For informed consent, a patient must do all of the following EXCEPT

(A) sign a document consenting to the procedure
(B) understand what will happen if he or she does not consent
(C) understand the diagnosis
(D) understand the benefits of the procedure
(E) understand that he or she can withdraw consent at any time

148. All of the following are true about psychopathology among the elderly in the United States EXCEPT

(A) depression is more common among the elderly than in the general population
(B) anxiety caused by insecurity is common
(C) changes in sleep patterns are more common among the elderly than in the general population
(D) suicide is less common among the elderly than in the general population
(E) most elderly people have a positive feeling about their lives

149. Which one of the following statements does NOT accurately describe catabolic reactions?

(A) They provide energy that can be used for work
(B) They have a net requirement for energy in order to proceed
(C) They use oxidized nicotinamide adenine dinucleotide (NAD$^+$) as a cofactor
(D) They produce reduced nicotinamide adenine dinucleotide (NADH) or reduced nicotinamide adenine dinucleotide phosphate (NADPH) as a product
(E) They occur in the absence of a suitable catalyst

150. All of the following are true about biofeedback EXCEPT

(A) the patient must be motivated to learn
(B) it involves learning control over physiologic activities
(C) it is an extension of classical conditioning
(D) it has been used to treat peptic ulcer
(E) it has been used to treat tension headache

151. T lymphocytes generally do NOT play a major role in

(A) eradication of virally infected cells
(B) delayed-type hypersensitivity reactions
(C) allograft rejection
(D) anti-tumor responses
(E) control of *Streptococcus pneumoniae*

152. Immunoglobulin G (IgG) is able to perform all of the following EXCEPT

(A) fixing complement
(B) neutralizing toxins and viruses
(C) opsonizing bacteria
(D) functioning in antibody-dependent cell-mediated cytotoxicity
(E) stimulating mast cell/basophil degranulation

153. Which of the following conditions is LEAST likely to be associated with alcoholism?

(A) Folate deficiency
(B) Hyperglycemia
(C) Sideroblastic anemia
(D) Ketoacidosis
(E) Increased synthesis of very low density lipoproteins

154. Viruses that can cause viremia and cross the placenta to infect the fetus include all of the following EXCEPT

(A) rubella
(B) hepatitis B
(C) cytomegalovirus
(D) herpes simplex
(E) respiratory syncytial virus

155. The number of medical malpractice suits are increasing yearly. The LEAST likely reason for this is

(A) physicians are making more mistakes
(B) patients are becoming more suspicious of physicians
(C) doctor–patient relationships are becoming more distant
(D) patients have higher expectations of doctors
(E) the increased number of patients under managed care

DIRECTIONS:

Each set of matching questions in this section consists of a list of four to twenty-six lettered options (some of which may be in figures) followed by several numbered items. For each numbered item, select the ONE lettered option that is most closely associated with it. To avoid spending too much time on matching sets with a large number of options, it is generally advisable to begin each set by reading the list of options. Then for each item in the set, try to generate the correct answer and locate it in the option list, rather than evaluating each option individually. Each lettered option may be selected once, more than once, or not at all.

Questions 156-160

Match the following diseases with the most appropriate metabolite.

(A) Glucocerebroside
(B) Sphingomyelin
(C) GM2 ganglioside
(D) Sulfatide
(E) Galactocerebroside
(F) Ceramide trihexoside
(G) Dermatan and heparan sulfate

156. Sex-linked recessive disease characterized by angiokeratomas, hypertension, and renal failure

157. Autosomal recessive disease characterized by massive hepatosplenomegaly, macrophages with a fibrillary appearing material in the cytoplasm, and an increase in total acid phosphatase

158. Autosomal recessive disease characterized by abnormal myelination, globoid bodies in the central nervous system, and psychomotor retardation

159. Autosomal recessive disease characterized by abnormal myelin, mental retardation, peripheral neuropathy, and metachromatic staining of tissue

160. Autosomal recessive disease characterized by severe mental retardation, hepatosplenomegaly, foamy macrophages, and zebra bodies visible upon electron microscopy

Questions 161-165

Select the enzyme involved in drug metabolism that applies to the following descriptions.

(A) Microsomal mixed function oxidase
(B) Nonmicrosomal dehydrogenase
(C) Plasma esterase
(D) Glucuronyl transferase
(E) N-acetyltransferase

161. Low levels of this enzyme in neonates contributes to gray baby syndrome after chloramphenicol administration

162. Requires cytochrome P-450, NADP, and molecular oxygen

163. Variations in activity of this enzyme are responsible for the distribution of isoniazid half-life shown in the accompanying figure

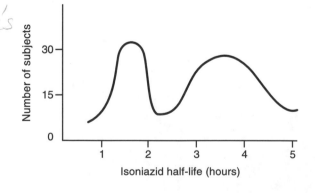

164. This enzyme accounts for rapid catabolism of aspirin

165. This enzyme is saturated by low doses of ethanol

Questions 166-170

For each scenario, select the most likely form of drug antagonism.

(A) Chemical antagonism
(B) Physiologic antagonism
(C) Competitive antagonism
(D) Noncompetitive antagonism
(E) Therapeutic antagonism

166. Tetracyclines reduce the antibacterial effect of penicillin when concurrently administered to patients with pneumococcal infections

167. Phenoxybenzamine forms covalent bonds with α-adrenergic receptors, producing a long-lasting effect on blood pressure

168. Protamine sulfate can be used to treat hemorrhage that results from an overdose of heparin

169. Propranolol inhibits tachycardia caused by excessive epinephrine administration

170. Epinephrine counteracts bronchospasm and hypotension in patients with severe allergic reactions

Questions 171-174

Match the viruses listed below with the appropriate description.

(A) A DNA enveloped virus
(B) A DNA nonenveloped virus
(C) An RNA enveloped virus
(D) An RNA nonenveloped virus

171. HIV   Retrovirus RNA — C

172. Human papilloma virus   PAPOVA — Naked DNA   B

173. Varicella-zoster virus   HERPES — A

174. Poliovirus — PICORNA — D

CPR

Questions 175-180

The accompanying schematic represents pyruvate and the tricarboxylic acid cycle. Match the following descriptions with the appropriate letter in the diagram.

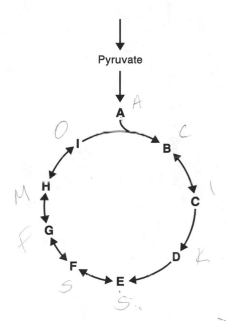

175. The α-keto analog of glutamic acid   D

176. Formed in a reaction catalyzed by an enzyme complex that promotes three catalytic conversions, using five different cofactors, and containing two regulatory enzymes   A

177. A substrate used for heme synthesis   E   your pee has

178. A product of the urea cycle   fumes

179. A substrate for and activator of fatty acid synthesis   B

180. A negative modulator of phosphofructokinase   B

ANSWER KEY

1. C	31. A	61. E	91. C	121. E	151. E
2. B	32. B	62. B	92. C	122. B	152. E
3. B	33. B	63. B	93. D	123. A	153. B
4. E	34. A	64. C	94. D	124. D	154. E
5. E	35. E	65. C	95. C	125. B	155. A
6. A	36. A	66. E	96. A	126. D	156. F
7. D	37. D	67. B	97. D	127. D	157. A
8. E	38. C	68. E	98. B	128. D	158. E
9. B	39. E	69. E	99. D	129. A	159. D
10. D	40. B	70. A	100. E	130. E	160. B
11. E	41. E	71. B	101. C	131. E	161. D
12. B	42. B	72. E	102. A	132. A	162. A
13. C	43. A	73. B	103. D	133. C	163. E
14. C	44. B	74. C	104. D	134. D	164. C
15. C	45. B	75. D	105. A	135. B	165. B
16. B	46. D	76. C	106. A	136. E	166. E
17. D	47. C	77. E	107. A	137. C	167. D
18. A	48. E	78. B	108. D	138. D	168. A
19. E	49. A	79. C	109. D	139. D	169. C
20. B	50. B	80. A	110. C	140. C	170. B
21. B	51. B	81. B	111. C	141. C	171. C
22. D	52. E	82. A	112. E	142. C	172. B
23. C	53. D	83. E	113. A	143. E	173. A
24. A	54. D	84. E	114. C	144. D	174. D
25. B	55. C	85. C	115. D	145. C	175. D
26. E	56. A	86. E	116. B	146. E	176. A
27. C	57. A	87. D	117. D	147. A	177. E
28. E	58. A	88. A	118. A	148. D	178. G
29. B	59. D	89. C	119. C	149. B	179. B
30. D	60. B	90. B	120. E	150. C	180. B

ANSWERS AND EXPLANATIONS

1. The answer is C. *(Behavioral science)*
Second marriages are more likely than first marriages to end in divorce. Second marriages are no more likely than first marriages to involve an older man and a younger woman, or to result in children.

2. The answer is B. *(Microbiology)*
The human immunodeficiency virus (HIV) is a retrovirus. As such, it contains two copies of a positive-sense RNA genome (i.e., one with the same nucleotide base composition as messenger RNA). For replication of HIV to occur, the reverse transcriptase (RNA-dependent DNA polymerase) must produce a double-stranded DNA copy of the viral genome. That DNA provirus is then inserted into the host cell's chromosome. Only then, can the host cell's RNA polymerase produce appropriate messenger RNA to facilitate viral replication. Reverse transcriptase is also involved in the replication cycle of hepatitis B virus. A pregenome RNA molecule is first produced and encapsulated into newly synthesized core particles. It serves as a template for the hepatitis B reverse transcriptase encoded within the polymerase gene. An enzyme removes the RNA template from the RNA–DNA hybrid, resulting in a negative-stranded DNA chain. The virally-contained DNA polymerase produces a partial positive-stranded DNA strand to complete the DNA genome found within the mature hepatitis B virion. The negative strand is complete and nicked, while the positive strand is incomplete. The DNA has a circular shape. Hepatitis A virus is an enterovirus, similar to poliovirus. As such, it contains an RNA genome that can function directly as messenger RNA. Hepatitis C and D virus do not have or need reverse transcriptase in their replication cycles.

3-4. The answers are: 3-B, 4-E. *(Behavioral science)*
Katie's change in behavior is an example of positive reinforcement. In this example, she has obviously received a reward (attention from her mother) for her behavior of running into the street because the behavior is increased. If Katie's behavior had increased because of the removal of an aversive stimulus, this would have been an example of negative reinforcement. If Katie's running into the street behavior had decreased

after the spanking, the spanking would be defined as punishment. Shaping involves rewarding increasingly closer approximations of a wanted behavior, and extinction is the disappearance of a learned behavior when a reward is withheld.

If Katie's running into the street is not rewarded by attention (spanking) from her mother, extinction (disappearance of a learned behavior when the reward or reinforcement is withheld) will occur and the behavior will cease.

5. The answer is E. *(Biochemistry)*
The catabolism of most amino acids begins with the transfer of the α-amino group to α-ketoglutarate to form glutamate. The original amino acid becomes converted to the corresponding α-keto acid. This reaction is catalyzed by enzymes called aminotransferases or transaminases. These amino groups are eventually incorporated into urea and excreted in the urine.

6. The answer is A. *(Microbiology)*
Equine encephalitis viruses are transmitted by mosquitoes. These viruses are togaviruses and include eastern equine, western equine, and Venezuelan equine encephalitis viruses. The flavivirus that causes St. Louis encephalitis is also transmitted by mosquitoes. These viral encephalitis types often have a high case-fatality rate, and are spread by mosquitoes with distinct ecologic distributions.

Varicella (a herpesvirus) presents as a systemic infection with viremia. Encephalitis occurs in 1 per 1000 cases. These viruses are transmitted person-to-person by inhalation of virus-containing droplets. Rubeola (measles) is a paramyxovirus that also is spread by inhalation of virus-containing droplets. Encephalitis is a postinfectious complication, with potentially serious consequences. The mortality rate of measles-related encephalitis is 15%, and 25% of survivors show sequelae. Hantavirus is a bunyavirus that causes a pulmonary disease syndrome. No insect vector is involved in its transmission. The rabies virus (rhabdovirus) is transmitted primarily by animal bites.

7. The answer is D. *(Pathology)*
Lead is the only heavy metal that is visibly deposited in the epiphysis of growing bones. Heavy metals produce

acute or chronic intoxication and include lead, arsenic, and mercury. In general, all of the heavy metals involve the central nervous system, gastrointestinal system, and the kidneys. Arsenic is responsible for most cases of acute heavy metal poisoning, and lead is responsible for the most cases of chronic intoxication. In general, urine tests are more useful than blood tests in screening for heavy metal poisoning.

8. The answer is E. *(Microbiology)*
In acute hepatitis B viral (HBV) infections, the time frames for hepatitis B surface antigen (HBsAg) and antibody to HBsAg (anti-HBsAg) are well established (see diagram). HBV core antigen (HBcAg) is produced early (months 1–2) in the infection. HBsAg rises, and then falls, between 1 month and 5 months after infection. Although production of anti-HBsAg begins at the time of infection, it typically is not detectable until month 6 or 7 because available HBsAg combines with it. If HBsAg and anti-HBsAg are measured between month 4 and months 6–7, false-negative results may occur. During this period, however, high levels of antibody to the HB core antigen (anti-HBcAg) are produced, and hence a serologic test for anti-HBcAg would be positive.

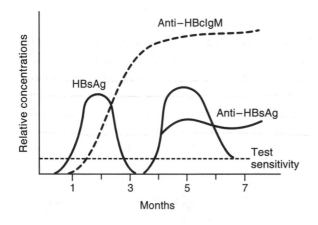

9. The answer is B. *(Biochemistry)*
Pyridoxal phosphate, a derivative of vitamin B_6, is required by all of the aminotransferases. During the reaction catalyzed by these enzymes, the amino group removed from an amino acid becomes covalently attached to pyridoxal phosphate before being transferred to an α-keto acid to form another amino acid.

The coenzyme biotin is required in carboxylation reactions. NAD^+, $NADP^+$, and FAD are involved in oxidation–reduction reactions.

10. The answer is D. *(Microbiology)*
Retroviruses contain two copies of a positive-sense RNA and a reverse transcriptase enzyme within the virion. Positive-sense RNA has the same configuration of base pairs as messenger RNA (mRNA). That is, the viral genome may function directly as mRNA in the infected cell, and effect protein translation at the cell's ribosomes (as polioviruses do, for example). Retroviruses must have a double-stranded DNA copy of the single-stranded, positive-sense RNA genome made and incorporated into the host's DNA chromosome before viral growth can occur. Because RNA is the template from which DNA is made, the reverse transcriptase is an RNA-dependent DNA polymerase.

DNA-dependent RNA polymerase is the type of enzyme that makes mRNA in human cell metabolism (RNA polymerase II). DNA-dependent DNA polymerase, also in human cells, is responsible for replication of cellular DNA when the cell divides.

A double-stranded RNA–dependent RNA polymerase is the type of enzyme coded for and used by reoviruses. These possess segmented, double-stranded RNA genomes. Such an enzyme is necessary to produce viral mRNA in the normal viral growth cycle.

Single-stranded RNA–dependent RNA polymerases are coded for and used by negative-sense (i.e., opposite base configuration to mRNA) viruses, such as influenza viruses and paramyxoviruses. This enzyme is responsible for mRNA production, as well as for genome replication.

11. The answer is E. *(Pathology)*
Multifactorial inheritance refers to the presence of small mutations enhanced by the effect of exposure to certain environmental factors. Obesity contributing to the clinical expression of type II diabetes mellitus is an example of multifactorial inheritance. Increased adipose tissue normally down-regulates the production of insulin receptors, which contributes to the development of glucose intolerance and diabetes mellitus.

12. The answer is B. *(Microbiology)*
Hepatitis B virus (HBV) contains double-stranded DNA. The DNA is in a circular form, with one strand

nicked and the other strand incomplete (one-half to two-thirds its normal length). The DNA is contained within an inner protein core (HBcAg), which, in turn, is surrounded by an outer surface protein (HbsAg). HBsAg is the material used in the licensed HBV vaccine. Originally, HbsAg was isolated from the serum of individuals who were actively producing HBV virions. Later, the HbsAg gene was transferred to a yeast. Both products are excellent antigens and produce protective antibodies in 95% to 96% of individuals who are vaccinated.

Because the vaccine consists of only HBV surface antigen and no other viral component, no antibodies could be made against HBV core or epsilon antigens, viral DNA, or the viral DNA polymerase.

13. The answer is C.   (Biochemistry)
Aspartate aminotransferase and alanine aminotransferase levels are elevated in the plasma in diseases of the liver. These enzymes normally are found inside cells, but are released into the plasma when liver damage occurs. Creatine kinase 2 (MB), lactate dehydrogenase, and glutamate oxaloacetate transaminase become elevated following myocardial infarction. Levels of dihydrofolate reductase are not useful for the diagnosis of either heart or liver damage.

14. The answer is C.   (Microbiology)
Bacterial flagella are thread-like appendages, composed entirely of protein. They are organs of locomotion. Three types of arrangements of flagella have been observed: monotrichous describes a single, polar flagellum; lophotrichous describes a clump of multiple polar flagella; and peritrichous describes several flagella distributed over the entire cell. Polytrichous is not a term that refers to flagellar arrangement.

15. The answer is C.   (Pathology)
Nodular skin lesions that are positive for S-100 antigen implies a tumor of neural crest origin that is metastatic. A neuroblastoma derived from the adrenal medulla, which is of neural crest origin, is the most likely primary site. This protein is also present in malignant melanomas, neurofibromas, schwannomas, and other adrenal medulla tumors. Neuroblastomas are commonly associated with hypertension. Patients under 2 year of age have a better prognosis than older children.

They commonly metastasize to the bone marrow, liver, and skin.

16. The answer is B.   (Microbiology)
Pneumococci (Streptococcus pneumoniae) are normal inhabitants of the human upper respiratory tract and can cause several diseases. Pneumococci are gram-positive diplococci that have a capsule of polysaccharide that is antigenic and permits typing with specific antisera.

Mixing encapsulated bacteria such as pneumococci with specific antibodies causes the capsules to swell. This reaction, called the quellung test, is useful for rapid identification and typing of the organisms in sputum or in cultures. Eighty-four distinct types of pneumonococcal polysaccharide capsules have been distinguished using the quellung reaction.

Enterococcus faecalis are normally isolated and identified by cultural procedures. Staphylococcus epidermidis normally do not produce capsules. Neisseria gonorrhoeae produce small capsules or none. Gardnerella vaginalis is nonencapsulated.

17. The answer is D.   (Biochemistry)
Most of the nitrogen-containing amino groups from degraded amino acids become incorporated into urea. In the first step of amino acid degradation, the amino group is incorporated into glutamate. Some of the glutamate breaks down to release ammonia, while most of the remainder transfers the amino group to aspartate. Ammonia and aspartate feed into the urea cycle, where the two amino groups combine with carbon dioxide to form urea, which is then transported to the kidneys and excreted in the urine. Creatinine is a derivative of muscle creatine that is excreted in the urine. Uric acid is the degradation product of purines.

18. The answer is A.   (Microbiology)
When describing genomes in general, two terms are used. Diploid means that two identical molecules (e.g., DNA or RNA) are present. Haploid means that one copy of the RNA or DNA molecule is present. Retroviruses are diploid. They have two identical single-stranded, positive-sense RNA molecules within each virion. All other viruses are haploid.

19. The answer is E.   *(Pathology)*
The pedigree depicts a sex-linked dominant inheritance pattern. Sex-linked dominant diseases are more common in females because they have two X chromosomes. This inheritance pattern is characterized by an absence of male-to-male transmission. However, an affected male transmits the disease to 100% of his daughters.

	X*	Y	
X	X*X	XY	X*Y: affected male
X	X*X	XY	X*X: affected female

The sons and the daughters of an affected heterozygous female (X*X) each have a 50% chance of inheriting the disease.

	X	Y	
X*	X*X	X*Y	XY: normal male X*Y: affected male
X	XX	XY	XX: normal female X*X: affected female

In the pedigree depicted in the question, note that both males and females are involved and that affected females transmit the disease to 50% of the males and 50% of females. The affected males transmit the disease to all of their daughters and to none of their sons. Vitamin-D–resistant rickets is an example of a sex-linked dominant disease.

20. The answer is B.   *(Microbiology)*
Hepatitis B (HBV) viral vaccine consists of the HBV surface antigen (HbsAg). The original Food and Drug Administration (FDA)–approved vaccine consisted of HbsAg purified from serum of individuals with active hepatitis B. The gene for HbsAG was excised using recombinant DNA technology and placed into a yeast. This HbsAg is identical to the original product except for minor chemical side chains. It has FDA approval

and is equal in vaccine efficiency as the original product, imparting protection to 95% to 96% of those vaccinated.

The vaccines for hepatitis A, rabies, and influenza A; and the Salk vaccine for poliomyelitis, are made of killed viruses. The general procedure for these vaccines is to grow large numbers of the desired viruses, concentrate them, and inactivate them with chemicals such as formaldehyde that do minimal damage to the viral structural proteins. Immunity is often brief, with booster shots necessary to ensure long-term protection. Cell-mediated immune response to these vaccines is generally poor. The Sabin vaccine for polio immunization is a live, attenuated product. Attenuated viruses do not cause disease, but do replicate in the body in a normal manner. Both the humoral and cell-mediated immune responses to this vaccine are excellent, imparting long-term protection.

21. The answer is B.   *(Biochemistry)*
Glutamate dehydrogenase breaks down glutamate to form ammonia and α-ketoglutarate. Aspartate aminotransferase transfers the amino group from glutamate to oxaloacetate to form aspartate. Ammonia and aspartate both feed into the urea cycle to supply the nitrogen used to synthesize urea. Argininosuccinate synthase, argininosuccinate lyase, and arginase are enzymes that catalyze other steps of the urea cycle.

22. The answer is D.   *(Microbiology)*
Hepatitis D virus (HDV), the delta agent, can replicate only when it is in a host cell that is co-infected by hepatitis B virus (HBV). Several mechanisms exist whereby defective mutants may be developed (e.g., deletion mutations). No nondefective isolates of HDV have been recovered.

HDV is an unclassified RNA virus with an inner protein layer (delta antigen) and an outer coat of HBV surface antigen. It may present as either an acute or a chronic infection. A serologic test is available for diagnosis. An individual with a successful HBV vaccination would be immune to infection by HDV.

Hepatitis A virus (HAV) is an RNA-containing picornavirus. It is transmitted by the oral–fecal route, presents only as acute or subclinical infection, and has no chronic carriers.

Hepatitis C virus (HCV) is an RNA-containing flavivirus, formerly termed non-A, non-B (NANB) hepatitis–transfusion associated. About half of HCV patients develop chronic infections.

Hepatitis E virus (HEV) is transmitted by the oral–fecal route and used to be termed NANB–enterically transmitted hepatitis. It is a small, positive-sense RNA genome with the biophysical properties of caliciviruses. No serologic test is available.

23. The answer is C.   (*Microbiology*)
Immunoglobulin M (IgM) is the B cell antigen receptor and is the most common class of antibody found embedded in the cytoplasmic membrane of resting B lymphocytes. When attached to the cell, it is a monomer. The variable (V) region of each IgM is specific for a particular epitope on an antigenic molecule. The binding of antigen to surface IgM, together with other activating signals, results in differentiation of the B cell into a plasma cell, which secretes IgM in pentameric form.

IgD is embedded in the surface of some B cells that also bear surface IgM. However, its function is not entirely clear. Although the binding of antigen to surface IgD appears to transmit signals similar to those seen after IgM binding, the expression of IgD stops once cell activation takes place.

24. The answer is A.   (*Biochemistry*)
Carbamoyl phosphate for the urea cycle is synthesized from ammonia and carbon dioxide by the enzyme carbamoyl phosphate synthetase I. Carbamoyl phosphate reacts with ornithine to form citrulline. Aspartate combines with citrulline to form argininosuccinate, which breaks down to form arginine. The enzyme arginase releases urea from arginine and again forms ornithine to begin the cycle again.

25. The answer is B.   (*Pathology*)
Electron microscopy reveals Weibel-Palade bodies in endothelial cells of angiosarcomas. These contain adhesion molecules (GMP-140) that help in the adhesion of leukocytes to the endothelial surface in inflammation. Epithelial tumors contain tonofilaments. Small-cell carcinoma of the lung, neuroblastomas, and carcinoid tumors have neurosecretory granules. Rhabdomyosarcomas have both thick and thin myofilaments. Histocytosis X (malignant histiocytic tumor) contains Birbeck granules in Langerhan's cells (histiocytes).

26. The answer is E.   (*Biochemistry*)
Arachidonic acid is usually esterified on the second position of glycerol in membrane-bound phospholipids and is liberated by the action of phospholipase A_2. This reaction is inhibited by cortisol and other corticosteroids, but not by the nonsteroidal anti-inflammatory drugs (NSAIDs). The liberated arachidonic acid can be acted upon either by 5-lipooxygenase to form leukotrienes, or by cyclooxygenase to form thromboxane A_2 and prostaglandins of the 2 series. NSAIDs inhibit this reaction: the action of aspirin is irreversible and that of the other NSAIDs is reversible. Thus, cortisol inhibits the synthesis of leukotriene A_4, thromboxane A_2, and prostaglandins PGE_2, $PGF_{2\alpha}$, and PGI_2, but NSAIDs do not inhibit leukotriene synthesis.

Prostaglandins are paracrine hormones, not telecrine hormones. Paracrine hormones act only a short distance from their site of synthesis. Telecrine hormones act at distant sites, and generally are transported to their site of action via the blood stream.

27. The answer is C.   (*Pathology*)
The most common benign tumor in women is a leiomyoma, and most of these are located in the myometrium of the uterus. Leiomyomas are composed of benign smooth muscle tissue that, unlike other types of muscle, is a stable tissue that has the capacity to enter the cell cycle and divide under the stimulus of estrogen. Another unusual feature is the lack of a capsule, which is unlike most benign tumors.

28. The answer is E.   (*Biochemistry*)
Ketogenic amino acids are broken down to produce acetoacetate, acetyl coenzyme A (CoA), or acetoacetyl CoA. Glucogenic amino acids are broken down to form pyruvate or an intermediate of the citric acid cycle that can be used for gluconeogenesis. Leucine and lysine are the only two amino acids that are ketogenic, but not glucogenic. Tyrosine, isoleucine, phenylalanine, and tryptophan are both ketogenic and glucogenic. Glutamate and valine are glucogenic only.

29. The answer is B.   (*Microbiology*)
Isotype switching from IgM to IgG involves the excision of the DNA that codes for the $C\mu$ region and

subsequent joining of the pre-rearranged VDJ segments to a C gene segment for IgG (Cγ). The plasmacyte can no longer secrete IgM, only IgG.

30. The answer is D.   *(Biochemistry)*
Albinism results from an inherited deficiency in the synthesis of the pigment melanin, which is found primarily in eyes, hair, and skin. The first step in the formation of melanin is the hydroxylation of tyrosine by the enzyme tyrosinase to form dopa. Tyrosinase is missing in classic, autosomal recessive albinism.

31. The answer is A.   *(Pathology)*
Testicular feminization, a sex-linked recessive disease, results from a defect in the androgen receptors. Testosterone and dihydrotestosterone in the developing male fetus (genotype XY) are not able to differentiate normal male accessory structures and external genitalia, so the external genitalia remain female (i.e., female phenotype). Because müllerian duct inhibitory factor is still made in the male fetus, müllerian structures (e.g., fallopian tubes, uterus) are not present. Testicles are present, and are most commonly located in the inguinal canals. A genotypic male who looks phenotypically like a female is called a male pseudohermaphrodite. Testicular feminization is the most common cause of male pseudohermaphroditism. These individuals are usually left female, but the testicles are removed because of an increased tendency for seminomas.

32. The answer is B.   *(Biochemistry)*
S-adenosylmethionine (SAM) serves as a donor of methyl groups in one-carbon metabolism. SAM is formed by the reaction of methionine with ATP. The methyl group attached to the sulfur atom is linked by a high-energy bond and can be transferred to other compounds during their metabolism. One-carbon groups at other oxidation states are usually supplied by a derivative of tetrahydrofolate.

33. The answer is B.   *(Microbiology)*
St. Louis encephalitis virus is a flavivirus. Flaviviruses are 40–50 nm in diameter and have a positive-sense RNA genome (i.e., same base composition as messenger RNA). The genome is a single-stranded, linear molecule. The virus is surrounded by a lipid envelope. It replicates in the cytoplasm of the cell and undergoes

an assembly within the endoplasmic reticulum. Other flaviviruses include yellow fever, dengue, and Japanese B encephalitis.

St. Louis encephalitis viruses are spread by *Culex* mosquitoes. The virus is normally found in nonhuman hosts. Although it is the most important arthropod-borne viral disease of humans in the United States, mortality rate is the lowest of the encephalitides viruses. Antibodies are detectable within a few days after the onset of illness. Immunity is considered to be permanent after a single infection. No specific antiviral treatment exists.

34. The answer is A.   *(Biochemistry)*
Maple syrup urine disease is caused by a deficiency of branched-chain α-keto acid dehydrogenase. This enzyme is involved in the catabolism of the branched-chain amino acids leucine, isoleucine, and valine. The sweet-smelling intermediates that accumulate in the urine give the disease its name. Neurologic problems are common in patients with this disease.

Phenylketonuria is caused by a deficiency of phenylalanine hydroxylase. Homocystinuria is caused by a deficiency of cystathionine synthetase. A deficiency of homogentisate oxidase results in alcaptonuria, and a lack of histidase causes histidinemia.

35. The answer is E.   *(Pathology)*
Testicular feminization is a sex-linked recessive trait. Cleft lip, hypertension, congenital heart disease, and coronary heart disease are examples of multifactorial (polygenic) inheritance, and result from multiple small mutations plus the effect of environment.

36. The answer is A.   *(Biochemistry)*
Long-chain fatty acids (more than 10 carbons) must be packaged into chylomicrons before being exported into the lymphatic circulation. To do so, the triacylglycerol molecule and cholesterol esters must first be resynthesized. This process is mediated by two enzymes: fatty acyl-CoA synthetase and acyl transferase. The synthetase uses coenzyme A (CoA) and ATP as cofactors. The ATP is broken down into AMP and inorganic pyrophosphate in the process. Thus, for each long-chain fatty acid that is re-esterified, two ATP equivalents are utilized. Because of this process, it requires more energy to digest and absorb a molecule

of a fat with long-chain fatty acids than one having short-chain fatty acids. The short-chain fatty acids liberated by the action of pancreatic lipase in a micelle are absorbed into the mucosal cell and then exported directly into the portal blood without further modification.

The mucosal cell must synthesize apolipoprotein B-48 in order to constitute and export the chylomicrons. Deficiency of apoprotein B-48 is called abetalipoproteinemia. It is characterized by malabsorption of lipids, low serum low-density lipoprotein values, hemolytic anemia, and retinitis pigmentosum.

Pancreatic lipase preferentially hydrolyses the ester linkage on carbons one and three of the triacylglycerol molecule. The primary products of hydrolysis are two free fatty acids and 2-monoacylglycerol. Pancreatic colipase is required to stabilize the lipase micelle complex. Very little predigestion occurs in the mouth or stomach.

Bile salts are required to emulsify lipids into small droplets called micelles, not chylomicrons. The micelles are then taken up by the mucosal cells where they are packaged into chylomicrons and exported into the lymphatic circulation. Formation of micelles is necessary for digestion by pancreatic lipase. In the absence of sufficient bile salt, a person will have steatorrhea (fatty stools) and may have deficiencies of vitamins A, D, E, and K.

37. The answer is D. *(Pathology)*
Fetal alcohol syndrome occurs in 2 out of every 1000 live births. Mental retardation is its most common manifestation. The syndrome occurs in 30% to 45% of the offspring of women who have more than 4 to 6 drinks per day. It results in the following abnormalities:

- maxillary hypoplasia
- intrauterine growth retardation
- mental retardation (average I.Q. 63; key finding)
- microcephaly
- short palpebral fissures
- atrial septal defects (least common finding)
- hypoglycemia at birth

38. The answer is C. *(Microbiology)*
In addition to the binding of the T-cell receptor (TCR) for antigen with the peptide–major histocompatibility complex (MHC) class II on the antigen-presenting cell (APC) surface, a number of accessory interactions must occur. The CD4 molecule, which is found on T helper lymphocytes, functions as a coreceptor. It binds directly to the class II MHC molecule on the APC, probably close to the cytoplasmic membrane surface. It does not bind to the peptide presented in the groove of the class II molecule.

CD2 is an adhesion molecule that binds to lymphocyte functional antigen-3 (LFA-3) on APCs. CD3, a five-chain complex found on virtually all T lymphocytes, is noncovalently associated with the TCR. During T cell activation, CD3 transmits signals from the TCR into the cytoplasm. It does not bind to MHC class I or II molecules. CD8 functions as a coreceptor for T cytotoxic lymphocytes. It binds directly to the MHC class I molecules on the APC and functions in a manner similar to CD4. CD10, also known as the common acute lymphoblastic leukemia antigen (CALLA), is a glycoprotein found primarily on human leukemia cells. It is also found on B cell precursors.

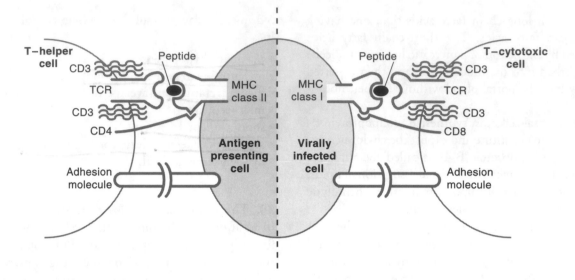

39. The answer is E. *(Biochemistry)*

Because oxidation of fatty acids is abnormal in whole tissue samples but normal in broken cell extracts, a system involving a cofactor or the impaired flow of a metabolite from one cell compartment into another should be expected. Carnitine acyltransferase carries fatty acid coenzyme A derivatives from the cytosol across the inner mitochondrial membrane into the mitochondrial matrix. The other enzymes listed should be equally active in a whole or broken cell system.

Congenital absence of carnitine acyltransferase, or of the enzymes that synthesize carnitine from lysine, causes a condition characterized by weakness following exercise. Pain and release of myoglobin and creatine phosphokinase into the blood are consequences of cell damage associated with the low ATP levels caused by the inability of the muscle cell to produce ATP from fatty acid. Although not uncovered in the physical examination, this boy would also be expected to suffer from a hypoglycemia after exercise, due to the dependence of his muscles on carbohydrate as the sole fuel source. This would further contribute to the child's listlessness.

40. The answer is B. *(Behavioral science)*

The 25-year-old medical student who remains asleep despite a ringing alarm clock is in the deepest stages of sleep, stages 3 and 4, which is delta sleep. Theta waves characterize stage 1 of sleep, the lightest stage of sleep. K complexes characterize stage 2. Beta waves and alpha waves characterize the alert-awake stage and the relaxed-awake stage, respectively.

41. The answer is E. *(Biochemistry)*

Acetyl coenzyme A (CoA) carboxylase, a liver enzyme, is the rate-limiting reaction in fatty acid synthesis. It becomes activated in the fed state when insulin levels are high. Citrate is a positive allosteric effector and fatty acyl CoA a negative allosteric effector. Mitochondrial citrate levels increase as isocitrate dehydrogenase becomes inactivated by the high-energy charge. The citrate is then transported into the cytoplasm where it both activates acetyl CoA carboxylase and is cleaved by citrate lyase to form acetyl CoA and oxaloacetic acid (OAA):

$$\text{citrate} \rightarrow \text{OAA} + \text{acetyl CoA}$$

OAA is reduced to malate by cytoplasmic malate dehydrogenase:

$$\text{OAA} + \text{NADH} + \text{H}^+ \rightarrow \text{malate} + \text{NAD}^+$$

Malate is oxidatively decarboxylated by a nicotinamide adenine dinucleotide phosphate (NADP)-dependent malate dehydrogenase (malic enzyme):

$$\text{malate} + \text{NADP}^+ \rightarrow \text{pyruvate} + \text{CO}_2 + \text{NADPH} + \text{H}^+$$

The cytoplasmic malate dehydrogenase uses cytoplasmic NADH (likely produced via aerobic glycolysis) to put reducing equivalents into oxaloacetic acid. The NADP-dependent malate dehydrogenase takes these hydranions from oxaloacetic acid to form NADPH, the cofactor required for fatty acid synthesis. Citrate thus plays a triple role in fatty acid synthesis: it activates the rate-limiting enzyme, it is the source of the required carbons, and it indirectly supplies the requisite reducing equivalents as NADPH. This couples the energy obtained in the triose dehydrogenase step of glycolysis to that needed for fatty acid synthesis.

42. The answer is B. *(Behavioral science)*
In a durable power of attorney, a person designates legal representatives to make decisions concerning his or her health care when he or she can no longer do so. In a living will, the patient gives directions for future care in the event that he or she can no longer do so. Involuntary treatment is provided for patients who are proven to be both mentally ill and dangerous to themselves or others. In informed consent, the patient is educated as to what to expect with any medical procedure. Managed care is a health care delivery system in which all aspects of a person's health care are coordinated by a group of providers to enhance cost effectiveness.

43. The answer is A. *(Biochemistry)*
In each step utilized, the free carboxyl carbon of malonyl coenzyme A is lost as CO_2. Therefore, no label is incorporated into fatty acid.

44. The answer is B. *(Microbiology)*
The Ouchterlony assay is sometimes called a double-diffusion assay because both the antibody and antigen diffuse toward each other through the agar gel. If binding occurs, the antigen and antibody form stable complexes at the zone of equivalence. Bands of precipitate usually can be visualized within 18–24 hours. The precipitin bands between wells 2 and 3 cross. This is evidence that the antigens in these wells are totally different from each other. The presence of precipitin bands here indicates that the patient has antibodies against the two antigens.

The smooth, continuous, curved band of precipitin between the center well and wells 1 and 2 indicates that the antigens in the two wells are identical. The results indicate that well 3 has two, but not more than two, different antigens against which the patient has antibodies. There are no bands of precipitate between the patient's serum and well 4. Therefore, the serum has no antibodies against antigen 4 that can be detected in this assay. There are no precipitin bands shown to indicate a relationship between antigens 2 and 4. The three classical precipitin band patterns are illustrated.

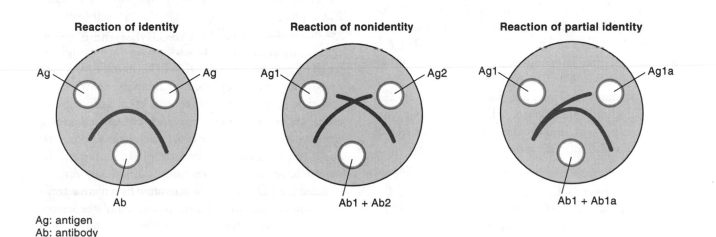

Ag: antigen
Ab: antibody

45. The answer is B. *(Biochemistry)*
ATP is urgently needed during muscle contraction. Nerve impulses cause membrane depolarization, which induces a release of calcium ions from the sarcoplasmic reticulum into muscle sarcoplasm. Some of these calcium ions bind to calmodulin. Calmodium is a calcium-binding protein that has many roles in regulating metabolism. One such role is as a subunit of phosphorylase kinase, which is activated by the binding of calcium to its calmodium subunit. This action allows phosphorylase to be activated without phosphorylase kinase being phosphorylated through the hormonally activated cyclic adenosine monophosphate (cAMP) cascade. When the muscle relaxes, the calcium returns to the sarcoplasm reticulum and phosphorylase kinase becomes inactive.

About 50% of serum calcium is bound to protein, but not to calmodulin. Calcium activates, not dampens, the activity of protein kinase C. Cellular calcium ion levels are increased by the action of hormones that induce the activation of phospholipase C, not A_2. Calcium channels have an important role in the contraction of heart muscle as evidenced by the role of calcium-channel blockers in medicine.

46. The answer is D. *(Microbiology)*
Interleukin-2 (IL-2), a globular protein previously known as T-cell growth factor, binds to high affinity receptors (IL-2R) on activated T lymphocytes and promotes T-cell proliferation. Lack of IL-2, or blocking of IL-2R with monoclonal antibodies, greatly reduces the ability of the cells to multiply. IL-2 is a lymphokine that is produced by activated T helper lymphocytes ($CD4^+$). It acts in both a paracrine and autocrine manner. The paracrine activity of IL-2 is especially critical for activated $CD8^+$ T cytotoxic lymphocyte expansion, because these cells generally secrete little or no IL-2 of their own.

47. The answer is C. *(Biochemistry)*
Palmitoleic acid has 16 carbons. It therefore will be cycled 7 times during β-oxidation, producing 8 two-carbon fragments. Normally, each cycle will produce 1 reduced nicotinamide adenine dinucleotide (NADH) and 1 reduced flavin adenine dinucleotide ($FADH_2$). The NADH is formed when the hydroxy intermediate is oxidized to the keto form. The $FADH_2$ is produced

when a double bond is inserted into the molecule. Because palmitoleic acid already has one double bond, $FADH_2$ is not produced in the cycle involving the double bond. Thus β-oxidation will produce 7 NADHs and 6 $FADH_2$s. Because there are 16 carbons, 8 acetyl CoAs will also result. In a tightly coupled system, each NADH will generate 3 ATPs, for a total of 21; each $FADH_2$ will generate 2 ATPS, for a total of 12; and each acetyl CoA will produce 12 ATPs, for a total of 96. Thus, a grand total of 129 ATPs will be generated. However, because the starting molecule is the free acid, it will have to be activated to the CoA derivative by the thiokinase reaction. This requires 2 ATPS, so the net energy yield is 127 ATPs.

48. The answer is E. *(Behavioral science)*
The patient himself must give consent for the surgery. Married or self-supporting minors are considered emancipated minors: they have the rights of adults and do not require parental consent for medical or surgical procedures.

49. The answer is A. *(Biochemistry)*
Superoxide, hydrogen peroxide, and other oxidizing agents induce the peroxidation of polyunsaturated fatty acids in membranes and other lipoidal structures, including those of low-density lipoproteins (LDLs). Macrophages possess high levels of nonspecific scavenger receptor activity. These receptors recognize oxidatively damaged LDL particles, causing the macrophage to engulf the oxidized LDLs. LDL particles that are not oxidized are recognized by an apoprotein B-100–specific receptor that mediates endocytosis of the particle. This receptor-mediated endocytosis activates a negative feedback mechanism, which reduces synthesis and further uptake of cholesterol. In contrast, the magrophage's scavenger receptor–induced engulfment of oxidized LDL does not activate this negative feedback effect, and the cholesterol accumulates in the cell. Excess cholesterol converts the macrophage into a foam cell, which tends to accumulate under the endothelial layer of the inner walls of arteries and becomes a site for the formation of plaques. Vitamin E inhibits this pathological process by protecting the polyunsaturated lipid from the initiating oxidation.

50. The answer is B. *(Microbiology)*
Hepatitis B virus is the only agent listed known to contain a virally coded DNA polymerase within the virion itself. Although Epstein-Barr virus probably replicates its genome by means of a virally coded enzyme, the DNA polymerase does not act directly on the DNA genome within the virion particle. Hepatitis C virus has a positive-sense RNA genome (identical to messenger RNA) and therefore does not need a virion RNA polymerase. Adenoviruses and parvoviruses contain DNA and replicate their genomes as part of the normal life cycle within the host cell. Adenovirus replicates its genome by means of a virally coded enzyme, and parvovirus replication is dependent upon functions supplied by replicating host cells or by coinfecting helper viruses.

51. The answer is B. *(Biochemistry)*
The three ketone bodies are acetoacetate, 3-hydroxybutyrate, and acetone. Ketone bodies are synthesized in the liver when the rate of fatty acid β-oxidation exceeds the rate of acetyl coenzyme A (CoA) oxidation in the tricarboxylic acid cycle. This occurs when the insulin to glucagon ratio is low, as in diabetic ketoacidosis or prolonged fasting. The resulting mobilization of fatty acids provides the liver with excess fatty acid as substrate. The acetyl CoA formed from the β-oxidation of these fatty acids activates phosphoenolpyruvate (PEP) carboxykinase, promoting the conversion of oxaloacetic acid to PEP, resulting in a relative deficiency of oxaloacetate and inhibiting citrate formation from acetyl CoA. The excess acetyl CoA is converted to acetoacetyl CoA by the action of thiolase. This newly synthesized acetoacetyl CoA (or acetoacetyl CoA formed as a byproduct of β-oxidation) combines with another molecule of acetyl CoA in a reaction catalyzed by 3-hydroxy-3-methylglutaryl-CoA synthase to form 3-hydroxy-3-methylglutaryl CoA (HMG CoA). HMG CoA lyase then cleaves an acetyl CoA, forming acetoacetate, which either spontaneously breaks down to form acetone or is reduced to 3-hydroxybutyrate.

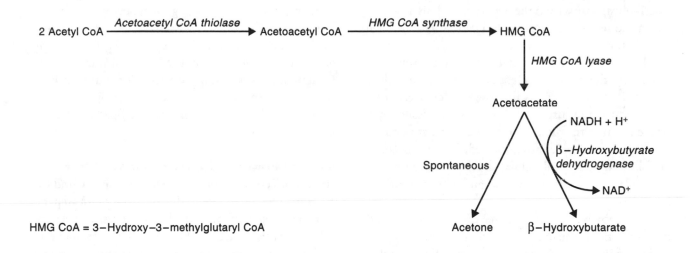

HMG CoA = 3−Hydroxy−3−methylglutaryl CoA

Acetone is not metabolized by any tissue in the body. It is, however, volatile and accounts for the fruity smell associated with uncontrolled diabetics and the fasting state. The liver can not use any of the ketone bodies as fuel, but muscle, brain, and some other peripheral tissues can use both acetoacetate and 3-hydroxybutyrate. Red cells can only use glucose as a fuel.

52. The answer is E. *(Behavioral science)*
For the claim of malpractice to be upheld in court, the family must prove that the doctor deviated from the established standard of care in that community. Malpractice is a tort or civil wrong; it is not a crime. The family does not have to prove that the doctor intended to cause the patient harm. Doctors' educa-

tion and charges for treatment are not directly relevant to malpractice.

53. The answer is D. *(Biochemistry)*
Low aldolase B activity in a liver biopsy sample is definitive evidence of hereditary fructose intolerance, which is an autosomal recessive inborn error of metabolism.

The infant did well as long as milk provided the sugar in the diet. Milk sugar (lactose) is converted into glucose and galactose in the gut by lactase, a brush border disaccharidase. Most baby foods are sweetened with table sugar (sucrose) or fructose-enriched corn syrup, and fruits and fruit juices are rich in free fructose. Fructose passes from the gut to the liver via the portal vein. In the liver, it is phosphorylated to yield fructose 1-phosphate, trapping the fructose intracellularly. The fructose 1-phosphate is split into two 3-carbon intermediates, glyceraldehyde and dihydroxyacetone phosphate (DHAP) by aldolase B (liver aldolase). Fructose intolerance is caused by a deficiency of aldolase B, which results in the accumulation of fructose 1-phosphate within the hepatocyte. This accumulation induces hypoglycemia and causes liver damage and cirrhosis.

The physician that recommends a fructose tolerance test is on the right track, because the history does suggest that the baby has fructose intolerance. However, because the suspected disease is manifested by a severe reaction to fructose in the diet, a fructose tolerance test would be contraindicated, because it could be followed by hypoglycemia, shock, and even death.

Aldolase B is a liver enzyme and is not found in fibroblasts.

If the baby is on a fructose-free diet, fructose would not be found in the urine. Chromatographic determination of urinary fructose could be a logical test if it is conducted during the time symptoms are observed.

Detecting a reducing sugar (any sugar having a free aldehydic or ketonic radical) in the urine during the acute phase is a good screening test, but it does not provide a definitive diagnosis of fructose intolerance. Many reducing sugars, including glucose, fructose, lactose, and pentoses, give a positive reducing reaction. Moreover, in hereditary fructokinase deficiency (essential fructosuria), fructose is not phosphorylated by the liver. This leads to a benign, asymptomatic condition in which fructose is excreted in the urine.

The use of a sugar reducing test in the urine (e.g., Clinitest) as the sole diagnostic tool in a case of fructose intolerance could result in a false diagnosis of diabetes, essential fructosuria, or other maladies. Simultaneous use of two dipsticks—one impregnated with glucose oxidase (and therefore specific for glucose) and the other for total reducing sugars—would greatly increase the chances of an accurate diagnosis.

54. The answer is D. *(Microbiology)*
Staphlococcus aureus is the most medically important species of the *Staphylococcus* genus and is distinguished from other species in the genus by its ability to produce coagulase. This enzyme has the ability to clot citrated plasma and is an important contributor to the pathogenicity of the species.

S. aureus produces a fibrin clot, or capsule, around each organism that inhibits phagocytosis by white blood cells. Protein A, the major protein of the cell wall, assists coagulase in this process. Protein A binds to the crystallizable fragment (Fc) portion of immunoglobulin G molecules, preventing the binding of complement, thereby inhibiting phagocytosis by white blood cells. Coagulase contributes to the formation of the typical abscess lesion of *S. aureus* by blocking access to the organism by the host's immune system. Coagulase makes it more difficult for antimicrobials to penetrate the abscess, as well.

None of the other organisms listed produces coagulase.

55. The answer is C. *(Biochemistry)*
Immunoelectrophoresis, zone electrophoresis, and the Western blot test involve the electrophoretic separation of proteins. In immunoelectrophoresis, an electrical current is added to facilitate the movement of antibodies and antigens through an agar gel, cellulose nitrate, or other solid matrix. Proteins move in an electrical field according to their size and charge. Applications of immunoelectrophoresis include the demonstration of paraproteins in serum, light chains in urine (Bence-Jones protein), and elevated protein levels in cerebrospinal fluid.

Zone electrophoresis involves the separation of proteins in an electrical field without application of antibodies. The proteins in a gel or other matrix can be stained and scanned in a densitometer, which converts the protein bands into peaks. In the Western blot test (the standard confirmatory test for antibodies against HIV-1), proteins are electrophoretically separated, "blotted" onto nitrocellulose paper, and serum is subsequently added. The Northern blot test is performed for the analysis of RNA, whereas the Southern blot test is used for DNA analysis.

56. The answer is A. *(Behavioral science)*
In sublimation, an unacceptable instinctual drive is rerouted to a socially acceptable action. In this case, the aggressive impulses of this individual were channeled to the acceptable action of stealing bases and getting paid for it.

57. The answer is A. *(Biochemistry)*
Methotrexate, aminopterin, and other folate analogs directly inhibit the enzyme dihydrofolate reductase, which is responsible for the reduction of folate to its active form, tetrahydrofolate. Tetrahydrofolate serves as a carrier of single-carbon groups in metabolism and is necessary for de novo purine biosynthesis and for thymidine monophosphate (TMP) biosynthesis. Inhibitors of nucleotide synthesis are used as anticancer agents, because fast-growing cancer cells have an increased demand for nucleotides to support their rapid growth.

Thymidylate synthase is indirectly inhibited by methotrexate because its mechanism of action requires involvement of a tetrahydrofolate derivative. Xanthine oxidase, phosphoribosyl pyrophosphate (PRPP) synthase, and hypoxanthine-guanine phosphoribosyltransferase (HGPRT) are involved in purine metabolism and are unaffected by methotrexate.

58. The answer is A. *(Behavioral science)*
Factors that increase the risk of suicide, in order of highest to lowest risk, are as follows: age more than 45 years, alcohol or drug abuse, prior suicide attempts, male gender, serious prior psychiatric illness, recent divorce or death of a spouse, serious medical illness, unemployment, and unmarried status.

59. The answer is D. *(Biochemistry)*
Although DNA and ribosomal RNA are often methylated, and eukaryotic messenger RNA undergoes extensive processing, transfer RNA contains the largest number of modified and unusual bases. Transfer RNA

also has extensive intrachain base pairing. Its function is to carry amino acids to the ribosome, and to serve as an adaptor molecule, helping to translate the base sequence present in messenger RNA into an amino acid sequence of a protein molecule.

60. The answer is B. *(Behavioral science)*
Almost half of children between the ages of 3 and 6 years have imaginary companions that help to decrease loneliness and anxiety. Nightmares are common in children of this age. Parallel play (i.e., playing alongside of one another) is common in children up to the age of four; after this age children tend to play cooperatively. Preschool children do not fully understand the meaning of death and may expect that a dead relative will come back to life.

61. The answer is E. *(Biochemistry)*
DNA fragments produced as a result of cleavage by two different restriction endonucleases can anneal and ligate if the two enzymes produce the same "sticky ends." These sticky ends are self-complementary because they are derived from palindromes. *Bsp*120I (G↓GGCCC) produces sticky ends with the sequence GGCC at the 5′ end of each DNA strand. *Eag* I (C↓GGCCG) produces this same sticky end, even though the entire recognition sequence is not identical. *Stu* I (AGG↓CCT), *Hae* III (GG↓CC), and *Sma* I (CCC↓GGG) all produce blunt ends, which cannot anneal to anything. *Apa* I (GGGCC↓C), although recognizing the same sequence as *Bsp*120I, cuts it differently, producing sticky ends at the 3′ end of each strand (note the position of the arrow, which indicates the position of cleavage).

62. The answer is B. *(Pharmacology)*
Rifampin is one of several drugs that induce the synthesis of hepatic drug-metabolizing enzymes and thereby accelerate the metabolism of other concurrently administered drugs. Other enzyme inducers include phenobarbital, phenytoin, and griseofulvin. Rifampin decreases the anticoagulant effect of warfarin by this mechanism, and decreases prothrombin time, because prothrombin time is increased by warfarin. Antithrombin III is activated by heparin rather than warfarin.

63. The answer is B. *(Behavioral science)*
The ego maintains a relationship to the external world by controlling the expression of instinctual (i.e., id) drives and by being flexible to life's frustrations. The id represents sexual and aggressive drives and is not influenced by external reality. The superego is the conscience, which incorporates the individual's moral values. The id, ego, and superego are part of Freud's structural theory of the mind. The unconscious, preconscious, and conscious are parts of Freud's topographic theory of the mind developed early in his career. In this theory, the unconscious mind contains repressed thoughts and feelings, the preconscious contains memories, and the conscious mind uses attention to become aware of stimuli from the outside world.

64. The answer is C. *(Biochemistry)*
Synthesis of all nucleic acid strands is accomplished in the 5′ to 3′ direction, with respect to the newly synthesized strand. Removal of RNA primers also occurs in the 5′ to 3′ direction, as a result of the action of a 5′ to 3′ exonuclease, which in bacteria is part of the activity of DNA Polymerase I. Proofreading is accomplished by the 3′ to 5′ exonuclease activity of bacterial DNA polymerases. This enzymatic activity is used to eliminate mistakes made during DNA synthesis by immediately removing nucleotides that are unable to base pair properly with the template strand of DNA.

65. The answer is C. *(Behavioral science)*
An individual with a mental age of 8 years and a chronological age of 10 years has an IQ of 80. The IQ formula is mental age (MA) divided by chronological age (CA) times 100: $8 \div 10 \times 100 = 80$.

66. The answer is E. *(Pharmacology)*
Drug potency is inversely related to the dose required to produce an effect. The relative potency of drugs is determined by the doses required to produce the same magnitude of effect and can be determined from the ratio of equivalent doses. In this case, $60:4 = 15$.

The pharmacologic potency of a drug does not indicate anything about its duration of action, toxicity, margin of safety, or volume of distribution.

67. The answer is B. *(Behavioral science)*
The MMPI is an objective personality test. An objective test is based on questions that can be easily scored and statistically analyzed. Projective tests, such as the Rorschach, TAT, and SCT, require the subject and the grader to interpret the questions. The Luria Nebraska is a test of neuropsychological performance.

68. The answer is E. *(Biochemistry)*
Repressor proteins are regulator proteins that regulate initiation of transcription in bacterial operons by binding to the DNA base sequence called the operator. When bound to the operator, the repressor protein prevents effective binding and initiation of transcription of RNA polymerase. Inducers are small molecules that bind to certain repressor proteins, causing them to fall off of the operator site. Corepressors are small molecules that bind to certain other repressor proteins, stimulating their binding to the operator. Promoters are binding sites on DNA for RNA polymerase. Enhancers are DNA sequences in eukaryotes that are involved in regulation of transcription.

69. The answer is E. *(Behavioral science)*
Extinction is the disappearance of a behavior when it is not rewarded. The pattern of reinforcement least resistant to extinction (i.e., the behavior disappears fastest when it is not rewarded) is continuous. In continuous reinforcement, the organism is rewarded every time the behavior is shown; for example, putting a dollar in a vending machine and receiving a cup of coffee. The pattern of reinforcement most resistant to extinction (i.e., the behavior disappears slowest when it is not rewarded) is variable ratio. In variable ratio reinforcement, the organism receives a reward after a random and unpredictable number of responses; for example, putting coins into a slot machine.

70. The answer is A. *(Behavioral science)*
The most common cause of disability in the elderly is musculoskeletal and joint disease. Depression occurs to some extent in about 15% of the elderly; 3% suffer more severe major depression. Alzheimer disease occurs in about 10% of the elderly population. Although debilitating, ulcers and Parkinson disease are not as widespread as musculoskeletal and joint disease among the elderly.

71. The answer is B. *(Pharmacology)*
Pharmacologic tolerance is defined as an increase in the dose required to produce a defined magnitude of effect. It is accompanied by a shift of the log-dose response curve to the right and an increase in the median effective dose. It may be caused by pharmacodynamic changes, such as a decreased number of drug receptors, or by pharmacokinetic changes, such as increased drug clearance and decreased plasma half-life.

72. The answer is E. *(Behavioral science)*
Denial is the least mature of these defense mechanisms. Less mature defense mechanisms are used primarily by children and adolescents, by people with psychiatric disturbances, and by people under severe stress. Mature defense mechanisms such as altruism, suppression, sublimation, and humor are used by normal, healthy individuals to deal with the stresses of everyday life.

73. The answer is B. *(Behavioral science)*
For the reference interval in this question to encompass 95% of the normal population, two standard deviations (% mg/dL) added to and subtracted from the mean of the test establishes the upper and lower limits of the reference interval.

Standard deviation is a measure of reliability (i.e., precision) of a test. The lower the standard deviation of a test, the more reliable it is. Most laboratories use two standard deviations from the mean of a test in order to establish the reference interval. Using 95% of the population for the reference interval, 5% of normal people will have a test result outside that range. This is considered a false-positive test result.

74. The answer is C. *(Behavioral science)*
About 20% of children in the United States live in a family structure in which the mother stays at home and the father works.

75-77. The answers are: 75-D, 76-C, 77-E. *(Biochemistry)*
In the fasting state, glucagon and catecholamine levels increase. This, in turn, activates hormone-sensitive lipase in the adipocyte, resulting in the liberation of free fatty acids and glycerol into the serum. Fatty acids are transported to the tissues and utilized as fuel via β-oxidation in the mitochondria. Glycerol is converted to glycerol 3-phosphate in the liver and used as a substrate for gluconeogenesis.

Pancreatic lipase is used in digestion. Acetyl CoA carboxylase, propionyl CoA carboxylase, and palmitoyl synthetase are anabolic enzymes used in lipid synthesis. These are normally inactive under fasting conditions, and active in the fed state.

Gluconeogenesis is stimulated by fasting. To permit gluconeogenesis to occur without inducing futile cycles (i.e., the utilization of gluconeogenic intermediates by glycolytic enzymes) the three irreversible steps of glycolysis must be inhibited. The key enzymes that catalyze these steps of glycolysis are hexokinase (glucokinase in the liver), phosphofructokinase-1, and pyruvate kinase.

Liver pyruvate kinase would be decreased in the fasting state because it is inhibited by direct phosphorylation by protein kinase A. Protein kinase A is activated by 3′,5′-cyclic AMP (cAMP), which is increased as a result of glucagon, the key hormone of the fasting state.

Protein kinase A also phosphorylates seryl residues on phosphofructokinase-2, thus phosphorylated phosphofructokinase levels increase rather than decrease. Phosphorylated phosphofructokinase-2 is inactive as a kinase but is active as a phosphatase. Therefore, in the fasting state, this enzyme no longer synthesizes fructose 2,6-bisphosphate (the key activator of the rate-limiting enzyme of glycolysis, phosphofructokinase-1), but rather breaks it down to form fructose 6-phosphate, thereby inhibiting glycolysis. Fructose 1,6-bisphosphate is an allosteric activator of liver pyruvate kinase in the glycolytic pathway. Therefore, the decrease in concentration of this compound further inhibits pyruvate kinase.

Muscle and adipocytes have an insulin-dependent glucose transporter. Therefore, under fasting conditions, with low insulin levels, this transporter is inhibited in these tissues. Glucose transport across the cellular membranes of brain cells, hepatocytes, and red blood cells is not directly dependent upon insulin and the transport mechanism is unaffected by fasting. This arrangement results in a glucose-sparing effect because glucose becomes less available to muscle and adipocytes under fasting conditions. This makes more glucose available to the brain and red blood cells, both of which require glucose for fuel.

78. The answer is B.   *(Behavioral science)*
This student is using rationalization to explain her poor performance on the psychiatry examination.

79. The answer is C.   *(Anatomy)*
Taxol is a drug derived from the bark of yew trees, widely used as an anticancer drug. Microtubules add and remove tubulin subunits during the movement of chromosomes. Taxol binds tightly to microtubules, thus acting as a stabilizer. Taxol also causes free tubulin to assemble into microtubules.

Nucleoli numbers usually increase in cancer cells but taxol does not react with these structures. Chromatin is not affected by taxol. Microfilaments play key roles in cell division (cytokinesis) but do not move chromosomes and they are not affected by taxol. Intermediate filaments, the third component of the cytoskeleton, are not influenced by taxol and seem to have no role in chromosome movement.

80. The answer is A.   *(Behavioral science)*
A normal newborn infant curls its hand around an object that is put in it. This is the palmar grasp reflex. This reflex, present at birth, disappears at approximately 2 months of age.

81. The answer is B.   *(Microbiology)*
As influenza viruses are inhaled, the viral protein neuraminidase degrades the protective mucous layer of the respiratory tract, allowing the virus to gain direct access to cells. Viremia rarely occurs, and usual disease manifestations result from necrosis of the superficial layers of the respiratory tract epithelium. Secretory IgA is the primary immunoglobulin that is deposited in tissues that are initially infected by viruses. Mucous membrane of the upper respiratory tract contains relatively large amounts of IgA. Interferon is produced and secreted locally, within hours of infection, by virus-infected cells. Interferon signals for production of an anti-viral protein (AVP) in newly infected cells. AVP directly interferes with viral messenger RNA activity and results in fewer viruses being produced.

Passive immunity mechanisms include the use of preformed antibodies. Although preformed antibodies against influenza viruses are present in immune serum globulin (gamma globulin) preparations, the use of these materials are not recommended for influenza

control. Recommended procedures include the use of amantadine and/or current, inactivated vaccine for people considered to be at greatest risk of influenza infection. Both are administered early in the influenza season, before the recipient encounters the virus.

Although stomach acids destroy influenza viruses, this is not a significant means of protection from infection. Antigenic drift refers to minor antigenic changes on the nucleocapsid. Macrophage engulfment is involved in the destruction and elimination of virally infected cells.

82. The answer is A.   *(Behavioral science)*
The Babinski reflex, in which the large toe extends upward when the sole of the foot is stroked, is normal in children from birth to 1 year of age. Presence of this reflex in older children indicates a neurologic problem.

83. The answer is E.   *(Biochemistry)*
Reduced nicotinamide adenine dinucleotide phosphate (NADPH) and reduced nicotinamide adenine dinucleotide (NADH) have equivalent potential energies and in theory each could be converted into three ATPs. However, NADPH is almost exclusively used extra-mitochondrially to support synthesis or to maintain the reducing atmosphere of the cytoplasm by keeping glutathione and other molecules in the reduced state. There are no transporters for NADPH or NADH, and neither can traverse the inner mitochondrial membrane. There are, however, two mechanisms by which the reducing equivalents carried by NADH can be transported into the mitochondrial matrix. They are the α-glycerol phosphate shuttle and the malate-aspartate shuttle. The former produces only two ATP equivalents and the latter produces three.

There are no analogous mechanisms to carry NADPH reducing equivalents across the mitochondrial membrane. Therefore, because the reduction of NADP$^+$ to form NADPH occurs in the cytoplasm, most of the cell's NADPH is found in the cytoplasm, where the ratio of NADPH to NADP ratio normally is very high. In contrast, most NADH is produced in the mitochondrial matrix, where it can send its reducing equivalents through the oxidative phosphorylation system to be converted into ATP.

84. The answer is E. *(Behavioral science)*
The defense mechanism of identification is used by this baseball manager in his coaching techniques.

85. The answer is C. *(Behavioral science)*
A union trust fund that contracts with physicians in private practice to provide health care to the fund's subscribers is known as a preferred provider organization (PPO). A health maintenance organization (HMO) is a prepaid insurance and service managed care plan in which physicians and other health care personnel are paid by salary to provide medical services to a group of people enrolled voluntarily who have paid an annual premium. An independent practice association (IPA) involves physicians in private practice who are hired by an HMO to provide services to HMO patients. A private insurance carrier pays for the medical costs of individuals or groups of individuals with whom it has contracts and who have paid specific yearly premiums. A diagnosis-related group (DRG) is an illness-classification system for determining the amount of reimbursement to hospitals for Medicare patients.

86. The answer is E. *(Behavioral science)*
Erikson described development in terms of stages that a person must resolve; if such resolution does not take place, all future stages are characterized by problems in emotional or social functioning. According to this theory, the stage of autonomy versus shame and doubt occurs in the toddler years. If autonomy is not achieved because of excessive parental control, the person feels that people look down on him or her (i.e., experiences shame) throughout life.

87. The answer is D. *(Behavioral science)*
Accidents are the leading cause of death among adolescents. Approximately 75% of these result from automobile accidents. Suicide and homicide are the second and third most common causes of death in adolescents.

88. The answer is A. *(Behavioral science)*
Piaget described development in terms of what a person can learn at each age. He described the period from birth to 2 years as the sensorimotor stage. In this stage, a child uses senses to learn, and then manipulates the environment using motor skills.

89. The answer is C. *(Biochemistry)*
Lithium and several hormones, including epinephrine in the liver, affect metabolic change by influencing the phosphoinositol cycle, which regulates intracellular calcium ion levels. Calcium ions, in turn, alter the activity of many enzymes, including protein kinase C, and also influence the action potential in conducting cells, such as neurons. Lithium affects intracellular calcium levels in the brain, and epinephrine affects intracellular calcium levels in the liver.

Lithium inhibits a phosphatase involved in the metabolism of 1,4,5-inositol trisphosphate (IP_3), an important second messenger (see the accompanying schematic).

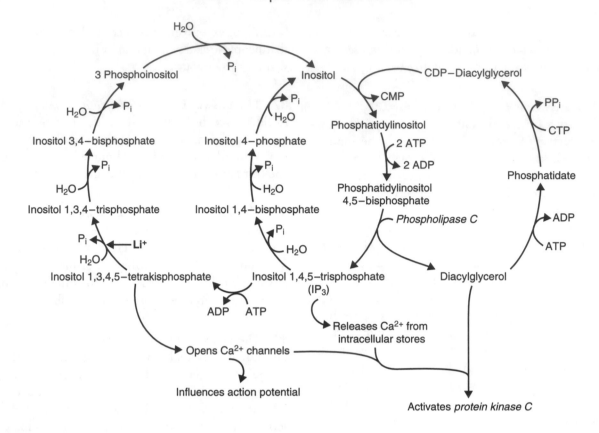

IP$_3$ affects the release of calcium ion from intracellular stores, thereby increasing the functional level of calcium in the cell. Diacylglycerol acts synergistically with calcium ion to activate protein kinase C.

IP$_3$ has a very short half-life. It is degraded by two alternative pathways. In one pathway, it is sequentially dephosphorylated to inositol. The intermediates in this path appear to have no regulatory significance. In the other pathway, it is first phosphorylated to form 1,3,4,5-inositol tetrakisphosphate. This compound induces the opening of calcium channels in the cell membrane. The phosphatase that causes hydrolysis of the 5-phosphate from this compound is inhibited by millimolar amounts of lithium ion (Li$^+$). This is the mode of action of this ion in the control of manic depression.

The 1,3,4-inositol trisphosphate formed from this inositol-sensitive hydrolysis is also sequentially hydrolyzed to inositol. The inositol formed from these two hydrolytic pathways is recycled by condensing with cytidine diphosphate–diacylglycerol to form phosphatidyl inositol, which is then re-phosphorylated

to re-form phosphatidyl inositol bisphosphate. The series of events is ready to be initiated again when another molecule of hormone binds to its receptor.

The plasma membranes of hepatocytes have an α-adrenergic receptor. Binding of epinephrine to this receptor activates phospholipase C, which, in turn, hydrolyzes phosphatidylinositol 4,5-bisphosphate to produce diacylglycerol and IP$_3$. The IP$_3$ induces the endoplasmic reticulum to release Ca^{2+}, which binds to the calmodulin subunit of phosphorylase kinase and to a calmodulin-dependent glycogen synthetase kinase. This calcium binding activates these kinases, resulting in the phosphorylation of both phosphorylase and glycogen synthetase. Phosphorylation activates phosphorylase and inhibits glycogen synthetase. This mechanism of promoting glycogenolysis is independent of the action mediated by glucagon.

90. The answer is B. *(Behavioral science)*
Memories that can be brought to mind easily are examples of preconscious thought. The unconscious contains repressed memories that are not available to

consciousness. The id represents instinctive aggressive and sexual drives, and the superego represents moral values and conscience.

91. The answer is C.   (Microbiology)

Fungi (yeasts and molds) are eukaryotic organisms, which means that they possess a membrane around their nuclear material. Bacteria, as prokaryotes, have their genomes diffused throughout the cytoplasm.

Both fungi and bacteria have cell walls. The fungal cell wall is chitin, and the bacterial cell wall is peptidoglycan. Fungi contain mitochondria but bacteria do not. Many of the energy-producing enzyme systems of bacteria reside in the cytoplasmic membrane.

Fungi have two forms of structure: yeasts, which are single oval cells that may bud to reproduce; and hyphae, which are long filaments or strands of cells. Most bacteria are single-celled organisms. Relatively few bacteria have the ability to branch or to grow in long chains.

Comparison of Bacteria and Fungi

Feature	Bacteria	Fungi
True cell	Yes	Yes
Nucleus type	Prokaryotic	Eukaryotic
Ribosome size	70S	80S
Mitochondria	No	Yes
Size (μm)	1–4	4–10
Cell wall contents	Peptidoglycan	Chitin
Replication method	Binary fission	Binary fission and budding
Flagella	Some	None

92. The answer is C.   (Behavioral science)

The topographic and structural theories of the mind are associated with Sigmund Freud. Piaget described development in terms of what a person can learn at each age. Spitz described the role of separation from the primary caregiver in development. Chess and Thomas described the role of temperament in the development of behavior. Erikson described development in terms of stages that an individual must resolve in order to proceed effectively to the next stage.

93. The answer is D.   (Biochemistry)

Disruption of the inner membrane of the mitochondrion produces five insoluble complexes (I–V), as well as several soluble molecules. Sequential addition of these complexes with purified fractions from the soluble phase has helped to determine the sequence and mechanisms involved in oxidative phosphorylation. Complexes I–IV each contain part of the electron transport system. Only complex V has ATPase activity and, in the intact system, is responsible for ATP synthesis. It does not bind oxygen. Complex IV is the terminal complex in the electron transport chain. It contains cytochrome $a+a_3$ (also known as cytochrome c oxidase), which normally reacts with oxygen. Cytochrome $a+a_3$ also reacts with cyanide (CN^-), carbon monoxide (CO) and sodium azide, all of which are potent inhibitors of oxidative phosphorylation.

Reduced nicotinamide adenine dinucleotide (NADH) dehydrogenase is part of complex I. Succinate dehydrogenase is part of complex II. Coenzyme Q is a soluble factor that serves to connect complexes I and II with complex III.

Relationships between these factors are shown in the accompanying diagram.

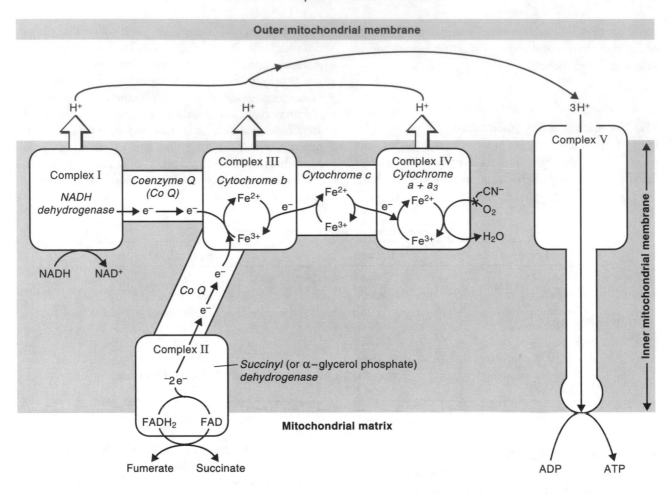

94. The answer is D. *(Anatomy)*

This is a plasma cell with an extensive array of rough endoplasmic reticulum. Ribosomes are bound to the membranes of endoplasmic reticulum, giving it a rough appearance and basophilic staining properties. Rough endoplasmic reticulum is prominent in cells specialized for protein secretion. Functions include segregation of protein for export or intracellular use, glycosylation of proteins, and multichain protein assembly.

The Golgi complex is visible as a clearer, paranuclear, membranous area. The lighter appearance results from a lack of associated ribosomes. The complex consists of stacks of membranes, vesicles, and vacuoles. Microtubules are linear structures that are smaller than rough endoplasmic reticulum. Collagen fibrils are assembled in the extracellular matrix. Smooth endoplasmic reticulum does not possess ribosomes.

95. The answer is C. *(Biochemistry)*

The standard free energy change $\Delta G^0 = -RT (\ln K_{eq})$, where R is the gas constant (1.987×10^{-3} kcal $\times$ deg^{-1} $\times$ mol^{-1}), T is temperature in degrees kelvin, and ln indicates the natural logarithm. It follows therefore that: if K_{eq} equals 1, ΔG^0 is zero (ln 1 = 0, -RT $\times$ 0 = 0); if K_{eq} is less than zero (the multiplicand of the concentration of products is less than that of substrates at equilibrium) ΔG^0 is positive, and: if K_{eq} is greater than zero (the multiplicand of the concentration of products is greater than that of substrates at equilibrium) ΔG^0 is negative. (Remember that the ln of a number less than zero is negative). Because by definition, a thermodynamically spontaneous reaction is one in which products accumulate relative to substrate, the ΔG^0 is negative for a thermodynamically feasible reaction. A major advantage of using standard free energy rather than the K_{eq} as a measure of the thermodynamic feasibility of a reaction is that the

ΔG^0 value is algebraically additive. This allows one to determine the feasibility of coupled reactions or even of a whole metabolic sequence. For example, the first two reactions in the glycolytic sequence:

1. Glucose + ATP → glucose 6-phosphate + ADP ΔG^0 = -4000 cal/mol

2. Glucose 6-phosphate → fructose 6-phosphate ΔG^0 = +400 cal/mol

1 + 2. Glucose + ATP → fructose 6-phosphate + ADP ΔG^0 = -3600 cal/mol

Another property resulting from the fact that $\Delta G^0 = -RT(\ln K_{eq})$ is that ΔG^0 is a constant at a given temperature. That is, R, T, and K_{eq} are constant, therefore their product, ΔG^0, is also constant and can not vary depending upon the concentration of substrate or reaction product. Moreover, ΔG^0 is defined as ΔG under standard conditions, in which all substrates and products are held constant, at 1 M; that is, in general, $\Delta G^0 = \Delta G - RT \ln [B] \div [A]$ and only when [B] and [A] are both equal to 1 M, does $\Delta G^0 = \Delta G$. This is a situation that will never occur in the real world. However, because the RT ln term is negatively added to (i.e., subtracted from) ΔG, ΔG^0 and ΔG will never be directly proportional.

96. The answer is A. (Microbiology)

The genes encoding γ/δ chains, as well as those encoding α/β chains, are expressed only by cells of the T lymphocyte lineage. The gene for the γ chain is located on chromosome 7, as is the gene for the β chain. The gene for the δ chain is located on chromosome 14, as is the gene for the α chain. The genetic mechanisms regulating the expression of γ/δ chains versus α/β chains are largely unknown. Although the vast majority of T-cell receptors (TCRs) for antigen consist of α/β chains, approximately 2%–5% of T cells express γ/δ chains instead. The γ/δ TCR differs from the α/β TCR in antigen specificity, pattern of CD4 and CD8 coreceptor expression, and biodistribution.

97. The answer is D. (Microbiology)

The enzyme-linked immunosorbent assay (ELISA) is used routinely for screening patient sera for many different antibodies (including antibodies against HIV-1) and antigens. The test, which is sensitive, safe, and requires only simple instrumentation, is illustrated in the figure. In the measurement of antibody, a known antigen (Ag) is attached to the bottom of wells in a microtiter plate and the patient's serum (Ab1) is added. After washing, a second antibody [anti-immunoglobulin (Ab2)] complexed to an enzyme (E) such as horseradish peroxidase, is added. The wells are washed again and a colorless substrate (open ovals) for the enzyme is added. The development of color (solid ovals) can be quantitated in a spectrophotometer and reflects the concentration of Ab1.

In immunofluorescence assays, fluorescent dyes (e.g., fluorescein and rhodamine) are bound to free amino groups on antibodies (or antigens) to serve as "markers" indicating that an antigen–antibody reaction has taken place. The dyes are detected by shining an ultraviolet light on them in a fluorescence microscope.

Flow cytometers analyze cells in single-celled suspensions for the presence of specific surface molecules (e.g., CD4 and CD8) to which fluorescent dye–antibody complexes have been attached. Cells flowing through a small orifice are hit with a laser beam of a certain wavelength, which causes the dye to fluoresce.

In radioimmunoassays (RIAs), radioactively labeled antigen and "cold" antigen compete for the same limited amount of antibody. Antigen–antibody complexes are isolated and the amount of bound radioactivity is counted. RIAs are highly sensitive tests and are used to measure insulin, other hormones, carcinoembryonic antigen, and drugs in serum.

Neutralization tests are performed to determine the presence of antibodies that can block toxin activity and virus infectivity in cell cultures or animals.

98. The answer is B. (Microbiology)

Cytokines are a diverse group of biologically active substances that are secreted by cells. Most of them are peptides or glycoproteins with very short half-lives (measured in minutes to hours). They exert their effects only locally. Nonetheless, these substances are extremely potent. A cytokine that affects nearby cells has paracrine activity, whereas one that acts on the cell that produced it has autocrine activity. The great majority of cytokines are synthesized *de novo* in response to specific stimuli.

99. The answer is D. *(Microbiology)*

The many substances that can interfere with viral replication are classified into two major groups: type I and type II. Type I IFNs are approximately 90% homologous in structure, and all bind to the same cell receptor molecule. They have significantly greater antiviral effects than type II IFN (IFN-γ). IFN-α, IFN-β, and IFN-ω belong in the type I category. (IFN-ω is a relatively new designation for a factor expressed by leukocytes; it is very similar to IFN-α.) IFNs act in a nonspecific manner; that is, IFN induced by one virus makes a cell refractory to infection by many different viruses. Type I IFNs can be synthesized by many different types of cells (including leukocytes) after viral infection. Infection with protozoa and fungi, as well as certain cytokines, can also induce their production.

100. The answer is E. *(Microbiology)*

Interleukin-10 (IL-10) was previously known as cytokine synthesis inhibitory factor. It has a profound inhibitory effect on the production of a number of cytokines, especially IL-2 and interferon-γ (IFN-γ), which are produced by the T_H-1 subset of T helper cells. The suppressive effect may be indirect (i.e., through the impairment of macrophage and dendritic cell accessory function). IL-10 favors humoral immune responses.

101. The answer is C. *(Microbiology)*

Tumor necrosis factor-α (TNF-α), a major immunomodulator produced by macrophages, was first described as a factor in the serum of lipopolysaccharide (LPS)-treated animals. It was later identified as cachectin, the mediator of the wasting syndrome seen in patients with overwhelming infections caused by gram-negative bacteria. LPS, which is present in the cell walls of these microorganisms, is an extremely potent TNF-α inducer.

Cachexia occurs in more than 50% of oncologic patients and is a significant factor in cancer-related

mortality. Cachexia is manifested as involuntary weight loss, anorexia, and atrophy of skeletal muscle and visceral organs. Although its etiology in cancer patients is undoubtedly multifactorial, it has recently been shown that many of these patients have high serum levels of TNF-α in the late stages of disease.

Wasting syndrome is one of the more than 20 "AIDS-defining conditions." Its etiology appears to be at least partly related to excessive production of TNF-α. Increased levels of the factor have been found in the sera of AIDS patients. Monocytic cells infected with HIV-1 secrete abnormally high amounts of TNF-α when stimulated in vitro. Because TNF-α has multiple detrimental effects on neuronal cells, it may also contribute to AIDS dementia.

102. The answer is A. *(Microbiology)*

Activated cytotoxic T lymphocytes develop granules that contain several types of molecules, including perforins. Perforins are high-molecular-weight proteoglycans that form a channel in the membrane of target cells. Monomers of perforin are released from the granules by exocytosis at the junctional space between the two cells. Upon contact with the target cell, they undergo a conformational change, become embedded in the cytoplasmic membrane, and, in the presence of Ca^{2+}, polymerize to form a cylindrical pore. The pore size is large enough to allow other substances released from the granules to enter easily. The target cells swell and are destroyed by osmotic lysis.

103. The answer is D. *(Microbiology)*

Some of the plasma cells generated after a first encounter with an antigen (the primary response) are thought to differentiate into long-lived memory B lymphocytes, which persist primarily in lymphoid follicles.

The antibody secreted by memory B cells is of higher average affinity than that produced by the cells during a primary response. This presumably results from immunoglobulin class switch and to somatic hypermutation in the variable domains of the immunoglobulin genes during a primary response. The affinity of the antibody continues to increase during secondary and subsequent exposures to the antigen.

104. The answer is D. *(Microbiology)*

The direct version of the Coombs test would be performed to determine if the infant has maternal IgG (anti-Rh) already bound to the erythrocytes in the cord blood. IgG antibodies are relatively small. When they coat large particles or cells, such as erythrocytes, they do not readily agglutinate them. In the direct Coombs test, anti-immunoglobulin (antibody against the Fc region of human IgG) is directly added to the infant's erythrocytes. The anti-immunoglobulin (also known as Coombs reagent) spans the distance between cells to form an agglutinating lattice that can be visualized in the test tube. The indirect Coombs test is a two-step procedure that identifies antibodies in the serum, rather than antibodies coating the red blood cells.

105. The answer is A. *(Microbiology)*
The complement fixation test is used in the diagnosis of psittacosis, other chlamydial infections, and a number of viral infections. Lysis of red blood cells in the test indicates that complement fixation did not occur in the first stage of the assay, which, in turn, indicates that the patient has no antibodies against *Chlamidia psittaci*. The test is performed in two stages as follows:

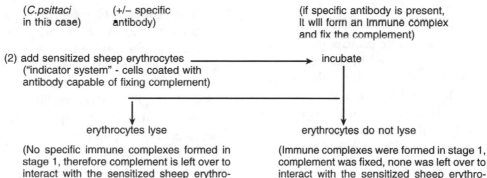

(1) known antigen + patient's serum + complement → incubate

    (*C.psittaci*   (+/– specific   (if specific antibody is present,
    in this case)   antibody)   it will form an immune complex
                                                  and fix the complement)

(2) add sensitized sheep erythrocytes ⟶ incubate
    ("indicator system" - cells coated with
    antibody capable of fixing complement)

                 erythrocytes lyse   erythrocytes do not lyse
    (No specific immune complexes formed in   (Immune complexes were formed in stage 1,
    stage 1, therefore complement is left over to   complement was fixed, none was left over to
    interact with the sensitized sheep erythro-   interact with the sensitized sheep erythro-
    cytes)   cytes)

The complement fixation test is not done to determine complement activity or the level of any specific component. The patient's serum is heat-inactivated at 56°C for 30 minutes to destroy complement prior to testing. A predetermined, known amount of complement (often from guinea pig) is then added to the test system in stage 1.

106. The answer is A. *(Microbiology)*
In the mixed lymphocyte culture (MLC) test, donor and recipient lymphocytes are incubated together with tritiated thymidine for several days. The test is performed to determine the degree of compatibility of the human leukocyte antigen (HLA) systems (particularly the HLA-D locus) of the donor and recipient. When lymphocytes of two HLA-disparate persons are mixed, the cells become large and blast-like, and begin synthesizing DNA. The tritiated thymidine is incorporated into the DNA. A high level of radioactivity within the cells signals histoincompatibility, whereas little or no radioactivity indicates histocompatibility.

107. The answer is A. *(Behavioral science)*
A man who enjoys watching a neighbor undressing in her apartment is a voyeur. Voyeurism is a sexual paraphilia. Like other paraphiliacs, voyeurs rarely seek help for their problem. Voyeurs are often married. While the voyeur gets sexual gratification out of sneaking observations of unclothed, unsuspecting women, he does not desire to meet or have sex with the victim, and he is also unlikely to rape the victim.

108. The answer is D. *(Microbiology)*
The α-hemolytic streptococci are the most important group of organisms responsible for subacute bacterial endocarditis, and they constitute the major group of facultative organisms in the oral cavity. The classic source of infection involves oral bacteria that have obtained entrance to the bloodstream as a result of dental manipulations. These organisms then colonize previously injured heart valves and grow. *Streptococcus salivarius* is a typical α-hemolytic oral streptococcus

that can be involved in this situation. Although group A streptococci (*S. pyogenes*) is the major direct cause of postinfectious rheumatic heart disease, the situation described involves a history of dental work within the last five weeks.

Haemophilis influenzae is a gram-negative rod. *S. faecaelis* is normally found in the intestinal tract and is found in very small numbers in the oral cavity on an intermittant basis. *S. agalactiae* is β-hemolytic and is a part of the normal vaginal flora. *Staphylococcus aureus* is a gram-positive coccus, but it is more likely to be involved in a rapidly acute clinical situation in which the time frame is days, rather than weeks.

109. The answer is D.   (Microbiology)
Interferons (IFNs) are host-coded proteins that inhibit viral replication and are produced by animals or cell cultures in response to viral infection or other induction. They are the cell's first defense against viral infection. Interferons are also cytokines, and play significant roles in modulating cellular and humoral immunity.

The three major groups of interferons are IFN-α, IFN-β, and IFN-γ. Interferons are produced in a virus-infected cell when repressed host genes are activated by products of the virus growth cycle. They are produced within hours of virus infection, well before the humoral immune system produces antibodies against the viruses. IFNs are released to the outside of the cell and attach to receptors on cells not yet infected by viruses. A signal is sent to the nucleus of the second cell, inducing the formation of an antiviral protein. The antiviral protein directly interferes with any viral messenger RNA metabolism that may result from viral infection of the second cell. This eliminates or supresses viral growth so that the virus load in the infected host (or cell culture) is lessened.

IFN's are species specific (i.e., human IFNs work best in human cells and mouse IFNs work best in mouse cells). However, interferons inhibit a broad range of viruses. There is no viral specificity, as is observed in immunoglobulins, which are specifically able to react with one type of virus. The mechanism of action of IFN is the production of antiviral protein, which directly interferes with viral messenger RNA metabolism. IFNs do not directly interfere with any host cell enzyme function that would be responsible for inhibition of virus growth within the host cell.

110. The answer is C.   (Microbiology)
Unstimulated B lymphocytes produce antibody molecules that have a hydrophobic domain at the carboxyl terminus of their heavy chains. This domain anchors the molecules in the cell membrane. Upon stimulation by antigen, the cell splices its heavy chain messenger RNA differently, so that the antibody has a hydrophilic region at the carboxyl terminus of its heavy chains. Because the membrane-anchoring domain is no longer present, the antibody is secreted from the cell. This is an example of how alternative splicing of messenger RNA can be used to produce two slightly different products from the same gene.

111. The answer is C.   (Microbiology)
A high concentration of immunoglobulin M (IgM) in the serum of a newborn is a sign that the infant has been infected before birth. IgM is the only class of antibody which can be synthesized by the fetus. This ability begins at about the fifth month of gestation. IgM is important in early defense, and it appears first in a primary response against many antigens. IgG is the most abundant class of antibody present in the serum of newborns, but it reflects the immunological status of the mother, not the infant. IgG, IgA, IgD, and IgE synthesis in the infant begins shortly after birth (although trace amounts of IgA may be produced before birth).

112. The answer is E.   (Pathology)
A nontender mass in the parotid gland is most likely a mixed tumor (pleomorphic adenoma). It is the most common overall salivary gland tumor, and the parotid gland is the most common location. The term mixed indicates that two types of tissue are present in the tumor, an epithelial component and a myxomatous, often cartilaginous-appearing, stroma. However, both types of tissue derive from the same cell layer, so it is not synonymous with a teratoma, which is a tumor derived from all three cell layers.

113. The answer is A.   (Pathology)
The pedigree represents a sex-linked recessive inheritance pattern, which is the mode of inheritance of Lesch-Nyhan syndrome. In sex-linked recessive disorders, only males are affected. Affected males pass the abnormal gene to their daughters, all of whom are

asymptomatic carriers. Affected males do not transmit the disease to their sons.

	X*	Y
X	X*X	XY
X	X*X	XY

XY: normal male
X*Y: affected male

XX: normal female
X*X: carrier female

The sons and daughters of asymptomatic female carriers each have a 50% chance of inheriting the abnormal gene. Unaffected males do not transmit the disease to any of their offspring.

	X	Y
X*	X*X	X*Y
X	XX	XY

It is remotely possible that female carriers (particularly those also carrying the gene for glucose-6-phosphate dehydrogenase deficiency) could have the normal X chromosome inactivated (rather than the X chromosome with the abnormal gene) and thus exhibit symptoms of the disease.

In the pedigree depicted in the question, note that because only carrier daughters (not shown) transmit the disease to their sons, a generation is skipped. If the carrier females are shown in the pedigree, it is as follows:

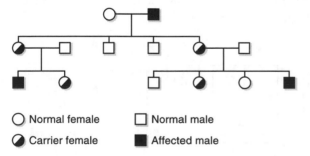

○ Normal female   □ Normal male
◑ Carrier female   ■ Affected male

Lesch-Nyhan syndrome results from a deficiency of hypoxanthine guanine phosphoribosyl transferase (HGPRT), which normally inhibits the action of 5-phosphoribosyl-1-pyrophosphate (PRPP) in purine synthesis. Deficiency of the HGPRT allows PRPP to increase the synthesis of uric acid, which causes hyperuricemia. Additional findings include mental retardation, self-mutilation, and involuntary movements.

114. The answer is C.   *(Pathology)*
Cardiac defects, gastrointestinal disease, mental retardation, and a predisposition for acute leukemia best characterizes the constellation of findings associated with Down syndrome. Down syndrome is most commonly associated with trisomy 21 (95% of cases), with the extra chromosome 21 coming from the mother.

115. The answer is D.   *(Pathology)*
The pedigree exhibits the concept of reduced penetrance, which primarily occurs in autosomal dominant diseases such as neurofibromatosis. When the frequency of expression of an autosomal dominant trait is below 100%, the trait is said to exhibit reduced penetrance. For example, 50% penetrance means that 50% of those who carry the gene express the disease and 50% do not express the disease. However, the 50% of those who do not express the trait are still capable of transmitting the disease to their offspring. In the pedigree depicted in the question, note that although both males and females express the disease, none of the three first-generation males express the disease. However, two of the males have offspring with the disease and one does not. This indicates that although penetrance in first-generation males was 0%, they were able to transmit the disease to their male and female offspring.

116. The answer is B.   *(Pathology)*
The pedigree is an example of an autosomal dominant inheritance pattern, which is consistent with congenital spherocytosis. Key features of autosomal dominant diseases include the following:

- Only one parent has to have the disease in order to transmit it to offspring, unless the disease is the result of a new mutation.
- An affected individual bears, on the average, both normal and affected offspring in equal proportion.

- Normal children of affected parents have normal offspring.
- Either males or females can inherit or transmit the disease.
- Autosomal dominant disease can express itself in a heterozygote or a homozygote condition.
- Homozygotes usually die in utero, because the disease is so severe.

The following diagrams depict some of the possible combinations of autosomal dominant inheritance.

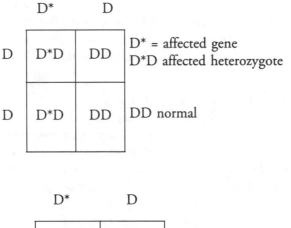

D* = affected gene
D*D affected heterozygote

DD normal

In the pedigree depicted in the question, note that the disease is present in both male and females, and that only one parent has to have the disease to transmit it to offspring.

117. The answer is D. (Pathology)
The pedigree is an example of an autosomal recessive inheritance pattern, which is consistent with sickle cell disease. Sickle cell disease is due to a substitution of valine for glutamic acid in the sixth position of the beta globin chain. It is the most common genetic hemolytic anemia among African-Americans. Key features of autosomal recessive disease include the following:

- Both parents must have the abnormal gene in order to transmit the disease to their children.

- Heterozygotes do not express the disease, and homozygotes do express the disease.
- Males and females are equally affected.
- The less frequent the mutant gene in the population, the greater the chance that affected individuals are the products of a consanguineous marriage.
- They are more commonly diagnosed in children than in adults.
- They generally involve enzyme defects (inborn errors of metabolism).

Each child has one chance in four of being affected if both parents are heterozygotes (asymptomatic carriers):

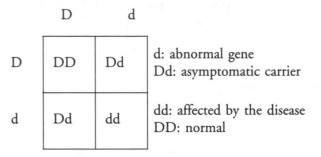

d: abnormal gene
Dd: asymptomatic carrier

dd: affected by the disease
DD: normal

Each child has two chances in four (50%) of being infected if one of the parents has the disease and the other is an asymptomatic carrier:

	D	d
d	Dd	dd
d	Dd	dd

Each child has a 100% chance of being affected if both parents have the disease:

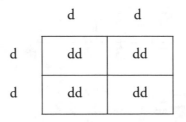

In the pedigree depicted in the question, the female is the initial carrier of the disease and married a normal male (see completed pedigree below). One of their two daughters is a carrier and married a carrier male resulting in 1 affected male, 2 carrier females, and 1 normal child

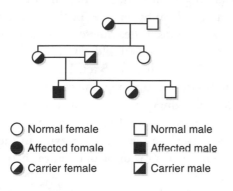

○ Normal female   □ Normal male
● Affected female   ■ Affected male
◐ Carrier female   ◪ Carrier male

Methionine → S-adenosylmethionine → S-adenosylhomocysteine → homocysteine

$$\text{homocysteine} \xrightarrow{\text{Cystathionine synthetase}} \text{cystathionine}$$

It resembles Marfan syndrome in some of its clinical features. The majority of patients affected by homocystinuria have arachnodactyly and a tendency for dislocated lens. Features that differentiate homocystinuria from Marfan syndrome are mental retardation, the tendency for thromboembolic phenomenon due to build-up of homocysteine, and osteoporosis.

Marfan syndrome is an autosomal dominant disease characterized by a defect in fibrillin, an important component of elastin. Areas affected include the skeleton, eyes, and cardiovascular system. Patients have eunuchoid skeletal proportions, in which the lower body is longer than the upper body, and arm span is greater than height. In addition, the patients have arachnodactyly (long fingers). Weakness of elastic tissue results in dislocated lens in the eye. Patients are predisposed to dissecting aortic aneurysms, which is the most common cause of death. The incidence of mitral valve prolapse is also increased.

119. The answer is C.   *(Pathology)*
Given the carrier rate for a genetic disease, the number of affected individuals in the population (prevalence) of a genetic disease can be calculated. If the carrier rate of sickle cell disease, an autosomal recessive disease, is 1 in 12, the number of black couples at risk is the carrier rate in males multiplied by the carrier rate in

118. The answer is A.   *(Pathology, Genetics)*
The similarity between homocystinuria and Marfan syndrome is an example of genetic heterogeneity. In genetic heterogeneity, mutations at several different loci produce the same genetic trait. For example, there are many different autosomal recessive diseases with different genetic abnormalities that result in nerve deafness. Homocystinuria is an autosomal recessive disease characterized by a deficiency of cystathionine synthetase:

females, or 1 in 144 ($1/12 \times 1/12$). Because sickle cell disease is autosomal recessive, there is a 1 in 4 chance of having a child with sickle cell disease. Therefore, $1/144 \times 1/4 = 1/576$.

120. The answer is E.   *(Pathology)*
The patient most likely died from the sudden infant death syndrome (SIDS), or crib death, the etiology of which is still unknown. The definition of SIDS is the sudden death of an infant under one year of age, in which the death remains unexplained even after a complete autopsy, examination of the death scene, and review of the previous clinical history (e.g., previous infection). The incidence is approximately 2/1000 live births. SIDS primarily occurs between 1 month and 1 year of age, with a peak age of 2 to 4 months. Death usually occurs while the child is sleeping (between midnight and 8 A.M.). The majority of patients have a history of minor upper respiratory infection.

The pathogenesis is still unknown. It is estimated that 10% of cases are the result of some inborn error of metabolism. Apnea and abnormal temperature control have been implicated and these may be related to prematurity and low birth weight, with possible neural development delay. Sleeping prone has also been implicated (nose and mouth are buried in soft mattress). The current recommendation is to place babies in a supine position on a hard mattress for sleeping.

121. The answer is E.   *(Biochemistry)*
The Clinitest reaction only detects reducing substances. Reducing sugars such as fructose, galactose, glucose, lactose, and pentose react with chemical agents in the Clinitest tablet (copper sulfate, sodium citrate, sodium carbonate, and sodium hydroxide) and produce a color reaction. Excess, undigested sucrose, a nonreducing sugar, in diarrheal fluid would not be detected by the Clinitest reaction. The Clinitest used to be the test of choice to screen the urine of diabetics for glucose, before glucose-specific reagent strips were developed. Screening the urine of newborns for reducing substances is useful in the detection of inborn errors of metabolism, such as fructokinase and galactokinase deficiencies. Ascorbic acid is a reducing agent, so it too reacts with Clinitest. Clinitest tablets are also used to test for reducing substances in stool in the presence of disaccharidase deficiencies (e.g., lactase deficiency).

In the absence of sucrase, sucrose cannot be broken down into fructose and glucose within the bowel. The increase in sucrose in the stool is acted upon by anaerobes in the colon. These anaerobes break down the sucrose into fatty acids, hydrogen gas, and carbon dioxide. Fatty acids are osmotically active and produce an osmotic diarrhea.

122. The answer is B.   *(Microbiology)*
Disinfection is removal or destruction of potentially pathogenic microorganisms. Surface-active agents such as detergents, substituted phenols, alcohols, heavy metals, and oxidizing agents can disinfect a surface. If a detergent is used simultaneously with an alcohol, the detergent would dissolve in the alcohol, which is an organic solvent, and would lose its surfactant properties.

123. The answer is A.   *(Pathology)*
Pluripotential stem cells divide into lymphoid stem cells for development of B and T cells, and into a trilineage myeloid stem cell from which all the other hematopoietic elements are derived (i.e., red blood cells, neutrophils, eosinophils, basophils, and platelets).

Severe combined immunodeficiency (SCID) is a heterogeneous group of conditions characterized by both B and T cell deficiencies. It includes both autosomal and sex-linked recessive diseases, and is more common in females. Classic SCID involves a defect in lymphoid progenitor cells, resulting in a deficiency of both B and T lymphocytes (A in the schematic). A deficiency of adenosine deaminase is a common variant that is associated with a build-up of adenine, which is toxic to B and T lymphocytes. Patients experience protracted diarrhea, vomiting, and cough, usually associated with pneumocystis pneumonia. Candida infections are also common. Recently, gene therapy has been used to replace the normal enzyme in these patients. A bone marrow transplant offers the best chance for cure.

Common variable immune deficiency (CVID) comprises a heterogeneous group of conditions in which patients experience recurring bacterial infections and decreased immunoglobulin levels. Onset is between 15 and 35 years of age. CVID is characterized by a failure of mature B cells to differentiate into plasma cells (D in the schematic). These cells are not able to secrete normal levels of immunoglobulin even when enhanced by CD4 T helper cells. Patients are prone to a variety of conditions, including diarrhea caused by giardia infection, autoimmune diseases, increased risk for lymphoid malignancies, malabsorption, lactose intolerance, pernicious anemia, and noncaseating granulomas at various body sites. Hypogammaglobulinemia is present, but unlike Bruton agammaglobulinemia, normal numbers of B cells are present peripherally and in the lymph nodes. Plasma cells, however, are not present.

Bruton agammaglobulinemia is a sex-linked recessive disease due to a failure of pre–B cells to differentiate into B cells (B in the schematic). All immunoglobulins are decreased, and lymph nodes lack germinal centers and plasma cells. Patients are particularly susceptible to infections resulting from *Streptococcus pneumoniae* or other encapsulated bacteria, but do well against viruses (except echoviruses) and fungi, which are usually handled by cellular immunity. Respiratory infections (i.e., sinusitis, pneumonia, otitis media) and skin infections (i.e., cellulitis, abscesses) usually predominate after the age of 4 months, when maternal immunoglobulins have subsided. In addition, there is a high incidence of autoimmune and immunoproliferative diseases (e.g., B- and T-cell lymphomas). Patients must be given intravenous infusions of immunoglobulin.

DiGeorge syndrome (thymic hypoplasia) is characterized by failure of the third and fourth pharyngeal pouches to develop, with subsequent absence of the parathyroid glands and thymus (*E* in the schematic). No distinct genetic predisposition is associated with the syndrome, and it is thought to be the result of malformation during the eighth week of intrauterine development. Patients have low-set ears, small jaws, and major cardiac vessel abnormalities (e.g., of the truncus arteriosus). The first clinical sign is hypoparathyroidism. Clinical presentation usually relates to cardiac failure due to vessel abnormalities or tetany due to hypoparathyroidism. Patients have varying susceptibilities to infection (e.g., septicemia), chronic candidiasis, and pneumocystis pneumonia. Patients are deficient in peripheral T cells, and T-cell function is defective. Thymus grafts have been utilized with some success in these patients.

Selective immunoglobulin A (IgA) deficiency occurs in 1 in 500 individuals and is the most common hereditary immunodeficiency. It may be either autosomal recessive or autosomal dominant. The disease is characterized by an intrinsic defect in the differentiation of immature B cells into mature B cells committed to synthesizing IgA (*C* in the schematic). Patients have decreased serum and secretory IgA, but serum IgG and IgM are normal. Many of these patients have selective IgG_2 and IgG_4 subclass deficiencies. IgA has a J chain attached to secretory IgA that prevents microorganisms and pollens from binding to epithelial cells. Patients may be asymptomatic, but the most common clinical manifestations of the deficiency are sinopulmonary infections. Patients may also experience diarrhea due to giardia infection. There is an increased incidence of allergies and autoimmune disease. Patients with anti-IgA antibodies are at increased risk for an anaphylactic reaction if they receive blood components containing IgA. Most patients do well with antibiotic therapy alone.

124. The answer is D.   *(Behavioral science)*
If she is mentally competent, this patient can refuse a cesarian section that is necessary to save her baby's life. Because the patient has this right, getting a court order to do the procedure, having the father consent to the procedure, or contacting a law enforcement or social service agency would not be appropriate. It is appropriate to consult a consultation liaison psychiatrist to speak to the patient about consenting to the cesarian; however, the patient has the final decision in this case.

125. The answer is B.   *(Behavioral science)*
In unipolar depression, REM sleep is characterized by a long first REM period, a short latency, and a shift in REM sleep from the end of the sleep cycle to the beginning of the night. In addition, more time is spent in REM sleep in major depression than when the individual is not depressed.

126. The answer is D.   *(Microbiology)*
Toxins produced by bacteria fall into into two groups: exotoxins and endotoxins. Endotoxins are part of the cell wall structure of gram-negative bacteria and are released when the organisms lyse. They are polysaccharide in nature and no toxoids can be formed from them. They are poorly antigenic.

Exotoxins are polypeptide (i.e., protein) in nature and are generally excellent antigens. Alteration by chemicals or heat produce toxoids. These modified forms lose pathogenicity, but retain antigenicity. They form excellent products for vaccines. Exotoxins are produced in the cell's cytoplasm and released either by an excretory process or by cell lysis. Many gram-positive and gram-negative bacteria produce exotoxins of significant medical importance. Examples include tetanus, botulism, and diphtheria (all gram positive) and the gram-negative neurotoxin produced by *Shigella dysenteriae*.

127. The answer is D.   *(Biochemistry)*
Alcohol stimulates the liver microsomal cytochrome P-450 mono-oxygenase system, which increases the metabolism of compounds (e.g., alcohol, drugs, vitamin D) normally handled by this system. This is one reason why alcoholics become more tolerant of alcohol the more they drink. When the cytochrome P-450 system is stimulated, synthesis of the enzyme γ-glutamyltransferase is increased, making this enzyme an excellent marker for following alcoholics in rehabilitation programs.

128. The answer is A. *(Microbiology)*
The extracellular fluid (ECF) volume constitutes approximately one-third of the total body water (TBW), or about 12–19 L. This compartment includes two subcompartments separated by the capillary membrane: blood plasma (intravascular fluid) and interstitial fluid. The ECF volume is measured with a test substance that does not penetrate the cells. Therefore, it has become common to measure the volume distribution of a specific substance and refer to it as, for example, the inulin space, if the test substance is inulin. All substances used to measure the ECF volume must cross capillaries and distribute at the same concentration in plasma and interstitial fluid.

129. The answer is A. *(Microbiology)*
Once a B cell has been "programmed" to secrete an antibody of a certain specificity, it is commited for life. The specificity of antibody secreted by a single plasmacyte or clone of genetically identical plasmacytes never changes.

130. The answer is E. *(Microbiology)*
Herpesviruses are DNA-containing viruses that are assembled in the nucleus of the host cell. After attachment and virion entry into the cytoplasm, the capsid releases the linear, double-stranded genome into the cytoplasm. It migrates to the nucleus and undergoes three stages of messenger RNA production and translation (cytoplasm). Virion maturation occurs in the nucleus, and the viruses acquire the envelopes from the nuclear membrane. Mature viruses are released by cell lysis.

Most of the growth cycle events of influenza viruses, measles, mumps, and retroviruses occur within the cytoplasm of the host cell. Influenza viruses and retroviruses use the host nucleus for some stages of their growth. All of these viruses, however, assemble final mature virions at the cytoplasmic membrane, where they are released by a budding process. At this time, they acquire their envelopes from the cytoplasmic, or plasma, membranes of the host cell.

131. The answer is E. *(Biochemistry)*
Dihydrofolate reductase catalyzes the reduction of inactive folate to the active compound tetrahydrofolate. Inhibition of this enzyme (e.g., by methotrexate)

would result in inhibition of any reaction requiring tetrahydrofolate. Derivatives of tetrahydrofolate are required for the synthesis of all purine nucleotides, including adenosine monophosphate (AMP), guanosine 5'-monophosphate (GMP), and inosine 5'-monophosphate (IMP). A tetrahydrofolate derivative is also required for the synthesis of the pyrimidine nucleotide thymidine monophosphate (TMP) by the enzyme thymidylate synthetase. Tetrahydrofolate is not involved in synthesis of the pyrimidine nucleotides uridine 5'-monophosphate (UMP) or cytidine monophosphate (CMP).

132. The answer is A. *(Microbiology)*
Polioviruses belong to the picornavirus family and are enteroviruses, along with coxsackie and enteric cytopathic human orphan (ECHO) viruses. These viruses are ingested via contaminated water or food and replicate in the oropharynx and intestinal tract. Viruses are excreted in feces.

The Salk (killed) and Sabin (live) vaccines are excellent, giving rise to long-term protection. Most natural infections are subclinical, giving rise to protective antibodies. All three polio types must be protected against. No permanent carrier state occurs following infection. Paralytic poliomyelitis occurs after a persistent viremia and subsequent brain stem involvement.

Polioviruses contain positive-sense, single-stranded RNA genomes, which can act directly as messenger RNA. Structural and polymerase proteins are produced from a post-translational cleavage of a large polyprotein translated from the viral genome.

133. The answer is C. *(Microbiology)*
The term "clonal" in monoclonal antibodies (MAbs) refers to the fact that a clone of genetically identical immunoglobulin-secreting cells are generated during the process of making MAbs. DNA cloning refers to production of multiple copies of DNA (e.g., the polymerase chain reaction).

All MAbs in a given batch bind to a single epitope. Their high specificity is considered to be a great advantage in interpreting results of in vitro assays and when used in vivo for a specific purpose. Polyclonal antibodies are derived from more than one activated B lymphocyte and have differing fine specificities.

During the production of MAbs, spleen cells and myeloma cells (malignant B cells) from an immunized mouse (or other animal) are fused together. Polyethylene glycol is a common agent used for fusion. Some of the spleen cells will be plasma cells activated by the immunizing antigen. The fusion results in an immortal MAb-secreting hybridoma cell. Supernatants of the fused cells are tested for antibody and the desired hybridomas are selected and propagated (cloned) in mass cultures. This technique allows for production of immunologically, chemically, and physically homogenous antibodies in virtually unlimited quantities.

Infusion of MAb (usually derived from mouse hybridomas) into a human results in human anti-mouse antibodies, which will form immune complexes with the MAb. In order to decrease the chance of this occurring, chimeric MAbs have been designed, in which the constant portion of both light and heavy chains is human and only the variable portion is murine. A few totally human hybridomas have also been developed.

134. The answer is D. *(Biochemistry)*
Sigma factor is a protein subunit of bacterial RNA polymerase that is involved in initiation of transcription in RNA synthesis. All other factors listed are involved in initiation of translation, or protein synthesis, in bacteria. AUG is the chain initiation codon. The 30S ribosomal subunit binds to the message and becomes aligned with the initiating codon. Formylmethionine is the amino acid used by bacteria to initiate protein synthesis in response to the first AUG. GTP provides the energy required for initiation, elongation, and termination of protein synthesis.

135. The answer is B. *(Microbiology)*
Potentially self-reactive B and T lymphocytes normally exist in the body. There are circulating B lymphocytes capable of producing autoantibodies against thyroid proteins and DNA. Studies also show autologous T-cell reactivity against pancreatic islet cells in normal animals.

136. The answer is E. *(Microbiology)*
Spores are a mechanism that allows bacteria to survive harsh environments that would kill vegetative forms. *Bacillus* and *Clostridium* organisms are gram-positive rods that are capable of forming spores when nutrients, such as sources of carbon and nitrogen, are depleted.

Spores contain DNA, a small amount of cytoplasm, cytoplasmic membrane, peptidoglycan, very little water, and a thick coat, which is resistant to heat, dehydration, radiation, and chemicals. Because they are within the confines of the bacteria, they do not take up a Gram stain.

The medical significance of spores is their extraordinary resistance to these forces. Although they are resistant to boiling, spores can be destroyed by autoclave conditions (121°C for 15 minutes).

Once formed, spores have essentially no metabolic activity. Dormancy can last for years. When returned to an environment with nutrients and water, enzymes degrade the coat and the spore germinates into a vegetative cell. Human disease results from vegetative cell growth or products.

137. The answer is C. *(Behavioral science)*
The divorce rate is higher for second than for first marriages. Overall, the divorce rate is at least 45% of marriages. Divorce is associated with marriage at a young age, and children of divorced parents have a higher divorce rate themselves. Most divorced people marry again; men are more likely to remarry than women.

138. The answer is D. *(Microbiology)*
A virus isolated from a stool specimen and containing double-stranded RNA (dsRNA) would be a rotavirus (reovirus group). The dsRNA is present in segments, and each segment codes for a different protein. The replication of the dsRNA is dependent upon a virion-contained, RNA-dependent RNA polymerase, which synthesizes viral messenger RNA. Because rotaviruses contain an RNA genome, there is no role for a DNA polymerase. This is not true for retroviruses, which use an RNA-dependent DNA polymerase to produce a DNA copy of the retroviral RNA genome.

Rotaviruses are ubiquitous and are the single most important world-wide cause of viral gastroenteritis in children, particularly during the winter months. While asymptomatic infections are common in infants younger than 6 months of age, reinfection does occur and may reflect the presence of multiple serotypes of virus. No evidence of genome (provirus) incorporation into the host cell chromosome has been reported.

139. The answer is D. *(Behavioral science)*
This child has experienced night terrors. Night terrors are a form of fright in which a person, usually a child, awakens in terror. Generally, the child cannot remember that he or she was aroused nor can the child remember a dream, despite careful questioning. Night terrors occur during slow-wave sleep, and may develop into sleepwalking episodes. They may be an early sign of temporal lobe epilepsy.

140. The answer is C. *(Microbiology)*
Latency is defined as a period of infection where whole or live viruses are not produced, except during intermittent episodes of acute disease, which are called recurrences. A chronic infection is one in which low, but detectable, numbers of viruses are produced by the host. Hepatitis A virus (HAV) is the only virus listed that does not develop a chronic or latent infection. It is an enterovirus, spread by fecal–oral transmission. It is endemic in most countries of the world and is often spread by ingestion of contaminated water. Many infections are subclinical and complete recovery occurs in most HAV infections. Chronic carrier situations do not occur in HAV infections.

All herpesviruses (cytomegalovirus and herpes simplex viruses) routinely develop latent infections. The causative agent for subacute sclerosing panencephalitis (SSPE) is a temperature-sensitive mutant of the rubeola, or measles, virus. The latency period of SSPE can be 10 to 20 years. Hepatitis B virus (HBV) is known to cause acute and chronic infections. In the case of HBV infection, chronic carrier status is determined when surface antigen is present for more than six months.

141. The answer is C. *(Microbiology)*
Measles virus (rubeola) infection can result in quite severe complications. Encephalitis occurs in 1/1000 cases, with a mortality rate of 10%. Permanent sequelae occur in 40% of such cases. Most fatalities that occur in measles complications arise from pneumonia.

Rotaviruses are the single most important worldwide cause of gastroenteritis in young children. Estimates of annual infection in children between the ages of 6 months and 5 years range from 0.5 to 1.0 billion, with an estimated 3.5 million deaths. Treatment consists of rehydration and electrolyte replacement.

Parainfluenza virus types 1 and 2 are major causes of croup, as well as pharyngitis. Respiratory syncytial virus is the most important cause of pneumonia and bronchiolitis in infants. The testes can be infected secondarily by mumps virus viremia. Unilateral orchitis, while painful, does not lead to sterility.

142. The answer is C. *(Behavioral science)*
Anorexia nervosa is not associated with mental retardation; anorexic individuals are often high academic achievers. Anorexia nervosa is characterized by the loss of 15% or more of body weight and by abnormal behavior in dealing with food; anorexic individuals are hungry but refuse to eat. It is more common during late adolescence, in upper socioeconomic groups, and in girls.

143. The answer is E. *(Microbiology)*
Adenoviruses routinely cause a wide variety of diseases, although approximately half of all such infections are asymptomatic. Upper respiratory tract infections include pharyngitis, pharyngoconjunctival fever, and acute respiratory disease (presenting as fever, sore throat, coryza, and conjunctivitis). Atypical pneumonia occurs in lower respiratory tract infection, with fever, cough, and patchy consolidation. Gastroenteritis with nonbloody diarrhea occurs mainly in children under 2 years of age.

Heterophil-negative mononucleosis is typically involved in cytomegalovirus and toxoplasmosis infections.

144. The answer is D. *(Behavioral science)*
Long-term nursing home care is not paid for by either part A or part B of Medicare. The patient is responsible for these expenses. Medicare B covers therapy, medical supplies, laboratory tests, outpatient hospital care, doctor bills, ambulance service, and medical equipment.

145. The answer is C. *(Behavioral science)*
Bipolar illness does not show any racial, ethnic, or gender differences in its occurrence. Obesity, hypertension, diabetes, and heart disease are more common in African-Americans than in white individuals.

146. The answer is E. *(Behavioral science)*
Of the listed individuals, the homeless schizophrenic man is least likely to be committed for involuntary

treatment. This is because a patient must be shown to be both mentally ill and a danger to himself or others in order to be committed for involuntary treatment. A depressed man who expresses an intent to commit suicide, a schizophrenic man who has threatened to kill his parents, a borderline patient who has threatened to kill his psychiatrist, and an Alzheimer patient who starts fires in his apartment all are at high risk for injury to themselves or others and are thus more likely to be committed for involuntary treatment.

147. The answer is A.   *(Behavioral science)*
For informed consent a patient must understand what will happen if he or she does not consent to a given procedure, understand the diagnosis, understand the benefits of the procedure, and understand that consent can be withdrawn at any time. A formal document, although desirable, is not strictly required for informed consent.

148. The answer is D.   *(Behavioral science)*
Suicide, depression, and changes in sleep patterns are more common among the elderly than in the general population. Anxiety arising from insecurities concerning health and strength arise easily in the elderly. Despite this, most people achieve a sense of ego integrity; that is, satisfaction and pride in one's past accomplishments in old age.

149. The answer is B.   *(Biochemistry)*
Catabolic processes are those that liberate energy. In general, these processes are convergent; that is, a large variety of substances yields relatively few end products. Catabolic reactions may simply involve the breakdown of macromolecules into smaller molecules, (i.e., digestion), or they may be coupled to anabolic reactions and do work, as in the glycolytic and citric acid (Krebs) cycle sequences, in which many different substrates yield the common end products: CO_2, H_2O, NADH, and ATP. Cofactors such as NADH, NADPH, and ATP are often intermediary products that couple a catabolic process to an anabolic one.

150. The answer is C.   *(Behavioral science)*
Biofeedback, in which learning is used to gain control over physiologic activities, is an extension of operant conditioning (i.e. learning by a system of rewards). In contrast, classical conditioning involves learning by association. For biofeedback to be effective, the patient must be motivated to learn and must receive continuous information about the physiologic parameter being conditioned. Biofeedback has been found to be effective in treating hypertension, tension and migraine headache, peptic ulcer, and Raynaud syndrome.

151. The answer is E.   *(Microbiology)*
Many pathogenic bacteria (e.g., *Streptococcus pneumoniae*) have a capsule composed of polysaccharide, which has a high molecular weight and contains multiple repeating antigenic determinants. Antigens of this type are T independent. B lymphocytes can be activated to secrete antibody without the assistance of T helper cells. The combination of antibodies complement activation, and phagocytes are generally considered to be of greater importance in control of bacterial infections than T lymphocytes.

152. The answer is E.   *(Microbiology)*
Type I hypersensitivity is mediated by immunoglobulin E (IgE), the homocytotropic antibody capable of binding to the host's own mast cells and basophils. Subsequent encounter with antigen causes cell surface–receptor aggregation, degranulation of the cell, and the release of pharmacologically active mediators.

IgG is the most versatile of all immunoglobulin classes and performs many functions. When bound to antigen, IgG can fix complement and activate the classical complement cascade. IgG is excellent for neutralization of toxins because of its high affinity for antigen. Toxins neutralized by IgG include those of *Clostridium tetani, Clostridium botulinum, Corynebacterium diphtheriae,* and the venom of snakes, spiders, and scorpions. It is the class of choice for passive immunization. IgG also neutralizes virus infectivity. Viruses infect cells by first attaching to them via surface glycoproteins. IgG directed against these molecules prevents virus attachment and, thus, also prevents infection.

IgG opsonizes bacteria and other foreign particles by binding to them via its two Fab arms. Macrophages and neutrophils are able to phagocytize opsonized particles much more readily than nonopsonized materials. Some particles, including most encapsulated bacteria, are not easily phagocytized until they are opsonized by IgG or one of the complement components. Macrophages and natural killer cells have receptors for the Fc region of IgG. These cells kill IgG-coated targets via antibody-dependent cell-mediated cytotoxicity.

153. The answer is B. *(Biochemistry)*
Hypoglycemia, rather than hyperglycemia, is likely in alcoholics, because the excess reduced nicotinamide adenine dinucleotide (NADH) that results from the metabolism of alcohol converts pyruvate into lactate. Because pyruvate is the key substrate for gluconeogenesis, fasting hypoglycemia should be expected.

154. The answer is E. *(Microbiology)*
Rubella virus, HIV, cytomegalovirus, herpes simplex, varicella-zoster, hepatitis B, and enteroviruses all have the ability of causing prenatal infections. Most maternal viral infections do not result in viremia and fetal involvement. However, if the virus does cross the placenta, serious damage may be done to the fetus.

Respiratory syncytial virus is the most significant respiratory virus of infants 6 months of age or less, causing the deaths of approximately 4500 infants per year. However, viremia of this virus has not been detected. Virus replication occurs primarily in the epithelial cells of the upper respiratory tract and may be spread to the lower respiratory tract by secretions.

Rubella virus and cytomegalovirus are currently the primary viruses responsible for congenital defects in humans. Hepatitis B, herpes simplex, varicella-zoster, measles, mumps, and some enteroviruses may occasionally cause congenital infections.

155. The answer is A. *(Behavioral science)*
Physicians are not more likely to make mistakes now than in the past. However, the number of medical malpractice suits are increasing yearly because doctor–patient relationships are becoming more distant, patients are becoming more suspicious of physicians, and patients have higher expectations of doctors.

156-160. The answers are: 156-F, 157-A, 158-E, 159-D, 160-B. *(Biochemistry)*
All of the diseases described are lysosomal storage diseases. These are a group of diseases in which certain degrading enzymes in the lysosomes are missing, thus leading to an accumulation of complex substrates, such as sphingolipids and glycosaminoglycans (mucopolysaccharides) in the lysosomes. Lysosomes contain hydrolytic enzymes that remain within the intracellular compartment.

Fabry disease is a sex-linked recessive disease resulting from an accumulation of ceramide trihexoside, caused by a deficiency of α-galactocerebrosidase A. It is characterized by angiokeratomas, hypertension, and renal failure.

Gaucher disease is an autosomal recessive disease resulting from an accumulation of glucocerebroside caused by a deficiency of glucocerebrosidase. It is characterized by massive hepatosplenomegaly, macrophages with a fibrillary-appearing material in the cytoplasm, and an increase in total acid phosphatase.

Krabbe disease is an autosomal recessive disease resulting from an accumulation of galactocerebroside caused by a deficiency of galactosylceramidase. It is characterized by abnormal myelination, globoid bodies in the central nervous system, and progressive psychomotor retardation.

Metachromatic leukodystrophy is an autosomal recessive disease resulting from an accumulation of sulfatide caused by a deficiency of arylsulfatase A. It is characterized by synthesis of abnormal myelin, mental retardation, peripheral neuropathy, and metachromatic staining of tissue due to the presence of sulfatides.

Niemann-Pick disease is an autosomal recessive disease resulting from an accumulation of sphingomyelin caused by a deficiency of sphingomyelinase. It is characterized by severe mental retardation, hepatosplenomegaly, foamy macrophages, and zebra bodies visible upon electron microscopy.

161-165. The answers are: 161-D, 162-A, 163-E, 164-C, 165-B. *(Pharmacology)*
Chloramphenicol is metabolized by glucuronidation and neonates lack sufficient glucuronyl transferase to metabolize the drug as rapidly as do older children and adults, thereby contributing to gray baby syndrome.

Microsomal drug oxidations catalyzed by the mixed function oxidases require cytochrome P-450, NADP cofactor, and molecular oxygen.

A genetic polymorphism affecting the amount of N-acetyltransferase results in the bimodal distribution of isoniazid and hydralazine half-lives and plasma drug concentrations.

Aspirin is rapidly hydrolyzed by plasma esterase to salicylic acid, which is then conjugated by phase II enzymes with glycine and glucuronide.

A nonmicrosomal enzyme, alcohol dehydrogenase, is responsible for the first step in ethanol metabolism and is easily saturated by low levels of ethanol, thereby contributing to zero-order ethanol kinetics except at very low plasma levels.

166-170. The answers are: 166-E, 167-D, 168-A, 169-C, 170-B. *(Pharmacology)*

Tetracyclines are bacteriostatic drugs that slow the growth of microbes and may reduce the therapeutic effectiveness of bactericidal drugs that are most active against bacteria in the log-growth phase. This is a form of therapeutic antagonism that is not related either to the direct interaction of these drugs with receptors or to physiologic mechanisms.

Phenoxybenzamine forms a reactive metabolite in vivo that covalently bonds to the α-adrenergic receptor, producing noncompetitive antagonism of α-agonists in which the antagonism is not surmountable. In contrast, drugs such as propranolol exhibit competitive antagonism: receptor binding is reversible and the antagonism is surmountable as concentrations of an agonist such as epinephrine are increased.

Protamine directly combines with and inactivates heparin, thus representing a form of chemical antagonism. Gastric antacids are another type of chemical antagonist.

Epinephrine can counteract the effects of histamine by producing physiologic effects that are opposite to the physiologic effects of histamine, thereby representing an example of physiologic antagonism.

171-174. The answers are: 171-C, 172-B, 173-A, 174-D. *(Microbiology)*

By definition, positive-sense RNA is identical to messenger RNA (mRNA), which can be directly translated into a protein by the ribosome. HIV contains two copies of a positive-sense RNA genome. The virus has a lipid envelope containing glycoprotein 120, which is the viral receptor. In order to grow a host cell, the reverse transcriptase must generate a double-stranded DNA copy of the RNA genome, which is incorporated into the host's chromosome.

Human papilloma viruses belong to the papovavirus group. They possess icosahedral symmetry, with no envelope. They are small (45–55 nm) and possess a circular genome of double-stranded DNA. The usual result of infection in humans is a benign tumor (i.e, a wart) of the surface epithelium. More serious manifestations include genital warts, laryngeal papillomas, and cervical carcinoma.

Varicella-zoster virus is a member of the herpesvirus group. These larger viruses all appear similar in electron micrographs. The virions possess double-stranded linear DNA molecules. The virus has a well-defined lipid envelope with glycoproteins that serve as receptors.

Polioviruses are picornaviruses of the enterovirus subgroup. Other members of this subgroup include coxsackie A and B, enteric cytopathic human orphan virus (ECHO), and hepatitis A virus. These are small icosahedral viruses possessing positive-sense RNA genomes. The single-stranded molecule serves directly as mRNA, producing a polypeptide that is later cleaved into structural proteins and enzymes (post-translational maturation). No lipid envelope is present.

175-180. The answers are: 175-D, 176-A, 177-E, 178-G, 179-B, 180-B. *(Biochemistry)*

Isocitrate (*C*) is converted to α-ketoglutarate (*D*), which is either transaminated, by any of a host of aminotransferases, or aminated by glutamate dehydrogenase to form glutamic acid.

Pyruvate dehydrogenase, which converts pyruvate to acetyl CoA (*A*), is an enzyme complex. It contains three catalytic components (pyruvate decarboxylase, dihydrolipoyl transacetylase, dihydrolipoyl dehydrogenase), uses five cofactors [thiamine pyrophosphate, lipoamide, flavin adenine dinucleotide (FAD), oxidized nicotinamide adenine dinucleotide (NAD^+), coenzyme A (CoA)], and has two regulatory enzymes: a kinase that inactivates the complex by phosphorylating it and a phosphatase that activates it by dephosphorylating it. The kinase is activated by reduced NAD (NADH) and acetyl CoA. This is an example of feedback inhibition by covalent modification. Neither the kinase nor the phosphatase are regulated hormonally. α-Ketoglutarate dehydrogenase is an enzyme complex that is similar to pyruvate dehydrogenase. It has three catalytic components that recognize α-ketoglutarate instead of pyruvate as the substrate, and produce succinyl CoA (*E*) instead of acetyl CoA. It uses the same five cofactors as pyruvate dehydrogenase, but does not have the regulatory component.

The energy of the thioester bond of succinyl CoA is conserved via the thiokinase reaction in which guanosine 5′ diphosphate (GDP) is phosphorylated to form guanosine 5′ triphosphate (GTP). The succinate product of this reaction is dehydrogenated to form fumarate (G), using FAD as a cofactor. Fumarate is also a product of the urea cycle. Fumarate is hydrated to form malate (H), and malate is dehydrogenated to form oxaloacetate (I).

When not used to produce energy, citrate (B) is transported out of the mitochondrion. In tissues other than liver it acts as an important modulator of phosphofructokinase-1, inhibiting glycolysis when the energy needs of the cell are met. In liver this inhibition is overridden by the hormonally regulated production of fructose 2,6-bisphosphate. This permits citrate to be synthesized from glucose even though the cell is satiated. This citrate is then available as substrate for cytoplasmic citrate lyase to form acetyl CoA, the basic building block used for fatty acid synthesis, and to activate acetyl CoA carboxylase, the rate-limiting reaction in fatty acid synthesis. Although acetyl CoA is a substrate for fatty acid synthesis, it does not activate acetyl CoA carboxylase, the rate-limiting enzyme of fatty acid synthesis.

Similarly, succinyl CoA is a substrate for heme synthesis, when not required by the cell for energy. The first step in heme synthesis is the condensation of succinyl CoA with glycine to form 5-aminolevalinate (ALA) in a reaction catalyzed by ALA synthase.

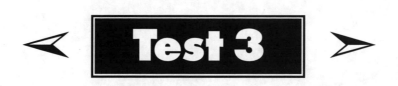

QUESTIONS

DIRECTIONS:

Each of the numbered items or incomplete statements in this section is followed by answers or by completions of the statement. Select the ONE lettered answer or completion that is BEST in each case.

1. Many Asians believe that the spiritual core of a person is located in the

(A) brain
(B) ears
(C) heart
(D) eyes
(E) throat

2. Autotrophic requirements are

(A) CO_2 as a carbon source
(B) NH_3 as a nitrogen source
(C) CO_2 and NH_3 together
(D) essential molecules that the bacteria are unable to synthesize
(E) glucose

3. δ-Aminolevulinate synthase catalyzes the rate-limiting step in the synthesis of

(A) catecholamines
(B) cholesterol
(C) porphyrins
(D) prostaglandins
(E) proline

4. When amphotericin B inhibits fungal growth, which mechanism is affected?

(A) Inhibition of cell-wall synthesis
(B) Inhibition of cytoplasmic membrane function
(C) Inhibition of nucleic acid metabolism
(D) Inhibition of protein synthesis
(E) Inhibition by metabolic analogues

5. A mother brings her 5-month-old infant to the physician for a well-baby checkup. At this time the physician should expect to see

(A) stranger anxiety
(B) a pincer grasp
(C) object permanence
(D) speech using meaningful words
(E) sitting with support

6. A patient with elevated levels of plasma phenylalanine, phenyllactate, phenylacetate, and phenylpyruvate, but a normal level of tetrahydrobiopterin is most likely to be genetically deficient in the enzyme

(A) dihydrobiopterin reductase
(B) dihydrobiopterin synthetase
(C) tryptophan hydroxylase
(D) phenylalanine hydroxylase
(E) tyrosine hydroxylase

7. When you conduct a physical examination on a 2-year-old boy, which of the following procedures is most effective?

(A) Ask the parent to leave the room so that you can handle the child better
(B) Ask the child's permission to do the examination before you begin
(C) Start the examination at the child's feet and work your way up toward the head
(D) Carefully explain to the child what you are going to do and why you are going to do it before you begin
(E) Ask the nurse to restrain the child for ease of examination

8. The nucleotide triplet CTC in the sixth position of the β-chain in DNA forms the complementary nucleotide on messenger RNA (mRNA) that codes for glutamic acid. A point mutation on the β-chain resulting in the nucleotide triplet CAC forms a complementary nucleotide on mRNA that codes for valine. In sickle cell anemia, you would expect the complementary nucleotide triplet on mRNA from 5' to 3' to read

(A) GAG
(B) CTC
(C) GTG
(D) CAC
(E) GUG

9. Which of the following factors most closely correlates with the ability to do abstract math?

(A) Previous exposure to mathematical concepts
(B) Cultural factors
(C) High intelligence quotient
(D) Acquisition of formal operational thought
(E) Female sex

10. Malignant cells characteristically

(A) have a shorter cell cycle than the normal cells in their parent tissue
(B) have the same DNA content as the normal cells in their parent tissue
(C) are contact inhibited in tissue culture
(D) take at least 30 doubling times before they become clinically detectable
(E) have complex biochemical systems

11. A normal child enjoys playing next to other children, but does not play cooperatively with them. This child is most likely to be age

(A) 1 year
(B) 2 years
(C) 4 years
(D) 6 years
(E) 8 years

12. A 25-year-old man with anemia and motor nerve disfunction has elevated levels of coproporphyrin III and δ-aminolevulinic acid (ALA) in the urine. This patient is most likely to have

(A) hyperammonemia
(B) alcaptonuria
(C) jaundice
(D) lead poisoning
(E) folate deficiency

13. In children, interactive or cooperative play typically begins at about age

(A) 1 year
(B) 2 years
(C) 4 years
(D) 6 years
(E) 8 years

14. The passive transfer of immunity is best exemplified by the

(A) administration of the oral polio vaccine
(B) inhalation of *Mycobacterium tuberculosis*
(C) injection of an antibiotic
(D) administration of a toxoid
(E) passage of immunoglobulin G (IgG) from mother to fetus

15. Which of the following parts of the mind develops at approximately the time a child starts first grade?

(A) Ego
(B) Unconscious
(C) Superego
(D) Conscious
(E) Id

16. Cysteine is considered a nonessential amino acid only in the presence of dietary

(A) methionine
(B) serine
(C) folate
(D) phenylalanine
(E) alanine

17. Which of the following tumors characteristically spreads by lymphatics, rather than by vessel invasion?

(A) Follicular carcinoma of the thyroid
(B) Renal adenocarcinoma
(C) Papillary carcinoma of the thyroid
(D) Hepatocellular carcinoma
(E) Osteogenic sarcoma

18. A protein to be secreted from the cell is most likely to have

(A) a hydrophilic signal sequence at its carboxyl terminus
(B) mannose-6-phosphate
(C) a hydrophobic signal sequence at its amino terminus
(D) a binding site for the mitochondrial membrane
(E) carbohydrate residues attached while still in the cytoplasm

19. Two hunters are found dead in a cabin. A half-empty bottle of whiskey is found on the table. On the outside of the cabin, an old bird's nest is noted to have blocked the exhaust system for a wood stove that had been used for warmth during the night? You would expect

(A) profound hypoxemia in both hunters
(B) a distinctive odor in the cabin
(C) visible cyanosis in both hunters
(D) a normal oxygen saturation calculated from the arterial PO_2
(E) that alcohol did not contribute to their death

20. Which of the following vaccines are composed of killed (inactivated) viruses?

(A) Influenza and Salk polio
(B) Respiratory syncytial virus and influenza
(C) Rubella and mumps
(D) Rubella and measles
(E) Sabin polio and parainfluenza

21. Which of the following associations is correct?

(A) Organophosphate poisoning—excessive lacrimation, muscle fasciculations, and decreased red blood cell cholinesterase
(B) Yellow phosphorus poisoning—centrilobular hepatic cell necrosis
(C) Oil of wintergreen ingestion—potential cause of profound metabolic alkalosis
(D) Ethylene glycol poisoning—metabolic acidosis complicated by blindness
(E) *Amanita* poisoning—inhibition of DNA polymerase

22. Proteins containing mannose-6-phosphate are most likely to be incorporated into the

(A) lysosome
(B) Golgi complex
(C) endoplasmic reticulum
(D) nucleus
(E) mitochondrion

23. Which of the following statements concerning radiation is correct?

(A) Lymphocytes are the most radiosensitive of the hematopoietic cells
(B) The longer the wavelength, the greater the penetration into tissue
(C) Stable cells are the most radiosensitive
(D) The central nervous system is most affected in patients receiving total body radiation
(E) Peak sensitivity of proliferating cells to radiation is the late S phase

24. Two weeks after a 5-year-old girl presents with a fever of unknown origin, her serum is assayed for antibodies against *Haemophilius influenzae*. The following results were obtained by the clinical laboratory using a precipitation test.

Serum

Undiluted	1:2	1:4	1:8	1:16	1:32	1:64	1:128	1:256	1:512
–	–	+	+	+	+	+	+	–	–

From this data, it can be correctly concluded that

(A) the patient needs to be immunized against *H. influenzae*

(B) the zone of equivalence is present at the 1:256 and 1:512 dilutions

(C) the patient has a 1:128 antibody titer against *H. influenzae*

(D) the positive results from 1:4 to 1:128 serum dilutions are false positives

(E) the titer cannot be determined from these results

25. Rank the following tissues in decreasing order of sensitivity to radiation.

1. Skeletal muscle
2. Gastrointestinal epithelium
3. Breast tissue
4. Lymphocytes

(A) 2-4-3-1

(B) 4-2-1-3

(C) 2-4-1-3

(D) 4-2-3-1

(E) 3-2-4-1

26. The mortality rate for African-American infants in the United States is approximately

(A) 1.5 times higher than that of white infants

(B) 2.5 times higher than that of white infants

(C) 4.0 times higher than that of white infants

(D) 6.0 times higher than that of white infants

(E) equal to that of white infants

27. Which of the following is more likely to occur in salt water, rather than fresh water drowning?

(A) Volume overload

(B) Faster death

(C) Hemolytic anemia

(D) Hypervolemia

(E) Hyponatremia

28. The greatest chance for long-term survival of an allograft would be expected with a

(A) kidney transplant

(B) heart transplant

(C) cornea transplant

(D) liver transplant

(E) pancreas transplant

29. Heat stroke differs from heat cramps or heat exhaustion in that it

(A) is associated with dehydration
(B) is associated with hypovolemia
(C) is associated with fever
(D) results in a hemorrhagic stroke
(E) is associated with a body temperature less than 40°C

30. In N-linked glycosylation, a core oligosaccharide is transferred to the polypeptide chain after first being attached to a molecule of

(A) serine
(B) phosphatidyl choline
(C) cholesterol
(D) dolichol
(E) threonine

31. Which of the following relationships regarding injury and its consequence is correct?

(A) Frostbite—profound vasoconstriction results in thrombosis of vessels and death of tissue
(B) Laser radiation—similar to a first degree burn in tissue
(C) Electrocution—voltage is more important than current
(D) Microwaves—possible association with acute leukemia and cataracts
(E) Automobile accidents—most common cause of death from 25 to 44 years of age

32. Tetanus immune globulin is used in the therapy of tetanus to neutralize

(A) circulating toxoid
(B) circulating toxin
(C) toxin fixed to nerve tissue
(D) toxoid fixed to nerve tissue
(E) circulating antibodies to tetanus

33. Which of the following relationships regarding drugs of abuse and their effects is correct?

(A) Cocaine—sympathomimetic drug predisposing to sudden cardiac death
(B) Heroin—stimulant associated with pulmonary edema
(C) Marijuana—depressant associated with delayed reaction time
(D) Phencyclidine (PCP)—depressant associated with aggressive behavior
(E) Lysergic acid diethylamide (LSD)—depressant associated with chromosomal breakage

34. Ethyl alcohol is used clinically as an antidote for both methanol and ethylene glycol poisoning. This treatment is effective because

(A) the K_m value of ethanol for alcohol dehydrogenase is much less than that of either of these poisons
(B) ethanol interferes with the conversion of the aldehydic product of ethylene glycol to oxalic acid
(C) ethanol inhibits the release of antidiuretic hormone (vasopressin) and thereby increases the rate of renal secretion of both poisons
(D) the metabolism of ethanol produces reduced nicotinamide adenine dinucleotide (NADH), which decreases the acidosis caused by either poison by promoting the conversion of lactic acid to pyruvic acid, which can then be oxidized
(E) the acetaldehyde produced by the reaction of ethanol with alcohol dehydrogenase competes with the toxic aldehydes produced by the two poisons, thereby reducing their reaction with vital organs

35. Which of the following effects is caused by both oral contraceptives and exogenous estrogens?

(A) No increased risk for endometrial cancer

(B) A decreased risk for ovarian cancer

(C) A decreased risk of malignant transformation of fibrocystic change

(D) An increased predisposition to liver (hepatic) cell adenomas

(E) An increased risk for gallbladder disease

36. A 55-year-old man takes his prescribed medication only intermittently and rarely follows his prescribed diet. The most likely reason for this man's behavior is

(A) he views his physician as distant and unfeeling

(B) he does not understand the doctor's instructions

(C) he does not remember the doctor's instructions

(D) he does not feel ill

(E) he does not understand how the medication can help him

37. In transplantation work-ups, patients who are found to have antihuman leukocyte antigen (anti–HLA) antibodies in their serum on a lymphocyte cross-match are

(A) in danger of having a graft versus host reaction

(B) likely to have an increased incidence of autoimmune disease

(C) no longer acceptable as candidates for an organ transplant

(D) at risk for a hyperacute rejection of an organ transplant

(E) likely to have a rejection of the donor graft by CD8 cytotoxic T cells

38. Methotrexate has been used with great success in the treatment of childhood leukemia. You have been asked to examine cancer cells taken from various patients for susceptibility to methotrexate. After the patients have been treated for several weeks with methotrexate, you recover leukemic white cells. You then prepare cell-free extracts and measure in vitro the interconversions listed as A through E below. In each study, the extracts are supplemented with the required substrates and cofactors, other than a folate derivative. Which of the following reactions would you expect to be markedly inhibited in cells from individuals in which the methotrexate is acting to suppress the cancer's growth?

(A) Tetrahydrofolate from dihydrofolate

(B) Choline from phosphatidylserine

(C) 5′-Phosphoribosyl 4-carboxamide 5-formidoimidazole from 5′-phosphoribosyl 4-carboxamide 5-aminoimidazole

(D) Pyrimidine ring synthesis

(E) Cysteine from methionine

39. Which of the following tests would be most beneficial in the diagnosis of a patient suspected of having chronic granulomatous disease of childhood?

(A) E rosette-forming assay

(B) Cell-mediated cytolysis

(C) Nitroblue tetrazolium (NBT) test

(D) Determination of CD4:CD8 ratio

(E) ^{51}Chromium (^{51}Cr) release assay

40. King George III of Great Britain suffered from intermittent bouts of acute abdominal pain, constipation, a feeling of marked weakness, and dementia. His urine darkened to a port wine color upon exposure to light. A urine sample would most likely be positive for

(A) porphobilinogen

(B) protoporphyrin

(C) coproporphyrin

(D) uroporphyrin

(E) bilirubin

41. A patient developed cellulitis on her foot. The infection failed to respond to penicillin G, but was successfully treated with dicloxacillin. The cellulitis was most likely caused by

(A) group A streptococci
(B) group B streptococci
(C) *Staphylococcus aureus*
(D) *Escherichia coli*
(E) *Pseudomonas aeruginosa*

42. Which of the following statements concerning glutathione (GSH) is true? Glutathione

(A) reductase is a selenium-containing enzyme that scavenges free radicals
(B) serves as a vehicle for the transport of amino acids into some cells
(C) peroxidase is used to maintain hemoglobin in the reduced state
(D) is present in most, if not all cells, in trace quantities
(E) transaminase adds a GSH moiety to a variety of compounds as a detoxification mechanism

43. Ribavirin is used to treat infections caused by

(A) rubeola
(B) rubella virus
(C) respiratory syncytial virus
(D) varicella–zoster virus
(E) cytomegalovirus

44. You are a family practitioner and have presided at the home delivery of an apparently well-developed, healthy baby boy. Upon visiting the infant and mother 4 days later, you notice a peculiar, maple sugar-like odor on the baby's diapers. You arrange for the baby to be seen in 2 days at the nearest university hospital for further tests. You also recommend that the

(A) mother stop nursing and put the baby on a cow's milk formula until the consultation
(B) mother stop nursing and put the baby on a sugar water and juice diet until the consultation
(C) baby's diet be supplemented with phenylacetic or benzoic acid until the consultation
(D) mother stop nursing and put the baby on a goat's milk formula until the consultation
(E) parents either switch brands of disposable diapers or change their diaper service, because the diapers they are using are leaving the odor

45. In individuals 2 to 18 years old, the Stanford-Binet Scale is most useful for evaluating

(A) cerebral dominance
(B) general intellectual ability
(C) perceptuomotor performance
(D) memory
(E) dyslexia

46. Various compounds are added to mitochondria having a tightly coupled oxidative phosphorylation system. Addition of which of the following substrates will generate the LEAST amount of adenosine triphosphate (ATP)?

(A) Malate
(B) Succinate
(C) Malate with rotenone
(D) Succinate with rotenone
(E) Malate with actinomycin D

47. Trisodium phosphonoformate (foscarnet) is a potent antiviral agent for treating herpes simplex infections. It works by affecting

(A) the viral RNA polymerase
(B) the viral DNA polymerase
(C) the viral reverse transcriptase
(D) the host-cellular DNA polymerase
(E) the host-cellular RNA polymerase

48. Which of the following statements best describes a G protein? All G proteins

(A) consist of an α, β, and γ subunit and the primary difference among them resides in the β subunit
(B) are associated with cellular membranes
(C) do not play a role in amplification of a hormonal signal
(D) play a role in regulating cyclic adenosine monophosphate (cAMP) levels
(E) have protein kinase activity

49. Cell-mediated immunity may be a factor in viral pathogenesis because cytotoxic T cells can destroy virally infected cells. In which of the following viral diseases is this process best demonstrated?

(A) Poliomyelitis
(B) Yellow fever
(C) Influenza
(D) Rabies
(E) Hepatitis B

50. A 4-year-old boy interrupts his mother every time she talks on the phone. The family pediatrician recommends that whenever the child interrupts her, the mother should pay no attention to him. The pediatrician has recommended

(A) intermittent reinforcement
(B) nonreinforcement
(C) positive reinforcement
(D) negative reinforcement
(E) punishment

51. A procedure commonly used to increase the immunogenicity of an antigen is

(A) conversion of the antigen into a superantigen
(B) employment of a very high dose of the antigen
(C) injection of the antigen, together with an adjuvant
(D) injection of a very low dose of the antigen
(E) attenuation of the microorganism

52. Prolonged antibiotic therapy may lead to superinfections caused by overgrowth of *Clostridium difficile*. Appropriate therapy for this infection consists of

(A) penicillin G
(B) tetracycline
(C) gentamicin
(D) sulfamethoxazole/trimethoprim
(E) metronidazole

53. Which of the following statements regarding the complement system is correct?

(A) It must go all the way to C9 when activated
(B) Its components are synthesized primarily by plasmacytes
(C) Immunization increases the production of its components
(D) It can be activated by antigen–immunoglobulin G (IgG) complexes
(E) Properdin is important in the classic and alternative pathways

54. The following are survival times recorded for five mice observed after chemotherapy: 2.4 months, 3.6 months, 4.6 months, 4.6 months, and 5.5 months. How would the statistics of the study be affected if the observed value of 5.5 months is recorded in error as 55 months?

(A) An increase in the mean
(B) An increase in the mode
(C) An increase in the median
(D) An increase in both the median and the mean
(E) An increase in the median, the mode, and the mean

55. Factors that are common to both the classic and alternative complement pathways are

(A) C1 inhibitor and C3
(B) C3 and C5
(C) factor B and C4
(D) C2 and C5
(E) factor D and C2

56. Bacterial resistance to fluoroquinolones, such as ciprofloxacin, is often mediated by

(A) enzymes that degrade fluoroquinolones
(B) enzymes that inactivate fluoroquinolones
(C) amplification of bacterial dihydrofolate reductase
(D) reduced fluoroquinolone binding to DNA gyrase
(E) changes in the bacterial cell wall peptidoglycan

57. The biologic consequences of anaphylatoxin generation include

(A) increased vascular permeability
(B) decreased neutrophil activity
(C) decreased macrophage mobility
(D) increased bacterial cell lysis
(E) increased opsonization

58. The three types of cancer that cause the most deaths among American women are (in descending order)

(A) breast, lung, colorectal
(B) breast, uterine, lung
(C) lung, breast, colorectal
(D) uterine, breast, colorectal
(E) lung, breast, uterine

59. Deficiency of which of the following complement components would most likely result in severe bacterial infections?

(A) CR1
(B) C3b
(C) C3a
(D) C4b2b
(E) C5b

60. A plasmid carrying a gene coding for β-lactamase is most likely to provide a bacterium with resistance to

(A) bacteriophage infection
(B) restriction endonucleases
(C) an antibiotic
(D) the hopping of transposons
(E) ultraviolet light

61. Which of the following statements is correct regarding complement?

(A) All bacteria can be destroyed when it is activated
(B) Virus infectivity is not affected by it
(C) It can be activated by acute-phase proteins
(D) It can result in removal of soluble immune complexes
(E) Heating serum increases its activity

62. Which of the following is the leading cause of death in the United States?

(A) Heart disease
(B) Cancer
(C) Stroke
(D) Accidental injuries
(E) Liver failure

63. Identify the toxic substance whose production by phagocytic cells is dependent upon the presence of oxygen.

(A) Lysozyme
(B) Defensin
(C) Tumor necrosis factor-α
(D) Nitric oxide
(E) Hydrolytic enzymes

64. Decreased binding to bacterial DNA-dependent RNA polymerase is often associated with resistance to

(A) rifampin
(B) trimethoprim
(C) ofloxacin
(D) vancomycin
(E) acyclovir

65. Which of the following genes is associated with a disease producing sacroiliitis, uveitis, and aortic regurgitation?

(A) DR2
(B) B27
(C) Dw14
(D) DR3
(E) DR4

66. Which of the following statements about Native Americans in the United States is true? They

(A) do not have a high suicide rate
(B) do not have a high alcoholism rate
(C) believe that mental and physical illness are interconnected
(D) do not believe in witchcraft
(E) have high socioeconomic status

67. The most important antigens in determining success or failure in organ transplantation are

(A) human leukocyte antigen (HLA)-A
(B) HLA-B
(C) HLA-C
(D) HLA-DP
(E) HLA-DR

68. Concomitant administration of which of the following drugs may increase the nephrotoxicity of gentamicin?

(A) Penicillin G
(B) Cephalothin
(C) Tetracycline
(D) Erythromycin
(E) Furosemide

69. A mentally competent 57-year-old patient refuses to have his gangrenous leg amputated. The first step the physician should take is to

(A) remove herself from the case
(B) tell the patient the consequences of refusing the amputation
(C) transfer the patient to another hospital
(D) obtain permission for the amputation from the patient's wife
(E) obtain permission for the amputation from the hospital board of directors

70. A patient is being administered 5% dextrose intravenously and is receiving no oral nutrition. Which of the following enzymes has no physiologic function in this situation?

(A) Glucokinase
(B) Hexokinase
(C) Phosphofructokinase 1
(D) Phosphoglycerate kinase
(E) Pyruvate kinase

71. Amikacin is not active against *Bacteroides fragilis* because of

(A) insufficient binding to ribosomal subunits
(B) limited uptake across the bacterial cell membrane
(C) rapid degradation by bacterial enzymes
(D) lack of activating enzymes in this organism
(E) the unique structure of the bacterial cell wall in this species

72. A certain drug has a 10% rate of side effects. A physician has two patients receiving this drug: patient 1 and patient 2. What is the probability that neither patient 1 nor patient 2 will develop side effects?

(A) 29%
(B) 36%
(C) 81%
(D) 90%
(E) 95%

73. Which of the following statements is true of both isoniazid and rifampin? They

(A) are active against *Mycobacterium leprae*
(B) are hepatotoxic
(C) impart an orange–red color to body fluids
(D) are metabolized by acetylation
(E) are active against meningococci

74. An important component of the model for the regulation of an operon that is regulated by attenuation involves alternate secondary structures that can form in

(A) DNA
(B) ribosomes
(C) the leader peptide
(D) messenger RNA (mRNA)
(E) the repressor protein

75. A child whose otitis media failed to respond to amoxicillin was successfully treated with amoxicillin plus clavulanate. The infection was most likely caused by

(A) *Pseudomonas aeruginosa*
(B) *Streptococcus pneumoniae*
(C) *Haemophilus influenzae*
(D) *Streptococcus pyogenes*
(E) *Mycoplasma pneumoniae*

76. Attenuation involves regulation by premature termination of which of the following processes?

(A) Protein synthesis
(B) Ribosome synthesis
(C) DNA synthesis
(D) Messenger RNA (mRNA) synthesis
(E) Histidine synthesis

77. Which of the following statements is true of both amoxicillin and methicillin? They are

(A) stable in gastric acid
(B) resistant to penicillinase
(C) eliminated by renal tubular secretion
(D) active against *Pseudomonas aeruginosa*
(E) coadministered with clavulanate

78. Which of the following conditions is most likely to be observed in a normal, 72-year-old man?

(A) Impaired consciousness
(B) Abnormal level of arousal
(C) Reduced speed of new learning
(D) Psychosis
(E) Depression

79. The committed step in a metabolic sequence is generally the one that is rate limiting and most highly regulated. The committed step in glycolysis is catalyzed by phosphofructokinase-1. In mammalian cells other than hepatocytes, its activity is synchronized to that of the tricarboxylic acid cycle by the concentrations of adenosine triphosphate (ATP) and citrate. In turn, the concentration of these mediators is largely determined by the activity of

(A) malate dehydrogenase
(B) succinyl coenzyme A (CoA) thiokinase
(C) isocitrate dehydrogenase
(D) fumarase
(E) pyruvate dehydrogenase

80. The current leading cause of death among teenagers in the United States is

(A) suicide
(B) cancer
(C) homicide
(D) cardiovascular disease
(E) accidents

81. You are a hematologist and a 2-year-old girl is referred to you. She has a chronic anemia with mild jaundice that has not responded to nutritional supplementation. Mild splenomegaly is present. Under the microscope, some of the cells appear to be echinocytes, but no spherocytes are observed. The reticulocyte count is abnormally high. Both parents are clinically normal and are first cousins of western European descent. The child most likely has hemolytic anemia caused by a deficiency of

(A) erythrocyte pyruvate kinase
(B) erythrocyte glucose 6-phosphate dehydrogenase
(C) erythrocyte membrane spectrin
(D) iron
(E) decay-accelerating factor (DAF)

82. A 54-year-old cancer patient who has undergone two chemotherapy sessions becomes dizzy when he enters the hospital for his third session. This is an example of

(A) operant conditioning
(B) classical conditioning
(C) extinction
(D) shaping
(E) depression

83. Which of the following processes affects the relative activity of an enzyme without changing the actual number of enzyme molecules present?

(A) Induction
(B) Repression
(C) Feedback inhibition
(D) Catabolite repression
(E) Attenuation

84. Which of the following facilities would be most suitable for an 80-year-old patient who requires restorative nursing case and assistance with self-care?

(A) A skilled nursing facility
(B) A residential care facility
(C) A hospice
(D) An intermediate care facility
(E) A halfway house

85. Individuals fund their own health care in which of the following countries?

(A) Canada
(B) England
(C) France
(D) Germany
(E) The United States

86. You are a family practitioner and are confronted with a patient who suffers from scaly dermatitis, grayish pallor, extreme lassitude, and muscle pains. Nutritional history reveals that this patient consumes 25 raw egg whites each day, eats no fruit or vegetables, and takes no vitamin supplements. In addition, he has been taking tetracycline to help clear up a bad case of acne. After putting him on a more traditional diet and supplying him with a multivitamin supplement, his symptoms subside. On the molecular level, this patient was unable to convert

(A) pyruvate to alanine
(B) pyruvate to oxaloacetate
(C) phospho*enol*pyruvate to pyruvate
(D) pyruvate to acetyl coenzyme A (CoA)
(E) pyruvate to lactate

87. In which of the following organizations are physicians paid a yearly salary to provide medical services to a group of people who have paid a yearly premium in advance?

(A) Health maintenance organizations
(B) Independent practice associations
(C) Preferred provider associations
(D) Hospices
(E) Residential care facilities

88. Patients in shock may have lactic acid acidosis, because the decreased delivery of oxygen to cells causes a backup of the tricarboxylic acid cycle and a build-up of acetyl coenzyme A (CoA), which in turn inhibits pyruvate dehydrogenase by a negative feedback mechanism. Since pyruvate cannot go to acetyl CoA, it is converted to lactate. It has been found that treatment with dichloroacetate accelerates the reversal of the lactic acid acidosis, because it is an inhibitor of pyruvate dehydrogenase kinase. Pyruvate dehydrogenase kinase is

(A) a cyclic adenosine monophosphate (cAMP)-dependent enzyme, and dichloroacetate acts by lowering cAMP levels
(B) a cAMP-dependent enzyme that regulates pyruvate dehydrogenase activity by phosphorylating it
(C) a subunit of the pyruvate dehydrogenase complex, and inhibits the dehydrogenase activity of the complex by phosphorylating it
(D) normally activated by pyruvate
(E) normally inhibited by acetyl CoA

89. An 82-year-old woman has lost 10 pounds and has become forgetful. She was recently diagnosed with breast cancer, and her best friend just died. This woman probably

(A) has Alzheimer disease
(B) is suffering from major depressive disorder
(C) is at decreased risk for suicide when compared with a young woman
(D) has a decreased IQ
(E) cannot be treated effectively with psychoactive drugs

90. Intermediate filaments (IFs) help link adjacent sarcomeres together in skeletal muscle. Which of the following proteins is an intermediate protein used diagnostically in pathologic cases to indicate muscle origin?

(A) Actin
(B) Desmin
(C) Actinin
(D) Clathrin
(E) Vimentin

91. Which of the following is characteristic of sexuality in healthy, aged men?

(A) More rapid erection
(B) Shorter refractory period
(C) Lack of interest in sex
(D) Need for increased direct genital stimulation
(E) Increased intensity of ejaculation

92. Which of the following types of genomes do measles and mumps viruses have?

(A) Positive sense DNA
(B) Negative sense DNA
(C) Positive sense RNA
(D) Negative sense RNA
(E) Nonsense RNA

93. In which of the following types of hospitals do most people in the United States receive medical care?

(A) Investor owned
(B) For-profit
(C) Voluntary
(D) Federally owned
(E) State owned

94. Which spore-forming bacteria listed below are associated with food poisoning?

(A) *Staphylococcus aureus* and *Clostridium difficile*
(B) *Clostridium tetani* and *Shigella flexneri*
(C) *Clostridium perfringens* and *Bacillus cereus*
(D) *Clostridium perfringens* and *Bacillus anthracis*
(E) *Salmonella enteritidis* and *Shigella sonnei*

95. The primary determinant of an individual's socioeconomic status is

(A) income
(B) occupation
(C) place of residence
(D) education level
(E) family situation

96. Glucose transport into cells is mediated by

(A) an insulin-dependent transporter in hepatocytes
(B) hexokinase in erythrocytes
(C) an insulin-dependent transporter in neurons in the brain
(D) a sodium ion cotransport system in muscle cells
(E) a sodium ion cotransport system in renal tubular cells

97. The most common cause of death in infants in the United States is

(A) congenital anomalies
(B) respiratory distress syndrome (RDS)
(C) sudden infant death syndrome (SIDS)
(D) leukemia
(E) cancer of the central nervous system

98. Identify the structures at the arrows in the figure that play a role in vesicle translocation.

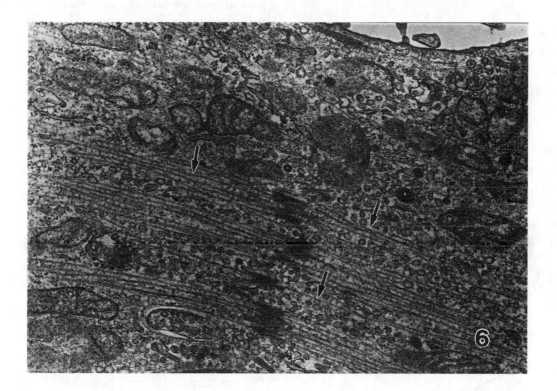

(A) Microtubules

(B) Stress fibers

(C) Microfilaments

(D) Myosin filaments

(E) Intermediate filaments

99. According to legal definition, for an act to be qualified as rape there must be evidence of

(A) penetration of the vulva

(B) penetration of the anus

(C) ejaculation

(D) struggling by the victim

(E) lack of previous sexual activity by the victim

100. Some bacteriologic culture media are used for both selective and differential purposes. Which of the following media may be considered differential, but not selective?

(A) Mannitol salt agar

(B) Blood agar plate

(C) Blood agar containing X and V factors

(D) Thayer-Martin agar

(E) Bile-esculin agar

101. Transvestites are best described as individuals who

(A) are also known as transsexuals
(B) are almost always homosexual
(C) usually have a defect in gender identity
(D) dress in women's clothes for sexual pleasure
(E) believe they were born the wrong sex

102. In the diagram below, various substances were added to a tightly coupled suspension of liver mitochondria in a buffered system containing phosphate, but no substrate or cofactor required to support oxidative phosphorylation. Liver mitochondria, substrate, adenosine diphosphate, 2,4-ditrophenol, and oligomycin were added (one substance per point) at the points labeled A–E on the accompanying diagram. Oligomycin was added at point

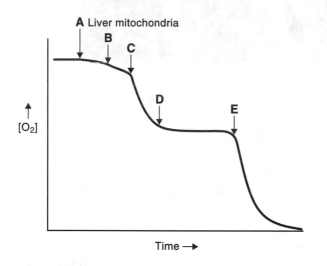

103. Compared with his sleep at age 20, the delta stage of sleep (stages 3 and 4) in an 80-year-old man

(A) decreases
(B) remains the same
(C) increases
(D) moves to the first half of the night
(E) is no longer necessary

104. Which of the following tests gives a "wheal and flare" response within minutes when a positive individual is injected with the appropriate antigen?

(A) Lepromin test
(B) Skin prick test
(C) Tuberculin test
(D) Patch test
(E) Schick test

105. Which of the following is the most open-ended question or statement?

(A) "Why didn't you come in sooner?"
(B) "What brings you here today?"
(C) "Tell me about the pain in your chest."
(D) "Have you been to a physician within the last year?"
(E) "Is there a history of heart disease in your family?"

106. Termination of translation in eukaryotes requires

(A) uncharged transfer RNA (tRNA)
(B) the codon AUG at the A site
(C) adenosine triphosphate (ATP)
(D) release factor
(E) binding of an aminoacyl-tRNA to the A site

107. Both the federal and state governments contribute to the cost of

(A) Medicaid
(B) Medicare
(C) Blue Cross
(D) Blue Shield
(E) Health maintenance organizations (HMOs)

108. Inverted terminal repetitions found in DNA virus genomes are significant because

(A) viral polymerases replicate the DNA more efficiently
(B) they prevent terminal cross-linking of strands
(C) they provide a target for antiviral chemotherapy
(D) they provide a mechanism for the formation of a circular genome
(E) they allow cellular polymerases to produce viral messenger RNA (mRNA)

109. A federally-funded program designed to provide coverage for the elderly, for people on social security disability, and for chronic dialysis patients is provided by

(A) Medicaid
(B) Medicare
(C) Blue Cross
(D) Blue Shield
(E) Health maintenance organizations (HMOs)

110. Which of the following statements concerning cholesterol and/or atherosclerosis is true?

(A) By inhibiting cholesterol 7 α-hydroxylase, vitamin C stimulates bile acid synthesis and tends to lower blood cholesterol levels
(B) Higher than normal levels of any serum lipoproteins are considered a risk factor for development of atherosclerosis
(C) Pharmacological doses of niacin lower blood cholesterol levels by inhibiting the activity of 3-hydroxy-3-methylglutaryl-coenzyme A (HMG-CoA) reductase
(D) Primary chylomicronemia is usually first managed by the appropriate use of drugs
(E) Diets containing sufficient quantities of "soluble" fibers, such as pectin, reduce cholesterol levels by a mechanism similar to that used by the cholesterol lowering drug cholestyramine

111. A 60-year-old man comes to your office complaining of gastric pain. He seems agitated, but does not speak. Which of the following statements will best encourage him to continue speaking?

(A) "Please continue."
(B) "How much liquor do you drink per week?"
(C) "Are you a heavy drinker?"
(D) "You should have come in 6 months ago."
(E) "Many people are upset by situations like this."

112. A secondary antibody response can be distinguished from a primary response because in a secondary response

(A) it takes a longer time to generate detectable antibody
(B) a higher dose of antigen is required to induce antibody production
(C) fewer memory cells are generated
(D) the major isotype of antibody produced is immunoglobulin G (IgG)
(E) antibody persists for a shorter period of time

113. Which of the following characteristics is representative of a benign, rather than a malignant, tumor?

(A) Lack of a capsule
(B) Increased nuclear/cytoplasmic ratio
(C) Immortality in tissue culture
(D) Presence of ABO antigens on the cell surface
(E) Atypical mitotic spindles

114. The most common cause of death in children between 1 and 4 years of age is

(A) drowning
(B) automobile accidents
(C) burns
(D) sudden infant death syndrome
(E) cancer

115. Third degree burns differ from first or second degree burns in that they

(A) lack pain sensation
(B) are partial thickness
(C) are associated with scarring
(D) are associated with blisters
(E) can reepithelialize from residual adnexal structures

116. Melanin synthesis is decreased in

(A) vitiligo
(B) Addison disease
(C) adrenogenital syndrome
(D) exposure to the sun
(E) phenylketonuria

117. A point mutation leading to the formation of a stop codon and premature termination of globin-chain synthesis is operative in

(A) α-thalassemia minor
(B) hemoglobin Bart disease
(C) hemoglobin H disease
(D) sickle cell disease
(E) β-thalassemia

118. Which of the following statements concerning sex chromosomes is correct?

(A) X chromosomes determine genetic sex
(B) Only paternally derived X chromosomes are inactivated in females
(C) Genes for testicular development reside on the Y chromosome
(D) Females transmit, but do not develop, sex-linked recessive diseases
(E) Females primarily have a single population of maternally derived X chromosomes

119. A post-pubertal male with mental retardation, everted ears, enlarged testicles, and a long face with a large mandible most likely has a defect characterized by

(A) triplet repeat mutations
(B) an XYY karyotype
(C) a single Barr body
(D) mutation in a mitochondrial gene
(E) a mutation with insertion of nucleotide bases into DNA

120. A newborn infant who has a positive Guthrie test should be placed on a diet with a low content of

(A) cysteine
(B) phenylalanine
(C) methionine
(D) tyrosine
(E) valine

121. *Mycoplasma pneumoniae* is sensitive to the action of which of the following antimicrobial agents?

(A) Penicillins
(B) Tetracyclines
(C) Cephalosporins
(D) Bacitracin
(E) Acyclovir

122. Biofeedback aimed at regulating peripheral temperature is most useful in the treatment of

(A) tension headache
(B) hypertension
(C) anal incontinence
(D) Raynaud disease
(E) asthma

123. By which mechanism do fimbriae or pili contribute to pathogenicity?

(A) Directly impede phagocytosis by white blood cells
(B) Bind the Fc portion of IgG molecules
(C) Allow bacterial movement in response to chemotaxis
(D) Allow tight adherence to tissue cells
(E) Provide genes for antibiotic resistance

DIRECTIONS:

Each of the numbered items or incomplete statements in this section is negatively phrased, as indicated by a capitalized word such as NOT, LEAST, or EXCEPT. Select the ONE lettered answer or completion that is BEST in each case.

124. All of the following are characteristic of children in single-parent households EXCEPT

(A) increased likelihood of divorce in adulthood
(B) criminal behavior
(C) high academic achievement
(D) drug abuse
(E) depression

125. Hyperuricemia is LEAST likely to be a result of

(A) treatment of acute leukemia
(B) overactivity of 5-phosphoribosyl-1-pyrophosphate (PRPP)
(C) high doses of aspirin
(D) underactivity of hypoxanthine-quanine phosphoribosyl transferase (HGPRT)
(E) thiazide therapy

126. Which of the following poison relationships is NOT correctly matched?

(A) Cyanide—almond smell to the breath
(B) Isopropanol—fruity breath and increased anion gap metabolic acidosis
(C) Arsenic—garlic breath
(D) Haloperidol—oculogyric crisis
(E) Strychnine—tetanic convulsions

127. Which of the following proteins does NOT contain heme as a prosthetic group?

(A) δ-Aminolevulinate synthase
(B) Catalase
(C) Cytochrome c
(D) Hemoglobin
(E) Myoglobin

128. All of the following statements concerning viral serotypes are correct EXCEPT that

(A) in nonenveloped nucleocapsid viruses, the serotype is determined by the surface proteins
(B) in enveloped viruses, the serotype is determined by the outer envelope proteins
(C) some viruses have multiple serotypes
(D) some viruses have a single serotype
(E) some viruses have an RNA polymerase that determines the serotype

129. An inherited deficiency of tetrahydrobiopterin production would be LEAST likely to inhibit synthesis of

(A) epinephrine
(B) norepinephrine
(C) phenylalanine
(D) serotonin
(E) tyrosine

130. Which of the following is LEAST likely to occur in patients who receive extensive burns from fires in homes?

(A) Cyanide poisoning
(B) Hypervolemia
(C) Adult respiratory distress syndrome
(D) Curling ulcers
(E) Carbon monoxide poisoning

131. A mucoid strain of a gram-negative bacillus was cultured from a cystic fibrosis patient with a chronic pulmonary infection. This infection could be empirically treated with any of the following EXCEPT

(A) ceftazidime
(B) ticarcillin
(C) aztreonam
(D) trimethoprim/sulfamethoxazole
(E) tobramycin

132. All of the following are virulence factors of group A streptococci EXCEPT

(A) hyaluronidase
(B) M protein
(C) erythrogenic toxins
(D) collagenase
(E) lipoteichoic acid

133. Which of the following statements about insulin is NOT correct? Insulin acts to

(A) increase the rate of synthesis of liver glucokinase
(B) enhance the rate of transport of amino acids into muscle
(C) increase activity of intracellular tyrosine kinase
(D) increase the transport of potassium from the serum into the cells
(E) increase the rate of transport of glucose into brain cells

134. All of the following statements concerning diphtheria toxin are true EXCEPT

(A) its production is mediated by lysogenic strains of bacteria
(B) fragment (polypeptide) A is responsible for inactivating elongation factor 2 of protein synthesis
(C) fragment (polypeptide) B is responsible for binding of the diphtheria toxin to cells
(D) the toxin used in the skin test (Schick test) transfers ADP ribose and turns off G_i protein
(E) the target organs are the heart and the peripheral nerves, leading to myocarditis and neuritis

135. All of the following antibiotics may produce ototoxicity EXCEPT

(A) erythromycin
(B) vancomycin
(C) tobramycin
(D) clindamycin
(E) gentamicin

136. All of the following molecules are either regulators or inhibitors of complement activity EXCEPT

(A) C4 binding protein
(B) factor H
(C) S protein
(D) C9
(E) factor I

137. A 10-year-old boy comes to your office for a physical. Which of the following statements is LEAST likely to be true about this boy?

(A) His conscience is almost completely formed
(B) He has the capacity for logical thought
(C) He identifies with his father
(D) His family is more important to him now than it was when he was age 5
(E) He prefers to play with boys rather than girls

138. All of the following statements regarding live vaccines are correct EXCEPT that they

(A) induce short-lived protection
(B) are more immunogenic than killed vaccines
(C) are attenuated
(D) can revert to virulence
(E) could be contaminated with another infectious agent

139. Receptors linked to guanosine triphosphate (GTP)-binding proteins whose activation leads to increased or decreased cyclic adenosine monophosphate (cAMP) production include all of the following EXCEPT

(A) nitric oxide
(B) β-adrenergic
(C) histamine H$_2$
(D) α$_2$-adrenergic
(E) dopamine

140. Attenuated viral vaccines are used for all of the following diseases EXCEPT

(A) mumps
(B) polio
(C) measles
(D) rubella
(E) influenza

141. All of the following are personality tests EXCEPT

(A) MMPI
(B) Rorschach Test
(C) Draw-a-Person Test
(D) Thematic Apperception Test
(E) WAIS-R

142. A breakdown in tolerance to self-antigens and the potential for autoimmune disease are associated with all of the following EXCEPT

(A) activation of T-suppressor lymphocytes
(B) enhanced expression of major histocompatibility complex (MHC) class II molecules
(C) infection with agents that have cross-reactive antigens
(D) release of sequestered antigens
(E) polyclonal activation of lymphocytes

143. All of the following statements correctly describe bacterial resistance to antibiotics EXCEPT that it

(A) may originate through spontaneous chromosomal mutations
(B) may occur by transfer of plasmids from one bacteria to another
(C) may involve selection of resistant organisms during antibiotic therapy
(D) usually requires specific defects in host cellular immunity
(E) may involve bacterial genes coding for resistance factors

144. Icosahedral viruses include all of the following EXCEPT

(A) parvovirus
(B) picornavirus
(C) paramyxovirus
(D) adenovirus
(E) herpesvirus

145. All of the following drugs inhibit bacterial cell wall synthesis EXCEPT

(A) spectinomycin
(B) vancomycin
(C) aztreonam
(D) cephalexin
(E) bacitracin

146. All of the following statements regarding haptens are correct EXCEPT

(A) they usually have a small molecular weight
(B) they can be immunogenic when coupled to a carrier molecule
(C) they are considered to be the same as epitopes
(D) they cannot activate T-helper cells on their own
(E) they cannot stimulate a secondary response on their own

147. Scientific evidence suggests that all of the following factors are involved in the etiology of male homosexuality EXCEPT

(A) genetics
(B) alterations in prenatal hormone levels
(C) alterations in adult hormone levels
(D) alterations in size of a hypothalamic nucleus

148. All of the following statements concerning the major histocompatibility complex (MHC) are true EXCEPT

(A) in humans it is known as the human leukocyte antigen complex
(B) the genes are scattered on different chromosomes
(C) it contains genes encoding class I, II, and III molecules
(D) it is polymorphic
(E) it is important in regulating immune responsiveness

149. All of the following components are required for the elongation phase of translation EXCEPT

(A) peptidyl transferase
(B) guanosine triphosphate (GTP)
(C) ribosomes
(D) messenger RNA (mRNA)
(E) formylmethionyl-transfer RNA (tRNA)

150. The immune defenses of the host against infectious agents can be avoided by all of the following EXCEPT

(A) antigenic variation
(B) presence of a capsule
(C) secretion of proteases
(D) antigenic mimicry
(E) blocking reduced nicotinamide adenine dinucleotide phosphate (NADPH) oxidase

151. During prolonged fasting, you would expect all of the following to occur EXCEPT

(A) an increase in glucagon and catecholamine levels, and a decrease in insulin levels
(B) an increase in hormone-sensitive lipase, and a decrease in lipoprotein lipase activity
(C) an increase in degradation of the steroid ring of cholesterol to acetyl coenzyme A (CoA), and a decrease in cholesterol synthesis from acetyl CoA
(D) an increase in phospho*enol*pyruvate carboxykinase activity, and a decrease in pyruvate kinase activity
(E) an increase in alanine–α-ketoglutarate aminotransferase activity, and a decrease in carbamoyl phosphate synthetase I activity

152. Which of the following statements regarding the deletion of self-reactive T-cell clones is NOT correct?

(A) It occurs in the thymus
(B) It involves the T-cell antigen receptor
(C) The process is most active in the elderly
(D) Self-reactive T cells become apoptotic
(E) $CD4^+CD8^+$ T-lymphocytes are killed

153. Which of the following is NOT an example of a germ cell tumor?

(A) Acute leukemia
(B) Cystic teratoma
(C) Seminoma
(D) Struma ovarii
(E) Yolk sac tumor

154. All of the following statements apply to major histocompatibility complex (MHC) class I molecules EXCEPT

(A) both chains are encoded by genes within the HLA
(B) they consist of an α chain plus $β_2$-microglobulin
(C) they are encoded in HLA-A, -B, and -C regions of DNA
(D) they are present on all nucleated cells
(E) they are important in T-cytotoxic lymphocyte activation

155. In the model below, a substrate (S) is converted irreversibly by various enzymes (E_1, E_2, and E_3) into intermediates (I_1 and I_2) before becoming the product (P). P exerts a negative feedback on enzyme E_1. If E_3 is deficient, you would expect all of the following EXCEPT a/an

$$E_1 \quad E_2 \quad E_3$$
$$S \rightarrow I_1 \rightarrow I_2 \rightarrow P$$

(A) increase in S
(B) increase in I_1
(C) increase in I_2
(D) activation of E_1
(E) decrease in P

156. Which of the following statements concerning major histocompatibility complex (MHC) class II molecules is NOT correct?

(A) They consist of two polypeptide chains
(B) They are expressed by B cells and macrophages
(C) Each molecule can bind only one type of peptide
(D) They are needed for antigen presentation to CD4$^+$ T cells
(E) One person can have up to six different class II molecules

157. A pediatrician is examining an infant who is 2 hours old. At this time the physician should expect to see all of the following in this infant EXCEPT

(A) visual tracking
(B) turning away from a noxious odor
(C) the rooting reflex
(D) the social smile
(E) the stepping reflex

158. All of the following statements concerning presentation of foreign peptides to lymphocytes are true EXCEPT

(A) immune responses against virtually all proteins require antigen presentation
(B) peptides are presented in the context of major histocompatibility complex (MHC) class I molecules
(C) peptides are presented in the context of MHC class II molecules
(D) presentation of peptides involves certain cell types
(E) all proteins are processed through the same intracellular pathway

159. Renal disease is LEAST likely to be a feature of

(A) mixed connective tissue disease
(B) multiple myeloma
(C) amyloidosis
(D) polyarteritis nodosa
(E) Sjögren syndrome

160. In Freudian theory, all of the following statements are true about the dream censor EXCEPT

(A) it is less active in naive individuals
(B) it integrates the latent dream with events that happened during the day
(C) it disguises the latent dream
(D) it operates according to the rules of primary process
(E) it works primarily on a conscious level

161. DNA viruses with no envelope include all the following groups EXCEPT

(A) adenoviruses
(B) papovaviruses
(C) parvoviruses
(D) poxviruses
(E) hepadnaviruses

DIRECTIONS:

Each set of matching questions in this section consists of a list of four to twenty-six lettered options (some of which may be in figures) followed by several numbered items. For each numbered item, select the ONE lettered option that is most closely associated with it. To avoid spending too much time on matching sets with a large number of options, it is generally advisable to begin each set by reading the list of options. Then for each item in the set, try to generate the correct answer and locate it in the option list, rather than evaluating each option individually. Each lettered option may be selected once, more than once, or not at all.

Questions 162-163

Match the compounds with the associated trait.

(A) Urobilin

(B) Heme

(C) Uric acid

(D) Iron

(E) Stercobilin

162. Responsible for the brown color of stools

163. Responsible for the yellow color of urine

Questions 164-168

Select the substance that has the designated role in signal transduction.

(A) Nitric oxide

(B) G_s

(C) G_i

(D) Diacylglycerol

(E) Phospholipase C

(F) Inositol triphosphate

(G) Cyclic adenosine monophosphate (cAMP)

(H) Cyclic guanosine monophosphate (GMP)

(I) Protein kinase C

164. Catalyzes formation of inositol triphosphate

165. Releases calcium from the sarcoplasmic reticulum

166. Activates cytoplasmic guanylyl cyclase

167. Activates protein kinases

168. Increases adenylyl cyclase activity

Questions 169-171

The letters A, B, C, D, and E designate regions of the titration curve of alanine shown below. Choose the appropriate region for each of the following items.

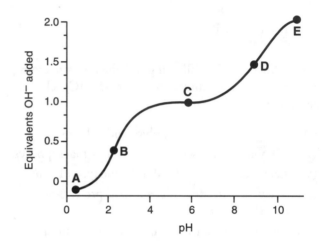

169. The isoelectric point

170. The region where alanine is fully protonated

171. The pK of the carboxyl group

Questions 172-176

Select the term that matches the following descriptions of pharmacologic properties.

(A) Partial agonist
(B) Full agonist
(C) Competitive antagonist
(D) Noncompetitive antagonist
(E) Potency
(F) Efficacy
(G) Tolerance
(H) Supersensitivity
(I) Desensitization
(J) Receptor down regulation

172. A drug attribute that is proportional to receptor affinity

173. Increasing doses are required to produce a specific magnitude of response

174. A drug that increases the median effective dose (ED_{50}) of an agonist but does not change the maximal response

175. Rapidly reversible decline in the response to an agonist drug during drug exposure

176. A condition that occurs when receptors are up-regulated

Questions 177-180

The DNA base sequence of the antitemplate strand for part of the normal β-globin gene is shown following, along with the base sequence found in five different mutant genes. Also shown is a copy of the genetic code. Match the description with the appropriate mutant gene.

The genetic code (codon assignments in messenger RNA)

First nucleotide	Second nucleotide				Third nucleotide
	U	**C**	**A**	**G**	
U	Phe	Ser	Tyr	Cys	U
	Phe	Ser	Tyr	Cys	C
	Leu	Ser	Term	Term	A
	Leu	Ser	Term	Trp	G
C	Leu	Pro	Hsi	Arg	U
	Leu	Pro	His	Arg	C
	Leu	Pro	Gln	Arg	A
	Leu	Pro	Gln	Arg	G
A	Ile	Thr	Asn	Ser	U
	Ile	Thr	Asn	Ser	C
	Ile	Thr	Lys	Arg	A
	Met	Thr	Lys	Arg	G
G	Val	Ala	Asp	Gly	U
	Val	Ala	Asp	Gly	C
	Val	Ala	Glu	Gly	A
	Val	Ala	Glu	Gly	G

	Codon number						
	3	**4**	**5**	**6**	**7**	**8**	**9**
Normal	CTG	ACT	CCT	GAG	GAG	AAG	TCT
(A) Mutant #1	CTG	ACT	CCT	GTG	GAG	AAG	TCT
(B) Mutant #2	CTG	ACT	CCT	GAG	GAG	TAG	TCT
(C) Mutant #3	CTG	ACG	CCT	GAG	GAG	AAG	TCT
(D) Mutant #4	CTG	ACT	CCT	GAG	GAG	ACG	TCT
(E) Mutant #5	CTG	AGT	CCT	GAG	GAG	AAG	TCT

177. During electrophoresis the protein product would migrate more slowly toward the positive electrode than the normal protein.

178. The protein product is completely normal.

179. A shortened protein is produced.

180. This segment of DNA would not be cut by the restriction enzyme MstII (recognition sequence: CCTNAGG).

ANSWER KEY

1. C	31. D	61. C	91. D	121. B	151. C
2. A	32. B	62. A	92. D	122. D	152. C
3. C	33. A	63. D	93. C	123. D	153. A
4. B	34. A	64. A	94. C	124. C	154. A
5. E	35. E	65. B	95. B	125. C	155. A
6. D	36. A	66. C	96. E	126. B	156. C
7. C	37. D	67. E	97. A	127. A	157. D
8. E	38. C	68. B	98. A	128. E	158. E
9. D	39. C	69. B	99. A	129. C	159. A
10. D	40. A	70. A	100. B	130. B	160. E
11. B	41. C	71. B	101. D	131. D	161. D
12. D	42. B	72. C	102. D	132. D	162. E
13. C	43. C	73. B	103. A	133. F	163. A
14. E	44. B	74. D	104. B	134. D	164. E
15. C	45. B	75. C	105. B	135. D	165. F
16. A	46. C	76. D	106. D	136. D	166. A
17. C	47. B	77. C	107. A	137. D	167. G
18. C	48. B	78. C	108. D	138. A	168. B
19. D	49. E	79. C	109. B	139. A	169. C
20. A	50. B	80. E	110. E	140. E	170. A
21. A	51. C	81. A	111. A	141. E	171. B
22. A	52. E	82. B	112. D	142. A	172. E
23. A	53. D	83. C	113. D	143. D	173. G
24. C	54. A	84. D	114. B	144. C	174. C
25. D	55. B	85. E	115. A	145. A	175. I
26. B	56. D	86. B	116. E	146. C	176. H
27. B	57. A	87. A	117. E	147. C	177. A
28. C	58. C	88. C	118. C	148. B	178. C
29. C	59. B	89. B	119. A	149. E	179. B
30. D	60. C	90. B	120. B	150. E	180. A

ANSWERS AND EXPLANATIONS

1. The answer is C. *(Behavioral science)*
Many Asians believe that the spiritual core of the person is located in the abdominal thoracic area, rather than the brain. Because of this belief, the concept of brain death and resulting organ transplantation are generally not accepted well in this group.

2. The answer is A. *(Microbiology)*
Nutrients in growth media must contain all the elements necessary for the biosynthesis of pathogenic microorganisms. This rule is especially true of media that are intended to have a selective (select for a specific group of bacteria) or differential (differentiate between a pathogenic and a normal or usual strain of a group) purpose.

Bacteria and plants use photosynthetic energy to reduce carbon dioxide expending water. The organisms that can use CO_2 as a sole source of carbon are termed **autotrophs.**

Chemolithotrophs are organisms that use an inorganic substrate, such as hydrogen or thiosulfate, as a reductant and CO_2 a carbon source. **Heterotrophs** require organic carbon for growth.

Many organisms possess the ability to assimilate nitrate (NO^-_3) and nitrite (NO^-_2) reductively by converting these forms to ammonia (NH_3). Dissimilation pathways are taken by microorganisms that use these ions as terminal electron acceptors in respiration. This process is known as denitrification, with the final product being nitrogen gas (N_2).

Fermentation is characterized by substrate phosphorylation, in which products such as glucose are involved for energy production.

Autotrophs should not be confused with auxotrophs. Auxotrophs are strains that require a nutrient that is not required by the parental or prototype strain. They are usually derived from mutants with defective synthetic capabilities.

3. The answer is C. *(Biochemistry)*
δ-Aminolevulinate synthase catalyzes the condensation of glycine and succinyl CoA to form δ-aminolevulinic acid (ALA). This reaction is the rate-limiting step in the synthesis of porphyrins such as heme. The synthesis of this enzyme is inhibited by hemin, which is formed from heme by the oxidation of the iron atom from Fe^{2+} to Fe^{3+}. Synthesis of this enzyme is increased by drugs such as phenobarbital, which aggravate symptoms associated with the porphyrins.

4. The answer is B. *(Microbiology)*
Amphotericin B is a complex polyene that has no inhibitory effect against bacteria, but strongly inhibits several pathogenic fungi. Amphotericin B binds to sterols on the fungal cell membrane and disturbs cytoplasmic membrane function. Given intravenously as micelles of sodium deoxycholate dissolved in dextrose solution, the drug is widely distributed in tissues. It does not penetrate well to the cerebrospinal fluid. Once attached to the fungal membrane, an amphotericin pore is introduced. Small molecules and ions are lost, eventually resulting in cell death. Mammalian cells are relatively resistant to amphotericin because it binds weakly to the cholesterol in mammalian cell membranes.

Amphotericin B is a broad-spectrum antifungal agent with activity against coccidioidomycosis, blastomycosis, histoplasmosis, sporotrichosis, cryptococcosis, mucormycosis, and candidiasis.

Amphotericin B does not work by any of the other four antimicrobial mechanisms of action.

5. The answer is E. *(Behavioral science)*
Sitting with support is normally seen in a 5-month-old infant. Stranger anxiety (fear of unfamiliar people) does not appear until approximately 7 months of age. A pincer grasp (using thumb and forefinger) appears at approximately 9 months of age, whereas object permanence (the ability to maintain a mental representation of an object although it can no longer be seen) occurs between 12 and 18 months of age. Using meaningful words is not commonly present until at least 12 months of age.

6. The answer is D. *(Biochemistry)*
Phenylketonuria (PKU) is a genetic disease caused by a deficiency of the enzyme phenylalanine hydroxylase. This deficiency causes the level of phenylalanine to become elevated. The excess phenylalanine is converted to phenyllactate, phenylacetate, and phenylpyruvate, compounds that are normally not produced in significant amounts. If tetrahydrobiopterin is present in normal amounts, the enzymes dihydrobiopterin

reductase and dihydrobiopterin synthetase must be functioning normally.

Some variants of PKU are caused by a deficiency in tetrahydrobiopterin production. In these variants, tyrosine hydroxylase, tryptophan hydroxylase, and phenylalanine hydroxylase are all inhibited because of the lack of their required cofactor. These variants have the symptoms of PKU but, in addition, cannot synthesize adequate amounts of melanin, the catecholamines, and serotonin.

7. The answer is C.   *(Behavioral science)*
In examining a 2-year-old child, start the examination at the child's feet and work your way up toward the head. Children are much more tolerant of having their feet touched than their head.

Because children at the age of 2 are fearful of separation from parents, having the parent in the room may help you handle the child. Children at 2 years of age do not fully understand what you are going to do or why you are going to do it, therefore, explaining your actions to the child would not be helpful. In addition, because the child's favorite word at the age of 2 is "no," asking the child's permission to do the examination before you begin will probably elicit that response. Asking the nurse to restrain the child would elicit fear in the child rather than make the examination easier.

8. The answer is E.   *(Biochemistry)*
The following schematics help to illustrate this example.

Normal β-chain on DNA

| C | T | C |

| G | A | G | - - - - - - - → | G | A | G | Codes for glutamic acid

(Complementary strand)

Messenger RNA

Sickle cell DNA

| C | (*A) | C | (*A is a point mutation in which adenine replaces thymidine)

| G | (T) | G | - - - - - - - → | G | (U) | G | Codes for valine

(Complementary strand)

Messenger RNA

Note that by changing the CTC triplet to a CAC, the messenger RNA (mRNA) changes from GAG, which normally codes for glutamic acid in the sixth position of the β-chain of hemoglobin, to GUG, which now codes for valine. This point mutation of a single base pair is responsible for sickle cell anemia.

9. The answer is D.   *(Behavioral science)*
The ability to do abstract mathematics is correlated with Piaget's stage of formal operations, which begins in adolescence at about age 17. An adolescent who acquires formal operational thought has gained the ability to think in abstract terms. Previous exposure to mathematical concepts, cultural factors, and high intelligence quotient are less related to the ability to do abstract math than is the acquisition of formal operational thought.

10. The answer is D.   *(Pathology)*
Malignant cells characteristically take at least 30 doubling times before they become clinically detectable. They commonly have a longer cell cycle than the normal cells in their parent tissue. Neoplasia is a problem due to an accumulation of cells over a period of time. Malignant cells have a greater DNA content than the normal cells in their parent tissue. This can be quantitated by flow cytometry for prognosis purposes. Diploid cells (multiples of 23 chromosomes) have a

better prognosis than aneuploid cells (uneven multiples). Malignant cells are not contact inhibited in tissue culture, and often pile up on top of each other. Malignant cells also have simple biochemical systems, with a predominantly anaerobic metabolism.

11. The answer is B.   (Behavioral science)
Parallel play, playing next to other children but not cooperatively with them, starts at about age 2 and continues to about age 4.

12. The answer is D.   (Biochemistry)
Lead inhibits the activity of δ-aminolevulinic acid (ALA) dehydrase and ferrochelatase, leading to an accumulation of ALA and coproporphyrin III in the urine. Inhibition of these enzymes for porphyrin biosynthesis blocks the synthesis of heme and brings about the anemia seen in these patients. Lead poisoning in adults causes motor nerve dysfunction, whereas lead poisoning in children can cause permanent central nervous system damage. Treatment must include removal of the source of lead from the patient's environment.

13. The answer is C.   (Behavioral science)
Interactive or cooperative play commences most typically at about age 4.

14. The answer is E.   (Microbiology)
Passage of immunoglobulin G (IgG) across the placenta is a good example of immunity that is passively acquired by the fetus. Passive immunization involves the transfer of preformed products of the immune system, and does not require active participation of the host. In contrast, active immunization does require participation of the host in order to generate protection.

IgG is the only isotype of antibody that can cross the placenta. All four subclasses are transferred, although transfer of IgG2 is the least efficient. Placental cells express receptors for the Fc portion of IgG to facilitate its transport. Newborns have a higher level of IgG than any other class. The maternal IgG declines over a period of several months, and is replaced by the infant's own IgG.

Breast-fed infants also become passively immunized by maternal IgA, which is present at high levels in colostrum (thin, milk-like fluid secreted by the mammary gland close to the time of birth) and milk. Milk also contains a moderate level of immunoglobulin M (IgM) and a low level of IgG.

Other examples of passive immunization include the administration of anti-Rh globulin to Rh-negative women and injection of antibodies against infectious agents, such as hepatitis A and B viruses, rabies virus, and cytomegalovirus.

Administration of the oral polio vaccine, or a toxoid, and the inhalation of a microorganism would result in protective immunity only after active participation of the host (i.e., the inoculated individual actively produces antibodies and cell-mediated immunity).

Administration of an antibiotic might be protective in killing or inhibiting the growth of the infectious agents; however, a microbicidal drug does not passively confer immunity.

15. The answer is C.   (Behavioral science)
The superego develops at approximately the time a child starts first grade (6 years of age). The superego controls id (the sexual and aggressive aspects of the mind) impulses and represents moral values and conscience. The ego (the personality) and the id develop at earlier ages. The unconscious and the conscious minds also develop at earlier ages.

16. The answer is A.   (Biochemistry)
An amino acid is considered nonessential if it can be synthesized in humans, whereas it is considered essential if it must be obtained from the diet. Cysteine is derived from the essential amino acid methionine; therefore, cysteine can be produced in the body only if adequate dietary methionine is available. The 10 essential amino acids are phenylalanine, valine, tryptophan, threonine, isoleucine, methionine, histidine, arginine, leucine, and lysine.

17. The answer is C.   (Pathology)
Papillary cancer of the thyroid characteristically spreads by lymphatics, rather than by vessel invasion.

Dissemination of tumor occurs by seeding within body cavities, lymphatic spread, or hematogenous spread. Seeding is commonly seen with colorectal cancers and ovarian cancers. Lymphatic invasion is more common in carcinomas than sarcomas. Lymphatic spread initially goes to the regional lymph nodes (subcapsular sinus is the first site), and from there into the systemic circulation via the thoracic duct. Hematogenous spread is favored by sarcomas (not exclusively), with spread to the lungs and liver a common finding. Carcinomas with a propensity for hematogenous invasion are: renal adenocarcinomas invading the renal vein, hepatocellular carcinomas invading the hepatic and portal veins, and follicular carcinomas of the thyroid, which commonly bypass the cervical lymph nodes and metastasize to the lungs and bone.

18. The answer is C. *(Biochemistry)*

A protein to be secreted from the cell usually has a hydrophobic region at its amino terminus, which causes the ribosome synthesizing that protein to become bound to the endoplasmic reticulum. The protein molecule enters the endoplasmic reticulum as it is being made. The signal sequence is cleaved off by the signal peptidase and carbohydrate residues are attached inside the endoplasmic reticulum. Additional carbohydrate residues are attached as the protein moves through the Golgi apparatus on its way to the outside of the cell. Proteins that are destined for the lysosomes are marked by the addition of mannose-6-phosphate.

19. The answer is D. *(Pathology)*

Carbon monoxide (CO) poisoning is a common accidental injury or method for suicide. Automobile exhaust is one of the most common sources of CO, as well as a blocked exhaust system for a wood stove, as in this case. Another source of CO is methylene chloride. CO is odorless.

CO has a high affinity for hemoglobin (Hgb) and results in a normal PaO_2, a decreased oxygen saturation (occupies the heme group rather than oxygen), and a decreased oxygen content, thus producing tissue hypoxia; however, if the oxygen saturation is calculated from the PaO_2, rather than directly measured, it is normal. Blood gas instruments without attached cooximeters calculate the oxygen saturation. Carboxyhemoglobin also shifts the oxygen dissociation curve to the left, which further reduces oxygen release by Hgb and ultimately to tissue. As a final insult, it also blocks cytochrome oxidase in the oxidative pathway.

The brain (globus pallidus in particular) and heart are primarily affected, but changes also occur in the liver (fatty change) and other organs. A cigarette smoker may have up to 8% to 10% carboxyhemoglobin in the blood. Patients with CO poisoning have a cherry red color to the skin and blood. The cherry red color blocks the presence of cyanosis, which should be present. Alcohol enhances the effects of CO poisoning and contributes to the death of the patient. The first symptom is headache. Concentrations above 60% generally result in death. Treatment involves the administration of 100% oxygen to displace the CO from Hgb, or the use of a hyperbaric oxygen chamber, which accomplishes the displacement of CO in a more timely manner.

20. The answer is A. *(Microbiology)*

Influenza vaccine consists of killed (inactivated) viruses grown in embryonated chicken eggs. The Salk polio vaccine consists of poliovirus types 1, 2, and 3 grown in cell culture, concentrated, and chemically inactivated. Killed vaccines appear to impart a limited type of immunity, because the viruses do not mimic a natural growth cycle in the host and stimulate only partial immune response against the virus. No secretory immunoglobulin A (IgA) is found in nasal or duodenal secretions, for example.

No approved vaccines currently exist for respiratory syncytial virus or parainfluenza viruses. Measles, mumps, and rubella viruses all have live, attenuated vaccines available. They are egg based vaccines, which could induce type I hypersensitivity reactions in patients with egg allergies.

21. The answer is A. *(Pathology)*

Organophosphates decrease red blood cell (RBC) cholinesterase levels. They are potent insecticides, which are readily absorbed through the skin, respiratory, and gastrointestinal systems. Poisonings are characterized by excessive autonomic system activity caused by an irreversible block of acetylcholine esterase, which causes an increase in acetylcholine, producing excessive lacrimation, excessive salivation, fecal incontinence, and constricted pupils.

Nicotinic effects, via inhibition of acetylcholine esterase activity, include muscle weakness, paralysis, and muscle fasciculations. Serum and RBC cholinesterase (pseudocholinesterase) levels are decreased with serum levels of cholinesterase decreased before the RBC levels. Atropine is the treatment of choice.

22. The answer is A.   (Biochemistry)
Mannose-6-phosphate is a carbohydrate that is often attached as a posttranslational modification to proteins that are to be incorporated into the lysosomes. Such glycosylation occurs as the protein molecule is processed through the endoplasmic reticulum and Golgi complex. Proteins that are destined for the mitochondria and nucleus are synthesized on free polysomes in the cytoplasm. Portions of their amino acid sequences serve to target them to the proper organelle.

23. The answer is A.   (Pathology)
Lymphocytes are the most radiosensitive of the hematopoietic cells. Trauma caused by ionizing radiation relates to the type of ionizing radiation. The shorter the wavelength, the greater the penetration into tissue (x-rays penetrate the body). Particulate radiation refers to radiation emitted by radioactive substances (e.g., alpha and beta particles, protons, deuterons). The overall effect of radiation on tissue is determined by the type of radiation involved, the dose, and the amount of tissue exposed to that dose.

Those cells that are labile and have a high turnover and mitotic index are most sensitive (e.g., hematopoietic cells, mucosal lining cells, germinal epithelium), while permanent cells or stable cells are of intermediate to low radiosensitivity. Cells are more susceptible to radiation when they are in the G2 phase (synthesizing the mitotic spindle) and in mitosis. They are least sensitive in the late S phase.

Radiation effects are mutagenic, genetic (affect DNA), and somatic. Leukemias/lymphomas lead the list of radiation-induced cancers. Total body irradiation produces certain identifiable syndromes, which occur after certain accumulative doses of radiation. The hematopoietic system is the most sensitive to total body irradiation. Peripheral leukopenias (particularly lymphocytes), thrombocytopenia, and bone marrow hypoplasia commonly occur, with an overall 20% to 50% mortality. The order of radiosensitivity of hematopoietic elements from greater to least sensitive is lymphocytes, granulocytes, platelets, and mature red blood cells (RBCs).

24. The answer is C.   (Microbiology)
The patient has antibodies against *Haemophilus influenzae* and the titer is 1:128. The titer is defined as the highest dilution of a specimen (e.g., serum, plasma, cerebrospinal fluid) at which there is still a positive reaction.

It is impossible to be certain if the antibodies are there because *H. influenzae* caused the fever of unknown origin, or if the patient has been infected with the bacterium sometime in the past. In order to establish that an infectious agent is the cause of a particular disease episode, a 4-fold rise in antibody titer from an acute to a convalescent serum sample is often used to make a definite diagnosis.

In the zone of equivalence, the proportion of antibody and antigen is optimal in relation to each other. They form an ever-growing lattice, which eventually comes out of solution as an insoluble precipitate.

The zone of equivalence is from 1:4 to 1:128. If there is antibody excess (prozone), efficient lattice formation cannot take place, and a false negative will occur. The false negative is shown for the patient's undiluted and 1:2 serum samples. This situation frequently occurs in secondary syphilis. Dilution of the patient's sample facilitates lattice formation and a positive reaction.

A negative result will also occur if there is antigen excess (postzone), as shown at the 1:256 and 1:512 serum dilutions.

25. The answer is D.   (Pathology)
Those cells that are labile and have a high turnover and mitotic index are most radiosensitive [e.g., hematopoietic cells (lymphocytes most radiosensitive of all cells), mucosal lining cells (gastrointestinal), germination epithelium], while those that are permanent cells (skeletal muscle) or stable cells (breast duct epithelium) are of intermediate to low radiosensitivity.

26. The answer is B.   (Behavioral science)
The mortality rate for African-American infants is about 2.4 times higher than for white infants. This is related to the fact that many African-American families have lower incomes than white families and thus may have less access to prenatal health services.

27. The answer is B. *(Pathology)*
Salt water drowning results in faster death than fresh water drowning. Salt water causes an osmotic shift of water into the alveolar spaces, with subsequent impaired oxygenation/ventilation and death (usually within 6 to 7 minutes). Patients have hypovolemia from these osmotic movements of fluid, and hemolysis is not a significant feature.

As it enters the lungs, fresh water destroys surfactant activity, leading to alveolar collapse and intrapulmonary shunting (perfusion without ventilation). Water is reabsorbed into the vascular system, producing volume overload with subsequent hyponatremia and hemolysis of red blood cells.

28. The answer is C. *(Microbiology)*
Of the grafts listed, cornea transplants have the longest survival time. Cells of the cornea do express HLA-A and HLA-B antigens, but their density is low compared with most other tissues. In addition, the cornea is considered to be an "immunologically privileged" site (i.e., blood vessels and lymphatics are lacking). There appears to be little or no interaction between corneal proteins and cells of the immune system.

HLA matching of donor and recipient is generally not done before cornea transplants. Topical and subconjunctival steroids are the conventional forms of immunosuppressive therapy used.

Other sites and tissues considered to be "immunologically privileged" include the brain, testes, and uterus.

As with most other types of allografts, rejection (if it is going to occur) of a transplanted cornea occurs most frequently during the first 3 to 6 months after transplantation.

A high success rate is also seen with bone allografts. Bone is often frozen or freeze-dried before transplantation. These procedures reduce its immunogenicity.

There are a few long-term survivors of kidney, heart, liver, and pancreas transplants, but the overall success rates are considerably lower than for cornea transplant patients.

29. The answer is C. *(Pathology)*
The key difference between heat stroke and heat cramps or exhaustion is the presence of fever.

Heat stroke is associated with a core body temperature above 40°C, and is subdivided into exertional and classic types. Neither type is associated with a hemorrhagic stroke. The exertional type is most commonly seen in people working or running outdoors in hot or humid climates. Characteristic findings include: hot, dry skin, with or without sweating; profound lactic acidosis; rhabdomyolysis with myoglobinuria; potential for acute tubular necrosis; and potential for disseminated intravascular coagulation.

The classic type is most commonly seen in chronically ill patients, alcoholics, very young patients, the elderly, or morbidly obese people in hot or humid weather. It can be precipitated by drugs that inhibit sweating (e.g., anticholinergics, phenothiazines).

The following chart distinguishes heat stroke from heat cramps and exhaustion.

	Dehydrated	Hypovolemic	Fever
Heat cramps	Yes	No	No
Heat exhaustion	Yes	Yes	No
Heat stroke	Yes	Yes	Yes

30. The answer is D. *(Biochemistry)*
N-linked glycosylation begins in the endoplasmic reticulum. A core oligosaccharide is synthesized attached to a molecule of the lipid dolichol. The oligosaccharide is transferred from dolichol to an asparagine residue of the polypeptide chain. The oligosaccharide is first trimmed and then modified by the addition of monosaccharide units as the protein molecule is processed through the endoplasmic reticulum and the Golgi apparatus.

31. The answer is D. *(Pathology)*
Microwaves have a possible association with the development of acute leukemia and cataracts.

Frostbite is a form of localized injury that results from exposure to freezing temperatures. It results in an initial vasoconstriction, occlusion of vessels by agglutinated red blood cells, thrombosis of vessels, nerve injury, and death of the tissue.

Laser radiation produces an intense area of localized heat that is equivalent to a third degree burn. It is used therapeutically (e.g., repair of retinal detachment, destruction of retinal microaneurysms) and in surgery.

Trauma caused by electrical energy occurs when the body acts as a conductor of electricity. Current flow is considered to be the most important factor in electrocution deaths. Because household voltage is usually constant at 120 volts, the biggest variable in the electrocution equation is the resistance of the human body. The body has an internal resistance of 500 ohms, with the skin having a high resistance. The hands and feet, because of a dry callous surface, have an even higher resistance than skin (1000 to 100,000 ohms).

Another factor that determines damage by an electrical current is the path taken through the body, which is always along the path of least resistance, rather than a direct line between two points. Blood is an excellent conductor, so electrical current flows through blood vessels in the body. A path of current from the left arm to the right leg is most dangerous, because it produces ventricular fibrillation. Death from low voltage is most commonly secondary to respiratory paralysis.

AIDS, not automobile accidents, is the most common cause of death between 25 and 44 years of age.

32. The answer is B.   *(Microbiology)*
Tetanus toxin (tetanospasmin) is released by vegetative *Clostridium tetani* organisms at the wound site. The toxin may reach the central nervous system by retrograde anoxal transport or via the bloodstream. Antibody to the tetanus toxin (active immunity by toxoid induction or passive immunity) will attach to and neutralize only free circulating toxin, thereby destroying the pathogenicity of the molecule. Toxin attached to receptors in the CNS can not be neutralized by antibodies.

The toxin's main mechanism of action is to prevent release of inhibitory factors (glycine), resulting in tonic contraction of voluntary muscles. Tetanus immunoglobulin confers passive immunity to nonimmunized patients who have dirty wounds.

33. The answer is A.   *(Pathology)*
Cocaine is a sympathomimetic drug predisposing to sudden cardiac death. It is an alkaloid from the cocoa plant and can be smoked, sniffed through the nose, ingested, or injected. Cocaine blocks the reuptake of the neurotransmitter dopamine and norepinephrine by the presynaptic axon, leading to excessive excitation of postsynaptic fibers or effector cells. It produces intensive craving rather than a true addiction; however, prolonged use can lead to physiologic dependence. As a sympathomimetic agent, it dilates the pupils (mydriasis), increases the heart rate and systolic pressure, and predisposes to ventricular arrhythmias and sudden death.

Heroin is a depressant drug that is closely related to morphine, codeine, and methadone, all of which are derived from the poppy plant. It is usually self-administered intravenously or subcutaneously ("skin popping," with a danger of tetanus) and is usually "cut" with some agent (quinine) to lessen its potency.

Marijuana contains a psychoactive stimulant called tetrahydrocannabinol (THC). Hashish is the extracted resin of marijuana, and has 5 to 10 times greater potency than the parent compound. Phencyclidine (PCP) is a stimulant associated with aggressive behavior. Lysergic acid diethylamide (LSD) is a hallucinogen associated with chromosomal breakage.

34. The answer is A.   *(Biochemistry)*
Ethanol is metabolized to acetate in a two-step process, each involving conversion of NAD^+ to NADH. The acetate is then converted to acetyl coenzyme A (CoA), which can be oxidized in the citric acid cycle, used to synthesize fatty acids, or converted to ketone bodies. See the following schema.

$$1 \quad \text{Ethanol} + NAD^+ \xrightarrow{\text{Alcohol dehydrogenase}} \text{acetaldehyde} + NADH$$

$$2 \quad \text{Acetaldehyde} + NAD^+ \xrightarrow{\text{Aldehyde dehydrogenase}} \text{acetate} + NADH$$

$$3 \quad \text{Acetate} + CoA + ATP \xrightarrow{\text{Acetyl CoA synthetase}} \text{acetyl CoA} + AMP + PP_i$$

A toxic substance, acetaldehyde, is formed in the first step catalyzed by alcohol dehydrogenase. This is normally rapidly oxidized to acetate in the second step catalyzed by acetaldehyde dehydrogenase. Methanol and ethylene glycol also serve as substrates for alcohol dehydrogenase. Methanol is converted by the same two enzymes, first to formaldehyde and then to formic acid. These are toxic substances that cause damage to the optic nerve and metabolic acidosis. Ethylene glycol is oxidized by alcohol dehydrogenase to oxalic acid, which tends to precipitate as calcium oxalate in the kidney tubules and causes renal failure. Ethylene glycol, methanol, and ethanol are all substrates for alcohol dehydrogenase; however, ethanol has the lowest K_m (highest affinity) and displaces the other two potential substrates from the active site, leaving them unmetabolised and eventually excreted.

Ethanol does inhibit the release of the antidiuretic hormone, and by increasing the rate of diuresis, does increase the rate of clearance of both poisons; however, this mechanism is of minor consequence.

All three compounds produce cytoplasmic NADH as they oxidize. The presence of excess cytoplasmic NADH upsets the redox balance in this compartment. In glycolysis, this excess NADH will drive the lactate dehydrogenase reaction from pyruvate toward lactate and 1,3-bisphosphoglycerate toward glyceraldehyde 3-phosphate. The glyceraldehyde 3-phosphate equilibrates with dihydroxy acetone phosphate (DHAP), which will be driven to form glycerol phosphate. This condenses with fatty acids formed from the excess acetyl CoA under the high energy conditions provided by the ethanol. The liver tries to package the excess fat as very low density lipoprotein (VLDL) packages, which tend to accumulate, producing a fatty liver and eventually cirrhosis. This process is exacerbated by the poor diet that often accompanies alcoholism. A particularly critical metabolite is choline, required for phosphotidylcholine (lecithin) synthesis; lecithin is needed to form VLDL. The choline can be ingested as such or synthesized *de novo*. The limiting factor in *de novo* synthesis is most often methyl groups, which are supplied in the form of the essential amino acid methionine.

35. The answer is E. *(Pathology)*
Both oral contraceptives and exogenous estrogens have an increased risk for gallbladder disease. Oral contraceptives contain ethinyl estradiol (estrogen) and a derivative of 19-nortestosterone as the progestational agent. The growing use of the minipill, which contains a lower amount of hormone, has led to a decrease in adverse problems.

36. The answer is A. *(Behavioral science)*
A 55-year-old man who takes his prescribed medication only intermittently and rarely follows his prescribed diet is noncompliant. The most likely reason for noncompliance, in this patient or any patient, is a poor doctor–patient relationship (i.e., he views the doctor as distant and unfeeling).

37. The answer is D. *(Pathology)*
Patients with antihuman leukocyte antigens (anti-HLA) have an increased risk for hyperacute rejection of an organ transplant, because the antigens react against the specific HLA antigens in the endothelial cells of the donor tissue, causing vessel injury and thrombosis.

There is no correlation between anti-HLA antibodies and a graft versus host reaction. There is also no likelihood of an increased incidence of autoimmune disease in the presence of anti-HLA antibodies, because the antibodies are derived from reactions against foreign antigens, not antigens in the host. Patients are still acceptable as candidates for an organ transplant, as long as the donor tissue is missing the HLA antigens the patient has antibodies against. Hyperacute rejection is primarily a humoral response (type II hypersensitivity), rather than a cellular rejection by CD8 cytotoxic T cells.

38. The answer is C. *(Biochemistry)*
The vitamin folate is activated in the liver, not white cells, by a two-step reduction, to dihydrofolate and then to the active tetrahydrofolate (THF). Methotrexate has approximately a 1000-fold greater affinity for dihydrofolate reductase than dihydrofolate; therefore, it inhibits the conversion of dihydrofolate to tetrahydrofolate. Tetrahydrofolate is distributed to the various tissues, where it plays a pivotal role in one-carbon metabolism, passing one carbon unit at various oxidative steps to a host of compounds. Critical reactions include the donation of carbons at the C2 and C8 (i.e., choice C, formation of 5′-phosphoribosyl 4-carboxamide 5-formidoimidazole from 5′-phosphoribosyl 4-carboxamide 5-aminoimidazole) during synthesis of the purine ring. Although the formation of 5′-phosphoribosyl 4-carboxamide 5-formidoimidazole from 5′-phosphoribosyl 4-carboxamide 5-aminoimidazole may seem trivial to remember, reading the choice

carefully shows that one-carbon metabolism is involved in this step. The only difference between the name of the substrate and the product is that the amino group of the former is replaced by a formido group, indicating the product did gain a formyl moiety. THF is involved in formate transfer reactions and THF cannot be formed in the presence of methotrexate.

In contrast, one carbon moieties are not incorporated into the pyrimidine ring; however, the reaction catalyzed by thymidylate synthase, conversion of deoxyuridine monophosphate (dUMP—a pyrimidine used in RNA) to deoxythymidine monophosphate (dTMP—a pyrimidine used in DNA), does. This reaction is also inhibited by 5-fluorouracil. Whereas the conversion of methionine from homocysteine requires the direct participation of N^5-methyltetrahydrofolate as well as that of methlycobalamin, a coenzyme derived from vitamin B_{12}, the transfer of methyl groups from methionine to various methyl acceptors, forming homocysteine does not. Homocysteine can then be catabolized to cysteine via homoserine.

These reactions are summarized in the following schema.

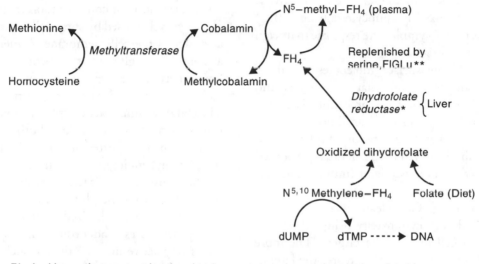

* Blocked by methotrexate, trimethoprim, 6—mercaptopurine, and cyclophosphamide
* Dihydrofolate reductase is inhibited by pterin analogues such as methotrexate
** FIGLu = foraminoglutamic acid, a product of histidine catabolism

Choline is synthesized from phosphotidylserine in a two-step sequence in which the seryl moiety is first decarboxylated to phosphotidylethanolamine, which is then methylated three times using S-adenosylmethionine (SAM) as the methyl-donating cofactor. SAM is synthesized from methionine using adenosine triphosphate (ATP) as a required cofactor in the following reaction sequence:

$$\text{L-methionine} + \text{ATP} \xrightarrow{\text{S-adenosylmethionine synthase}} \text{S-adenosylmethionine} + \text{PPi} + \text{Pi}$$

This reaction would not be greatly inhibited in a fully supplemented cell-free extract.

39. The answer is C. *(Microbiology)*
Patients with chronic granulomatous disease, a sex-linked recessive disease, are deficient in phagocyte function. The neutrophils/monocytes lack reduced nicotinamide adenine dinucleotide phosphate (NADPH) oxidase, a critical enzyme that is needed for the production of reactive oxygen intermediates (ROIs) responsible for the respiratory burst. Nitroblue tetrazolium (NBT) is a pale yellow dye that accepts

H$^+$ and is reduced as a result of NADPH oxidation to a blue intracellular precipitate. In the NBT test, peripheral blood neutrophils take up the dye after a stimulus (latex beads or other particles). Failure of the cells to reduce the NBT dye to a blue color is consistent with a diagnosis of chronic granulomatous disease.

E rosette-formation is a historically important assay for identification of human lymphocytes. T cells have a receptor (CD2) by which they are able to bind sheep erythrocytes (E). A lymphocyte with several erythrocytes attached to it has the appearance of a rosette.

There are several versions of cell-mediated cytolysis assays, the great majority of which are used to evaluate either T-cytotoxic or natural killer (NK) cell activity. An example is the mixed lymphocyte culture (MLC) test, which measures T-lymphocyte response to foreign histocompatibility antigens.

CD4 and CD8 are surface molecules found on T-lymphocyte subpopulations that have helper and cytotoxic activities. A common procedure is to use fluorescence-labelled monoclonal antibodies that are specific for each marker. Enumeration of cells labelled with either antibody can then be manually counted under a fluorescence microscope or (more accurately) in a flow cytometer.

The ^{51}chromium (^{51}Cr) release assay is a short-term assay for NK cell cytotoxicity using K562 cells (erythroleukemia cell line) as the targets. The more ^{51}Cr released from the targets, the greater the level of NK cell cytotoxicity.

40. The answer is A.   *(Biochemistry)*

The symptoms suggest that King George III suffered from acute intermittent porphyria, a disease diagnosed in two of his descendants. This diagnosis could have been confirmed by analysis of the urine for porphobilinogen, had a clinical laboratory been available. The darkening of the urine on exposure to light confirms the diagnosis, because oxidized porphobilinogen (porphobilin) has a dark color. Treatment would be administration of hemin, which inhibits δ-aminolevulinic acid (ALA) synthase and the accumulation of porphyrin intermediates.

41. The answer is C.   *(Pharmacology)*

Cellulitis is usually caused by group A streptococci or *Staphlococcus aureus*. Group A streptococci are sensitive

to penicillin V or G, but many staphylococci produce penicillinase, which inactivates these antibiotics. Penicillinase-producing staphylococci are usually sensitive to penicillinase-resistant penicillins (PRP) such as methicillin, nafcillin, oxacillin, and dicloxacillin. The PRP have a bulky R group that prevents binding to the active site of penicillinase. Of the penicillin-resistant penicillins, dicloxacillin and cloxacillin are preferred for oral therapy because of their superior oral bioavailability.

42. The answer is B.   *(Biochemistry)*

Glutathione is a tripeptide, γ-glutamylcysteinylglycine, present in high concentration in all cells. The γ-glutamyl cycle is used by some cells to transport amino acids across the cell membrane. A membrane-associated enzyme, γ-glutamyl transpeptidase forms peptide bonds between the glutamyl moiety of glutathione and the amino acid to be transported into the cell. The glutamyl-amino acid is split off from the cysteinylglycine part of the molecule as both are brought into the cell. The transported amino acid is then split from the glutamyl moiety, depositing the free amino acid on the cytosolic side of the membrane. 5-Oxyproline is produced from the glutamyl moiety, which has to be replaced or resynthesized, as does the glutathione. This process uses 3 adenosine triphosphates (ATPs), but is very active in some tissues, such as the kidney.

Glutathione reductase is the enzyme used to protect the red cell from oxidative stress and to reduce methemoglobin. Glutathione peroxidase is the selenium-containing enzyme used to scavenge free radicals and peroxides.

Glutathione is present in all cells in relatively large amounts, attesting to its importance in metabolism.

Glutathione S-transferase is a liver enzyme used in detoxification reactions. It forms a glutathione complex with the compound to be detoxified. There is no such enzyme as glutathione transaminase.

43. The answer is C.   *(Microbiology)*

Ribavirin is a nucleoside analog in which a triazole–carboxamide moiety is substituted in place of the normal purine precursor aminoimidazole–carboxamide. This drug inhibits the synthesis of guanine derivatives, which are essential for both DNA and RNA viruses. Ribavirin is delivered in an aerosal to treat infants with pneumonitis caused by respiratory syncytial virus and possibly influenza B and Hantavirus infections.

While there is some evidence that ribavirin might be a broad-spectrum antiviral agent, approved usage is as previously described.

The only other antivirals available for use to treat other viruses listed in the question are famciclovir or acyclovir for varicella–zoster, and ganciclovir for cytomegalovirus. No antiviral agents are currently useful against measles or rubella infections.

44. The answer is B. *(Biochemistry)*
Maple syrup urine disease is caused by a deficiency of branched-chain α-ketoacid dehydrogenase. Decreasing the amount of protein in the diet decreases the accumulation of branched-chain α-ketoacids and the concomitant acidosis. This dietary change diminishes the chance of retardation and/or death. The absence of protein in the diet for a few days will not have an adverse effect on the baby.

Changing from one type of milk to another will not reduce the intake of branched chain amino acids.

Addition of benzoic or phenylacetic acid is useful in the treatment of hyperammonemia, but has no place in the treatment of maple sugar disease. These compounds reduce the nitrogen load by forming a harmless glutamine conjugate, which is excreted in the urine.

Unfortunately, dirty diapers do not smell like maple sugar.

45. The answer is B. *(Behavioral science)*
The Stanford-Binet Scale is useful for evaluating general intellectual ability in individuals 2 to 18 years old. Cerebral dominance, perceptuomotor performance, memory, and presence or absence of dyslexia are evaluated in adults using neuropsychological tests such as the Halstead-Reitan and Luria-Nebraska test batteries.

46. The answer is C. *(Biochemistry)*
Rotenone is a site-specific inhibitor of electron transport. It acts at the level of complex I. Malate feeds electrons to reduced nicotinamide adenine dinucleotide (NADH), which in turn is passed into the electron transport system at the level of complex I, through

NADH dehydrogenase just before the blockage induced by this drug. Therefore, no electrons can be transported from NADH and no adenosine triphosphates (ATPs) are made. Succinate feeds in electrons from the reduced form of flavin adenine dinucleotide ($FADH_2$) at the level of complex II, through the action of succinyl dehydrogenase. Complex II passes its electrons to coenzyme Q at a point beyond the site of rotenone inhibition; therefore, rotenone has no inhibitory effect and 2 ATPs are produced per atom of oxygen consumed. (The number of ATPs produced per atom of oxygen used is often expressed as the number of phosphate ions taken up divided by the atoms of oxygen used. This is called the P/O ratio.) In the absence of any inhibitor, the P/O ratio for malate is 3 and for succinate 2.

Actinomycin D is an inhibitor of DNA synthesis, not oxidative phosphorylation. The inhibitor of electron transport is actinomycin A.

47. The answer is B. *(Microbiology)*
Trisodium phosphonoformate (foscarnet) inhibits herpes simplex virus (HSV) replication. Foscarnet is a potent inhibitor of HSV-induced DNA polymerase, and has little effect on known cellular DNA polymerases. Herpesvirus mutants resistant to the drug arise easily.

To a lesser extent, foscarnet also appears to inhibit the polymerase of hepatitis B virus and retroviruses.

Combinations of antivirals, including foscarnet, are currently prescribed to increase the clinical usefulness of the drugs.

48. The answer is B. *(Biochemistry)*
G proteins are membrane proteins that act as transducers by passing the signal conveyed to a receptor, via a hormone, to an enzyme that is located inside the membrane. This enzyme then alters the concentration of a second messenger, which induces the required intracellular response. There are many different types of G proteins; the primary difference among them is found in the α subunit, rather than the β or the γ subunits.

G proteins play an important role in signal amplification because one receptor can activate several G proteins, which in turn effects the activity of many enzymes, such as adenylate cyclase or phospholipase

C. These G proteins are divided into three major groups defined by their effect. G_S proteins activate adenylate cyclase, raising cyclic adenosine monophosphate (cAMP) levels; G_i proteins inhibit adenylate cyclase, lowering cAMP levels; and, G_p proteins activate phospholipase C, liberating inositol triphosphate and diacylgylcerol.

G proteins have no intrinsic protein kinase activity.

49. The answer is E. *(Microbiology)*
The most important mode of transmission of hepatitis B virus is via blood. From there, the virus infects hepatocytes. Immune attack by CD8 cytotoxic T cells against viral antigens on the infected hepatocytes appears to play an important role in pathogenesis by directly destroying the virally infected cells. This leads to hepatic cell necrosis.

Antigen–antibody complexes cause symptoms (e.g., arthralgia, urticaria) and some complications (e.g., glomerulonephritis and vasculitis) in chronic hepatitis.

Poliovirus, yellow fever virus, influenza, and rabies are capable of directly killing host cells without implicating cellular immunity. The lesions of yellow fever are caused by the localization and propagation of the virus in a particular organ. Death may occur from necrotic lesions in the liver and kidney.

Influenza viruses cause cellular destruction and desquamation of the mucosa of the respiratory tract. Humoral (antibody) responses are important in immunity to influenza, but the role of cell-mediated immune responses is unclear.

50. The answer is B. *(Behavioral science)*
In this scenario, the pediatrician has recommended extinguishing the interruptions by nonreinforcement. This means that the child's interrupting behavior will no longer be reinforced or rewarded by attention from the mother and will diminish over time. Intermittent, positive, and negative reinforcement all involve rewarding a desired behavior. Although punishing the child for the interruptions will be effective initially, the results of punishment are not as long lasting as the results of extinction.

51. The answer is C. *(Microbiology)*
Adjuvants are substances that increase the immunogenicity of an antigen when injected simultaneously.

One of the oldest of these is Freund complete adjuvant (FCA), which consists of killed mycobacteria suspended in a water-in-oil emulsion. The active part of the mycobacterial wall is muramyl dipeptide (MDP). MDP calls in and activates macrophages. This subsequently results in increased T- and B-lymphocyte functions. FCA is extremely potent and is not approved for humans (high fever and granuloma formation are possible side effects). Aluminum compounds (e.g., alum precipitate) are the most widely used adjuvants in humans. They are often added to inactivated, killed vaccines and to vaccines consisting of only part of the pathogenic agent, such as the diphtheria toxoid and tetanus toxoid.

Adjuvants act by prolonging the retention time of the antigen, by increasing the effective size of the antigen, and by increasing macrophage accumulation and antigen presentation.

A few antigens fall into the category of superantigens. These types of antigens activate a very large number of T lymphocytes (1% to 10%) without prior processing by an antigen-presenting cell. Superantigens bind directly to the major histocompatibility complex (MHC) molecules (outside of the peptide binding groove) and the Vβ region of the T-cell antigen receptor. Stimulation with a superantigen is nonspecific and can have disasterous consequences (e.g., massive production of cytokines, which may lead to systemic toxicity). Bacterial superantigens include *Staphylococcus aureus* toxins, which produce toxic shock syndrome and food poisoning, and the M protein of *Streptococcus pyogenes* (β-hemolytic streptococcus group A), which is associated with rheumatic fever. There is speculation that some HIV-1 proteins may act as superantigens.

A very high dose of antigen (or a very low dose) can lead to the induction of tolerance to that specific substance.

Attenuation of infectious agents reduces their pathogenicity. In the preparation of vaccines, care is taken so that their immunogenicity is not compromised.

52. The answer is E. *(Pharmacology)*
Superinfections caused by the anaerobic gram-positive bacillus, *Clostridium difficile,* may produce diarrhea and pseudomembranous colitis and are usually treated

with metronidazole or oral vancomycin. Vancomycin is not absorbed from the gut and remains in the intestinal tract to eradicate the infecting organism. Vancomycin must be given intravenously for systemic infections caused by methicillin-resistant staphylococci and for enterococcal infections in penicillin-allergic patients. Metronidazole is the drug of choice for *C. difficile* superinfection.

Gentamicin and other aminoglycosides are not effective against anaerobes because they require oxygen-dependent transport into bacteria. Although penicillin is used in the treatment of cellulitis caused by *Clostridium perfringens* (often with clindamycin or metronidazole), it is not effective against *C. difficile* enterocolitis.

53. The answer is D.   (*Microbiology*)
Immunoglobulin G (IgG; IgG1, IgG2, and IgG3 subclasses) and immunoglobulin M (IgM) are the two classes of antibodies that can activate complement. One molecule of IgM or two adjacent IgG molecules in an immune complex can activate the classic pathway. Immune complexes that are bound to the surface of a cell or particle are more efficient at fixing complement than soluble immune complexes. The binding of antibody to the antigen causes a conformational charge in the Fc portion of the antibody, so that C1q, the largest of the major components, can bind to it. C1q is a collagen-like protein with six globular heads connected to a common stem. It is multivalent and can bind more than one antibody molecule.

The complement system consists of approximately 25 proteins that are continuously present in the plasma in inactive form. The major components, C1qrs–C9, cascade in a sequential manner in which one component interacts with the next, either enzymatically or biochemically (cascade system). The remaining proteins of the system act in regulation and control. The kinin cascade, blood coagulation, and fibrinolysis are physiological processes that occur in an analogous manner.

54. The answer is A.   (*Behavioral science*)
Because all observations are added to obtain the mean or average, this is the measure of central tendency that would be most affected by an error that records 5.5

months as 55 months. Such an error would not alter either the median (middle score) or the mode (most commonly occuring score) in this set of scores.

55. The answer is B.   (*Microbiology*)
C1, C4, C2, and C1 inhibitor (C1INH) function in the classic, but not alternative, complement pathway, whereas factors B and D function only in the alternative. Both complement pathways have an initiation, amplification, and membrane attack phase. The latter two phases are common to both. The amplification phase begins with C3, the most abundant of the complement components, whereas the membrane attack phase begins with C5b. Thus, C3 and C5 are involved in both pathways.

C1INH destroys the activity of C1r and C1s and thus down-regulates the classic complement pathway. It also acts as an inhibitor of the kinin-generation pathway, the coagulation cascade, and the fibrinolytic system. C1INH is consumed while acting as an inhibitor.

A very low level of $C3(H_2O)$ is thought to be generated continuously and spontaneously. Factor B binds to this altered species of C3. Factor D, in turn, binds to the $C3(H_2O)$-factor-B complex and cleaves factor B. The remaining complex has C3 convertase activity in the alternative complement pathway.

There are two complement cascades, the classic (C1qrs, C4, C2, C3, C5, C6, C7, C8, and C9) and the alternative (C3, C5, C6, C7, C8, and C9). Properdin is important only in the alternative pathway. The convertase in this pathway (C3bBb) is highly unstable and dissociates rapidly. Properdin stabilizes the complex by binding to it, thus ensuring that the alternative cascade will proceed. C3 convertase in the classic pathway is C4b2b.

Immunization has no effect on complement synthesis and an immunologic stimulus is not required to induce the production of any of the components.

The liver is considered to be the major site of complement synthesis; however, a variety of cells are involved: hepatocytes (C3, C6, and C9), macrophages (C1q, C2, C4, and C5), splenocytes (C5 and C8), and intestinal epithelial cells (C1r and C1s).

The genes for C2, C4, and factor B are located within the class III region of the major histocompatibility complex (MHC) on the short arm of chromosome 6.

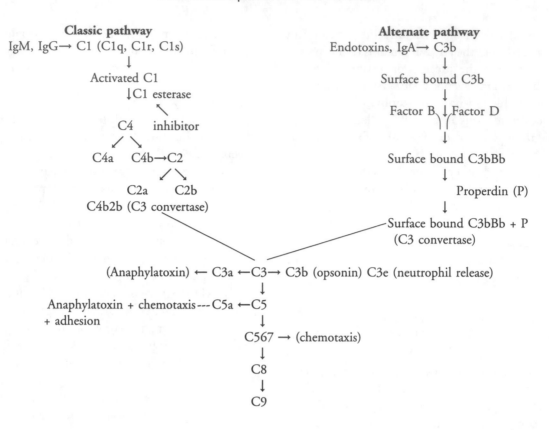

56. The answer is D. *(Pharmacology)*

Fluoroquinolones exert their antibacterial effects by inhibiting bacterial DNA gyrase (topoisomerase II), and resistance is often because of mutations in chromosomal genes that alter the structure of DNA gyrase and decrease fluoroquinolone binding. Resistance may also be associated with decreased drug permeation across the bacterial cell membranes. As yet, no quinolone-degrading or quinolone-inactivating resistance has been detected, and plasmid-mediated quinolone resistance has not been found. There is no association between bacterial cell wall structure or dihydrofolate reductase and fluoroquinolone resistance.

57. The answer is A. *(Microbiology)*

The cleavage of C3, C4, and C5 during complement activation generates C3a, C4a, and C5a, which are collectively referred to as anaphylatoxins. These small peptides (MW 8–11 kD) induce smooth muscle contraction and degranulation of mast cells and basophils with the subsequent release of histamine and other vasoactive molecules. C5a is by far the most potent of the three. C4a has the least activity.

The half-lives of C3a, C4a, and C5a are short because of removal of the terminal arginine by a carboxyl-peptidase enzyme that is present in plasma. An anaphylactic reaction caused by these substances occurs infrequently compared to an immunoglobulin E (IgE)-mediated hypersensitivity response (type I).

C5a has effects that are not shared by the other two cleavage products. It is also a potent chemoattractant for neutrophils and cells of the monocyte–macrophage series. These cells migrate toward the highest concentration of C5a.

In addition, C5a stimulates neutrophil adhesiveness, thereby causing them to aggregate. Oxidative metabolism and release of unstable oxygen radicals are dramatically increased in the cells.

Recent studies suggest that C5a may have direct effects on endothelial cells, which lead to increased vascular permeability independently of histamine release.

An important consequence of complement activation is the lysis of bacteria and other microorganisms; however, the anaphylatoxins do not participate in this defense mechanism. The binding of antibody (IgM or IgG1–3) to an antigen on the bacterial cell surface activates the classic complement cascade. A transmembrane channel is formed by the sequential attachment of C5b, C6, C7, C8, and C9. These latter components make up the membrane attack complex (MAC), which has a hydrophobic outer surface and a hydrophilic core. Small ions and water pass through the core, osmotic and chemical equilibrium is lost, and the cell swells and bursts.

Opsonization of bacteria and other cells occurs when C3b binds to them. C3b promotes their ingestion by phagocytes that have receptors for this cleavage product.

58. The answer is C. *(Behavioral science)*
Lung, breast, and colorectal cancer are the types of cancer responsible for the most deaths among American women.

59. The answer is B. *(Microbiology)*
C3b is an opsonin that is generated during complement activation. It can bind directly to cell membranes. When C3b attaches to bacteria, other particulate antigens, or immune complexes, their engulfment by phagocytic cells, which have receptors for C3b, occurs much more readily. Because the activation of C3 represents the amplification step in both the classic and alternative pathways, foreign materials generally become extensively coated with C3b, thus facilitating their removal from the body.

CR1 is a complement receptor (i.e., type 1 complement receptor), not an opsonin. It is a glycoprotein that has a high affinity for C3b. It can also bind to C4b, but with low affinity. CR1 is widely distributed and is expressed by monocytes, macrophages, neutrophils, eosinophils, erythrocytes, follicular dendritic cells, B lymphocytes, and some T lymphocytes.

Other complement receptors include CR2 (expressed by lymphoblastoid cells and B lymphocytes) and CR3 (expressed by phagocytic cells) These receptors bind primarily to several degradation products of C3b. CR2 is the receptor for the Epstein-Barr virus, which is the cause of infectious mononucleosis. CD3, a member of the integrin protein family, plays a significant role in cell adherence.

Activation of macrophages by C5a (or other agents) can increase the expression of CR1s from 5000 on resting phagocytes to 50,000. C5a also facilitates

phagocytosis by attracting neutrophils to the site of its generation.

C4b, which is attached rapidly and covalently to the target cell membrane, binds C2b to form C4b2b (C3 convertase). The most important function of this complex is to cleave large numbers of C3, not to opsonize.

C5b is the first component in the membrane attack complex (MAC). It attaches to cell membranes, but is highly unstable until the next component, C6, binds to it. It does not participate in opsonization.

Antibodies of the immunoglobulin G (IgG) class can also act as an opsonins. Macrophages and monocytes have high affinity receptors (FcγRI) for the Fc portion of the antibody. The rate of phagocytosis is dramatically enhanced by antibodies. In some cases, a 4000-fold higher rate of phagocytosis has been observed in the presence of antibody specific for an antigen compared with its absence.

60. The answer is C. *(Biochemistry)*
The β-lactamase gene encodes the enzyme β-lactamase, which catalyzes the hydrolysis of penicillins. Bacteria that produce this enzyme as a result of carrying such a resistance plasmid will be able to inactivate penicillins and, therefore, will be insensitive to them. If the plasmid is conjugative, resistance can be readily transmitted to other bacteria.

Restriction endonucleases are enzymes used by bacteria to degrade foreign DNA and, thus, protect themselves from bacteriophage infection. Neither transposition nor ultraviolet light damage are affected by β-lactamase.

61. The answer is C. *(Microbiology)*
Complement can be activated by interaction with certain acute-phase proteins that bind to bacteria, but not host cells. C-reactive protein is an acute phase–phase protein that binds to phosphorylcholine on bacterial cell surfaces and activates the complement cascade. This can result in lysis or opsonization of the microorganism. Phosphorylcholine is also found on mammalian cell membranes, but it is in a form that does not interact with C-reactive protein.

Mannose-binding protein (MBP) is another acute-phase protein that can activate complement. Its structure is similar to that of C1q. MBP binds directly to mannose residues on bacterial surfaces. It does not bind to mammalian cells, because the mannose of their carbohydrates are covered by other sugars.

Complement action can result in the destruction of many bacteria. This can occur within minutes after infection; however, there are some bacteria that are relatively resistant to direct complement action and must be eliminated in other ways.

Complement plays an important role in neutralizing the infectivity of enveloped viruses (e.g., influenza, herpes). Activation of complement can lead to lysis of the membranous viral envelope. In addition, C3b can bind to the envelope and thus disrupt the configuration of the glycoproteins by which the virus attaches to cells. C3b also enhances the aggregation of viruses in the presence of antibody.

Soluble immune complexes that are coated with C3b are more efficiently removed from the body than unbound complexes. This role of complement is especially striking in individuals who are unable to generate normal amounts of C3b as a result of deficiency in C1, C2, or C4.

Complement is heat-labile. It is readily inactivated by heating serum for 30 minutes at 56°C.

62. The answer is A.   (Behavioral science)
The leading causes of death in adult Americans in 1993 were heart disease (34%), cancer (23%), and stroke (7%), followed by chronic obstructive pulmonary diseases and accidents.

63. The answer is D.   (Microbiology)
An organism that is phagocytized is exposed to a wide range of different killing mechanisms. The generation of reactive nitrogen intermediates is a recently discovered oxygen-dependent pathway that may be especially important in microbial cell killing. Nitric oxide synthetase combines oxygen with the nitrogen of L-arginine to generate nitric oxide (NO). NO has broad antimicrobial toxicity. It is toxic to many bacterial, fungal, helminthic, and protozoal pathogens. In addition, it may be a mediator of macrophage and neutrophil cytotoxicity against tumor cells. It is also a very potent vasodilator.

The synthesis of tumor necrosis factor-α (TNF-α) by macrophages is not oxygen dependent; however, TNF-α, together with interferon-γ (IFN-γ) are

needed for optimal expression of NO. IFN-γ activates the pathway that leads to NO production and TNF-α greatly facilitates its release.

Lysozyme and the hydrolytic enzymes of macrophages and neutrophils mediate oxygen-independent microbial cell killing. Lysozyme is an enzyme that is found in many different cell types and body secretions. It can break the sugar backbone of the walls of both gram-positive and gram-negative bacteria.

Defensins are a group of toxic cationic peptides whose degradative properties are oxygen independent. They form ion-permeable channels in lipid bilayer membranes, and are most active at pH 7.0, or early after phagolysosome formation (before acidification). Defensins can kill bacteria (e.g., *Staphylococcus aureus, Pseudomonas aeruginosa, Escherichia coli*), fungi (e.g., *Cryptococcus neoformans*), and viruses (e.g., *Herpes simplex*).

The production of reactive oxygen intermediates (ROIs) is another important oxygen-dependent killing mechanism of phagocytes (in addition to the NO pathway). This process is triggered by an enzyme reduced nicotinamide adenine dinucleotide phosphate (NADPH oxidase) in the phagocyte membrane that reduces O_2 to superoxide (O_2-). This, in turn, generates other ROIs (hydroxyl radicals, singlet oxygen, and hydrogen peroxide).

$$NADPH + 2O_2 \xrightarrow{\text{NADPH oxidase}} NADP + 2O_2\text{-} + H^+$$

$$2O_2\text{-} + 2H^+ \xrightarrow{\text{Superoxide dismutase}} H_2O_2 + O_2$$

$$H_2O_2 + Cl^- \xrightarrow{\text{Myeloperoxidase}} H_2O + OCl^-$$

ROIs are powerful oxidizing agents that interact with lipid membranes.

64. The answer is A.   (Pharmacology)
Bacterial DNA-dependent RNA polymerase is inhibited by rifampin, a unique broadspectrum antibiotic that is often used in treating tuberculosis. Resistance is frequently caused by mutations that reduce the affinity of the enzyme for rifampin. Trimethoprim inhibits bacterial dihydrofolate reductase and fluoroquinolones, such as ofloxacin, inhibit bacterial DNA gyrase. Acyclovir inhibits viral DNA polymerase, whereas vancomycin inhibits cell-wall synthesis by binding to the D-alanyl-D-alanine precursor of the peptidoglycan.

65. The answer is B.　*(Pathology)*

Inheritance of B27 is strongly associated with the development of ankylosing spondylitis. The B27 gene codes for a human leukocyte antigen (HLA) located within the class I region of the major histocompatibility complex (MHC). Presence of B27 carries a relative risk factor of approximately 90 (i.e., approximately 90% of individuals who have the disease also have B27); however, an individual may have B27, but not the disease.

Alkylosing spondylitis, the prototype of all HLA-associated diseases, is a chronic progressive inflammatory disease of the spine and large joints, sacroiliitis, uveitis, and aortic regurgitation. The great majority of cases occur in males. Onset is insidious and usually begins in the second or third decade of life. Patients are seronegative for rheumatoid factor, thus the term seronegative spondyloarthropathy.

An association also exists between B27 and Reiter syndrome (an autoimmune disease consisting of arthritis, urethritis, and conjunctivitis) and psoriatic arthritis (an autoimmune erosive polyarthritis).

Inheritance of HLA-DR3 and DR4 is strongly associated with insulin-dependent (type I) diabetes mellitus, whereas HLA-DR2 has a negative association with the disease.

A relative risk factor of 47 is reported for HLA-Dw14 and juvenile rheumatoid arthritis, which usually occurs in children under the age of 16 years.

The role of the HLA in the development of autoimmune diseases is unclear. Undoubtedly, autoimmune diseases are not inherited according to simple mendelian segregation of alleles. Studies of identical twins, in which both have the same risk factor and only one develops the disease, indicate that environmental factors are also important.

The relative risk value reflects the chance that a person who is heterozygous for a particular allele will develop the disease. A risk factor of 1 indicates that incidence of the allele is the same in populations with or without the disease.

66. The answer is C.　*(Behavioral science)*

The distinction between mental and physical illness among Native Americans may be blurred; there is also a belief that witchcraft can result in illness. Native Americans have a high suicide rate and a high rate of alcoholism.

67. The answer is E.　*(Microbiology)*

Comparisons of graft survival and human leukocyte antigen (HLA) differences show that the likelihood of organ rejection is greatest when the donor and recipient do not match in the HLA-DR locus. For example, in heart transplantation, a 90% survival with one mismatch in the HLA-DR can drop to 65% when two antigens are mismatched. The reasons for this are unclear, but may be partly related to the fact that the HLA-DR codes for class II antigens.

Class II molecules are critical in antigen presentation to CD4$^+$ T-helper lymphocytes. These cells are the most important cells in graft rejection.

The HLAs are highly polymorphic. There are approximately 35 different class II (HLA-DP, HLA-DQ, and HLA-DR) and 80 different class I (HLA-A, HLA-B, and HLA-C) molecules that have been identified in humans. The chances of a 100% match in the HLA between two randomly selected individuals is very remote. Among siblings, there is a 25% chance for a perfect HLA match, 25% for no match, and a 50% chance for a 1 haplotype match.

Allelic differences within the HLA are very small (i.e., at most, the expressed antigens differ in only one or a few amino acids).

Serologic typing with a panel of cytotoxic antibodies against all known HLA antigens can be performed within a few hours. In the mixed lymphocyte culture (MLC, also known as mixed lymphocyte reaction or MLR), a low recipient antidonor response correlates with excellent graft survival; however, the test requires that donor and recipient cells be incubated together for about six days, which is not always possible (e.g., if it is a cadaveric donor, or in heart transplantation, in which time is of essence). The MLC is especially important in bone marrow transplantation, in which the risk for a graft versus host reaction is great.

Identity within the HLA does not guarantee graft survival. Transplanted tissue is also rejected because of differences in various minor histocompatibility loci; however, the rejection is less vigorous and can frequently be controlled with immunosuppressive drugs, such as cyclosporine.

68. The answer is B.　*(Pharmacology)*

Two interactions may occur between aminoglycosides, such as gentamicin, and parenteral cephalosporins, such as cephalothin. They may exhibit an additive or synergistic bactericidal effect against susceptible pathogens and they may potentiate the nephrotoxicity of each other. New cephalosporins cause less nephrotoxicity than the original cephalosporins, and evidence for increased nephrotoxicity is greater for the gentamicin–cephalothin combination than for other members of these groups. Furosemide may potentiate the auditory toxicity of aminoglycosides, both of which may cause hearing loss when given alone, but there is no evidence of increased nephrotoxicity with this combination of drugs.

69. The answer is B.   (Behavioral science)
If a patient refuses to have a gangrenous leg amputated, the first step the physician should take is to tell the patient the consequences of refusing the amputation. Because mentally competent patients can refuse medical treatment, permission obtained from a relative or from the hospital board of directors is irrelevant in this case. Transferring this patient to either another physician or another hospital will not change the outcome of this case.

70. The answer is A.   (Biochemistry)
Glucokinase is a high K_m enzyme (low affinity for glucose) designed to act when the liver is presented with the high glucose levels found in portal blood. It allows the liver to remove much of the glucose absorbed after a meal and prevents serum glucose levels from rising to high levels. In this case, the glucose administered intravenously goes into the general circulation and should not raise the blood glucose level to the point at which glucokinase activity becomes significant. The glucose will be phosphorylated in all tissues by hexokinase, which has a low K_m (high affinity for substrate). Unlike glucokinase, hexokinase acts on several hexoses and is inhibited by glucose 6-phosphate.

The other enzymes are all kinases involved in the glycolytic sequence. Their activity continues to be important in the patient's present condition.

71. The answer is B.   (Pharmacology)
Aminoglycosides such as gentamicin, tobramycin, and amikacin use an oxygen-dependent transport system to enter bacterial cells, where they bind to the 30S ribosomal subunit and cause misreading of messenger RNA.

72. The answer is C.   (Behavioral science)
The rate of side effects for this drug is 10%. The probability that neither patient will have side effects is obtained by multiplying the probability that patient 1 will not have side effects (100% - 10% = 90%) by the probability that patient 2 will not have side effects (100% - 10% = 90%). Thus, the probability that neither patient 1 nor patient 2 will develop side effects is calculated as 90% × 90% = 81%.

73. The answer is B.   (Pharmacology)
Isoniazid and rifampin are used together in treating tuberculosis, but only rifampin is active against *Mycobacterium leprae,* meningococci, staphylococci, and other nontubercular organisms. Both drugs are hepatotoxic, but only rifampin imparts an orange–red color to urine and other fluids. Isoniazid is metabolized by acetylation, whereas rifampin is metabolized by deacetylation.

74. The answer is D.   (Biochemistry)
In operons regulated by attenuation, messenger RNA (mRNA) synthesis is initiated at a constant rate. The 5′ portion of the message encodes a short leader peptide. The rate of synthesis of this leader peptide by the ribosome influences the secondary structures that form as a result of folding of the mRNA molecule. One of these alternate secondary structures is the attenuator—a transcriptional termination signal that, when formed, causes RNA polymerase to prematurely terminate mRNA synthesis. The attenuator forms in the mRNA molecule, not DNA. No repressor protein is involved in regulation by this mechanism.

75. The answer is C.   (Pharmacology)
Clavulanate protects amoxicillin from inactivation by bacterial β-lactamase, thereby increasing its effectiveness in infections caused by penicillinase-producing organisms that are otherwise susceptible to amoxicillin. Penicillinase-producing strains of *Haemophilus influenzae* have become more common and are often associated with cases of otitis media that do not respond to amoxicillin, but usually respond to amoxicillin plus clavulanate.

The most common pathogens causing otitis media are *Streptococcus pneumoniae* and *H. influenzae.* Most streptococci are sensitive to penicillins and usually do not produce penicillinase or require clavulanate therapy. Streptococcal resistance is usually caused by decreased binding of penicillin to streptococcal penicillin-binding proteins. *Pseudomonas* and *Mycoplasma* are not sensitive to amoxicillin, with or without clavulanate.

76. The answer is D.   *(Biochemistry)*
In operons regulated by attenuation, such as the histidine operon, messenger RNA (mRNA) synthesis is initiated at a constant rate. Regulation occurs at the level of premature termination of mRNA synthesis. In the presence of excess histidine, synthesis of the polycistronic message coding for the enzymes of the histidine biosynthetic pathway is stopped before the structural genes encoding the enzymes are reached. Lack of enzyme synthesis and histidine synthesis are secondary effects, caused by the failure to complete synthesis of the mRNA molecule. DNA synthesis and ribosome synthesis remain unaffected.

77. The answer is C.   *(Pharmacology)*
Both drugs are rapidly excreted by renal tubular secretion. Amoxicillin is stable in gastric acid and has high oral bioavailability, whereas methicillin is acid labile and must be injected. Amoxicillin is not resistant to penicillinase and is often coadministered with clavulanate, a penicillinase inhibitor. Methicillin is resistant to penicillinase and has been used to treat staphylococcal infections. Neither drug is active against *Pseudomonas aeruginosa.*

78. The answer is C.   *(Behavioral science)*
In aging, reduced speed of new learning may occur, although the IQ remains stable throughout life. Impaired consciousness and abnormal level of arousal occur in delirium. Psychosis and depression are pathologic conditions and are not seen in normal, aging people.

79. The answer is C.   *(Biochemistry)*
Isocitrate dehydrogenase is the main regulated step in the tricarboxylic acid cycle, in which it has a role analogous to that of phosphofructokinase-1 in glycolysis. It depends on adenosine diphosphate (ADP) for activity and is deactivated by reduced nicotinamide adenine dinucleotide (NADH) under conditions of high adenosine triphosphate (ATP) concentration (low ADP). When it is inactivated, citrate accumulates and is transported into the cytoplasm where, in most cells, it acts in conjunction with ATP to inhibit phosphofructokinase-1. In liver cells, this inhibitory effect is overridden by a hormonally induced (high insulin, low glucagon) increase in fructose 2,6-bisphosphate. In addition, the citrate is used as a substrate for fatty-acid synthesis.

80. The answer is E.   *(Behavioral science)*
The leading cause of death among teenagers in the United States is accidents. Approximately 75% of these deaths result from automobile accidents. Suicide and homocide are the second and third leading causes of death in teenagers. Cardiovascular disease is a relatively rare cause of death in this age group.

81. The answer is A.   *(Biochemistry)*
Pyruvate kinase deficiency is the most common cause of chronic hereditary hemolytic anemia because of an enzyme deficiency in the glycolytic pathway. It is inherited in an autosomal recessive fashion, which is consistent with the parents being first cousins and asymptomatic carriers of the defective gene. The red blood cell is particularly vulnerable to deficiencies of glycolytic enzymes, because anaerobic glycolysis is the only way they can produce energy. Usually, hemolytic anemia induced by pyruvate kinase deficiency produces relatively mild symptoms because the block is below the level of 2,3-diphosphoglycerate synthesis, causing this intermediate to accumulate. This compound reduces the affinity of hemoglobin for oxygen and permits the reduced number of red cells to function more effectively. Moreover, there is generally some degree of adaption to the anemia in the form of a reticulocytosis.

The western European ancestry of the patient suggests that it is not glucose 6-phosphate dehydrogenase deficiency. Furthermore, glucose 6-phosphate dehydrogenase deficiency is inherited in a sex-linked recessive manner. Hemolytic anemia only occurs after the cells are subjected to an oxidizing stress, generally an oxidative drug like primaquine.

The membrane protein, spectrin, is defective in hemolytic anemia associated with congenital spherocytosis. In this disease, red blood cells appear spherical rather than as biconcave disks because of the faulty membrane structure. Moreover, the mode of inheritance is autosomal dominant, so one of the parents would probably have the disease.

Iron deficiency or other defects in iron metabolism do not cause hemolytic anemia.

Decay-accelerating factor (DAF) is deficient in paroxysmal nocturnal hemoglobinuria (PNH), which is acquired hemloytic anemia associated with increased sensitivity to complement destruction. Normally, DAF accelerates the metabolism of complement. PNH produces intravascular hemolytic anemia at night when a decrease in blood pH enhances complement activation. Hemoglobinuria is noted in the first morning void.

82. The answer is B. *(Behavioral science)*
Classical conditioning is defined as learning by association. The patient has learned to associate the hospital (the conditioned stimulus) with the dizziness that results from chemotherapy (the unconditioned stimulus). In operant conditioning, a relationship is established between a stimulus and a response by a system of reward or reinforcement. Extinction is the disappearance of a learned behavior. Shaping involves rewarding closer and closer approximations of behavior, and modeling is learning by observation.

83. The answer is C. *(Biochemistry)*
Feedback inhibition involves regulation by negative allosteric effectors. The effectors are small molecules that bind to the enzyme, altering its affinity for substrate or its maximal catalytic activity. A feedback inhibitor is often the end product of a pathway, and inhibits an early, committed step in the pathway. All of the other processes listed are genetic regulatory mechanisms that control the actual number of enzyme molecules synthesized.

84. The answer is D. *(Behavioral Science)*
The type of nursing home designed to provide restorative nursing care and assistance with self-care is an intermediate care facility. A residential care facility is a type of nursing home that provides a sheltered

environment but no nursing care. In a hospice, physicians, nurses, social workers, and volunteers provide inpatient and outpatient supportive care to terminally ill patients. A skilled nursing facility has practical nurses 24 hours a day and registered nurses during daytime hours.

85. The answer is E. *(Behavioral science)*
Canada, England, France, and Germany have national health systems. With the exception of the United States, all developed countries provide some form of government-funded health care.

86. The answer is B. *(Biochemistry)*
The unusual diet contains large quantities of avidin, which binds to and prevents the absorption of biotin. Moreover, the patient is getting little biotin in his diet or from his bacterial flora, since he is taking tetracycline. Biotin is required for carboxylation reactions, namely the carboxylation of pyruvate to form oxaloacetate and of acetyl coenzyme A (CoA) to form malonyl CoA.

None of the other reactions utilize biotin. Phospho*enol*pyruvate is converted to pyruvate by the action of pyruvate kinase. The irreversible nature of this step makes it necessary for pyruvate to undergo a circuitous route when it is converted to phospho*enol*pyruvate.

The conversion of pyruvate to acetyl CoA, catalyzed by pyruvate dehydrogenase, uses thiamine as a cofactor.

The conversion of pyruvate to lactate, catalyzed by lactate dehydrogenase, uses reduced nicotinamide adenine dinucleotide (NADH) as a cofactor. Niacin (nicotinic acid, nicotinamide) is the vitamin prescursor of the pyridine ring of NAD^+.

87. The answer is A. *(Behavioral science)*
In a health maintenance organization (HMO), physicians are paid a yearly salary to provide medical services to a group of people who have paid a yearly premium in advance. A union trust fund, which contracts with physicians in private practice to provide health care to the fund's subscribers, is known as a preferred provider organization (PPO). In an independent practice association (IPA), physicians in private practice are hired by an HMO to provide services to HMO patients. A residential care facility is a type of nursing

home that provides a sheltered environment but no nursing care. Physicians, nurses, social workers, and volunteers provide inpatient and outpatient supportive care to terminally ill patients in a hospice.

88. The answer is C. *(Biochemistry)*
Pyruvate dehydrogenase is a large complex containing five different enzyme activities and five cofactors. Two of the five enzymes are regulators: a kinase and a phosphatase. Pyruvate dehydrogenase kinase phosphorylates the complex, which inactivates the ability of the enzyme to oxidatively decarboxylate pyruvate. This kinase is cyclic adenosine monophosphate (cAMP)-independent, but is activated by acetyl coenzyme A (CoA) and reduced nicotinamide adenine dinucleotide (NADH), accounting for the negative feedback action of these metabolites when they accumulate under energy-rich conditions or during β oxidation of fatty acids. By inhibiting the kinase with dichloroacetate, the pyruvate dehydrogenase activity is "jump started," even in the presence of accumulated acetyl CoA or NADH, so that lactate can once again be metabolized.

89. The answer is B. *(Behavioral science)*
This woman's recent losses and her weight change suggest that she is suffering from a major depressive disorder. In the elderly, depression is often characterized by cognitive disturbances, such as loss of memory. It is important to distinguish whether an elderly patient is depressed or is showing the early signs of dementia, because the former is highly treatable. Although elderly people are at increased risk for depression and suicide when compared with the younger population, depression in the elderly can be treated effectively with antidepressant medications or with electroconvulsive therapy (ECT). While aging is associated with slower rate of learning, IQ remains the same over the course of an individual's lifetime.

90. The answer is B. *(Anatomy)*
Desmin is the intermediate filament (IF) protein that polymerizes to form the desmin IF of skeletal muscle. It is found in smooth, skeletal, and cardiac muscle. The desmin IF links desmosomes of cardiac muscle, thus serving to stabilize cell junctions.

Actin is the protein of microfilaments—the smallest diameter filament of the cytoskeleton. Actinin is an actin-associated protein (an actin-bundling protein) that serves to cross-link actin bundles and anchor actin filaments to the cell membrane.

Clathrin forms a basket or cage around endocytotic vesicles.

Vimentin is a widely distributed IF protein present in many cells of mesodermal origin.

91. The answer is D. *(Behavioral science)*
In healthy, aged men, sexuality is characterized by increased need for direct genital stimulation. Sexuality in this group is also characterized by slower erection, longer refractory period, and decreased intensity of ejaculation. In spite of physical changes and societal attitudes, many elderly people are interested in and continue to engage in sexual activity.

92. The answer is D. *(Microbiology)*
Rubeola (measles) and mumps viruses belong to the paramyxovirus group, which also includes respiratory syncytial virus and parainfluenza viruses. These viruses have a negative sense, linear RNA as a genome. As such, the genome cannot act directly as messenger RNA (mRNA) and the virion contains an RNA-dependent RNA polymerase. This enzyme uses a virion genome as a template for viral mRNA production. In contrast to orthomyxoviruses (influenza viruses), which have a segmented genome and undergo frequent reassortment, paramyxoviruses do not have a segmented genome and do not reassort frequently. Reassortment refers to the fact that any virus with a segmented genome (influenza, reoviruses) may have any or all segments of the genome included in a progeny virus. The mechanism for this is currently not understood. Coinfection of one host cell by two related viruses (e.g., two influenzas) may have genome segments of both viruses included in progeny virions, thereby creating a new or hybrid influenza virus type. All members are antigenically stable.

93. The answer is C. *(Behavioral science)*
Most Americans receive medical care in voluntary hospitals. Only 12% of hospitals in the United States are for-profit, investor owned hospitals. State governments own and operate psychiatric hospitals, whereas

the federal government owns and operates Veteran Administration and military hospitals.

94. The answer is C.   *(Microbiology)*

Many of the organisms listed have the ability to cause some level of gastroenteritis (food poisoning). The spore-forming designation should identify the genera of *Clostridium* and *Bacillus*. *Bacillus cereus* is usually associated with spores on grains, such as rice, and may survive steaming and rapid frying. Spores germinate when rice is kept warm and vegetative organisms are ingested. The organism produces two enterotoxins, one that is heat labile and the other heat stable. *Clostridium perfringens*, normally thought of in myconecrosis (gas gangrene), has spores that are commonly located in soil and on food. They survive cooking, and the organisms routinely grow to large numbers in reheated foods, especially meat dishes. An enterotoxin (mechanism unknown) is produced.

95. The answer is B.   *(Behavioral science)*

Occupation is the primary determinant of socioeconomic status. This is followed by educational level and place of residence.

96. The answer is E.   *(Biochemistry)*

Glucose is transported into mucosal cells and out of the lumen of the renal tubules by a sodium-ion cotransport system. The insulin-dependent glucose transport systems are not present in hepatocytes or in the brain; they are most important in muscle and adipose cells. Hexokinase does not transport glucose across the membrane of any cell type. It does phosphorylate glucose once it is transported into the cell, thereby maintaining a concentration gradient.

97. The answer is A.   *(Behavioral science)*

The most common cause of death in infants in the United States is congenital anomalies. Respiratory distress syndrome (RDS) and sudden infant death syndrome (SIDS) are the second and third leading causes of death in infants.

98. The answer is A.   *(Anatomy)*

Microtubules are hollow tubes formed of the dimer tubulin. They can polymerize and depolymerize rapidly, and have many cellular functions, such as chromosome movement, vesicle translocation (especially in axons), ciliary and flagellar movement, organelle movement, and cell structural changes.

Stress fibers are aggregates of microfilaments, which function to maintain the structural integrity of the cell. They are usually oriented parallel to the long axis of the cell.

Microfilaments are actin filaments capable of polymerizing and depolymerizing, just like microtubules. They are small and are more readily seen in their aggregated (bundle) form. Intermediate filaments are intermediate in size between microfilaments and microtubules and are rope-like, weaving throughout the cytoplasm. They are not hollow.

99. The answer is A.   *(Behavioral science)*

By legal definition, rape is penetration of the vulva by the penis; erection and ejaculation do not have to occur. Nonconsenting penetration of the anus and oral–penile contact are legally defined as sodomy, not rape. In rape trials, the victim does not have to prove that she struggled against the rapist, and her previous sexual activities are not admissible as evidence.

100. The answer is B.   *(Microbiology)*

Culture techniques remain a major mechanism in the isolation and identification of specific microorganisms as etiologic agents of disease. While some bacteria may be isolated from a lesion or other clinical specimen in pure culture, more often the pathologic agent will need to be isolated from a mixture of many bacteria (including nonpathogenic normal flora). A selective medium contains an added chemical that will inhibit large numbers of unwanted bacteria (normal flora) and allow specific types to grow. For example, mannitol salt agar selects for *Staphylococcus*, Thayer-Martin agar selects for *Neisseria gonorrhoeae* and *N. meningitidis*, and bile-esculin agar is selective for enterococci (enteric streptococci). Differential medium will include a system to distinguish specific species within a selected group. The mannitol in mannitol salt agar will distinguish between *Staphylococcus epidermidis* (mannitol negative-nonpathogenic) and *S. aureus* (mannitol positive-pathogenic).

X and V factors are used to identify species of *Haemophilus*. Factor X is heme and factor V is nicotinamide (NAD) or other coenzymes. X and V are supplied to the culture system by being placed on paper strips on the agar surface.

Blood agar (5% sheep RBC enriched) is an enriched medium, supplying nutrients for a wide variety of microorganisms. It may serve as a base medium for selection or differentiation, but does not perform these functions by itself. For example, it can differentiate between types of hemolysis.

Hemolysis: Types and Examples

Type	Action on RBC	Example
Beta (clear zone)	Complete on destruction	*Streptococcus pyogenes*
Alpha	Incomplete destruction, hemoglobin released	*Streptococcus pneumoniae*
Gamma	No reaction	Group D, nonenterococcus

101. The answer is D.   *(Behavioral science)*
Transvestites are men who dress in women's clothes for sexual pleasure. They are heterosexual and have a male gender identity (sense of themselves as men). Transsexuals have a defect in gender identity and believe that they were born the wrong sex. Homosexuals are sexually and emotionally interested in people of the same sex.

102. The answer is D.   *(Biochemistry)*
The mitochondria are added at point A and substrate at point B. Little oxidation occurs, because this is a tightly coupled system and oxidation cannot occur without phosphorylation. The addition of the phosphate acceptor, adenosine diphosphate (ADP), at point C allows oxidation to start. Oligomycin is added at point D. Oligomycin is an inhibitor of adenosine triphosphate (ATP) synthetase. It prevents ADP from being phosphorylated to form ATP and creates a condition analogous to that which existed before the addition of ADP. That is, it also inhibits the flow of electrons through the electron transport chain and the utilization of oxygen. Oligomycin inhibits both oxidation and phosphorylation in a tightly coupled system by preventing ADP from being phosphorylated. The addition of 2,4-dinitrophenol at point E uncouples oxidation from phosphorylation and permits the unimpeded flow of electrons to start. The rate of oxygen consumption is actually greater than when ADP was phosphorylated because the system is doing no work.

103. The answer is A.   *(Behavioral science)*
Compared with his sleep at age 20, delta sleep in an 80-year-old man decreases. Quantities of both delta sleep and rapid eye movement (REM) sleep decrease with age, and elderly people report that they sleep less than when they were young.

104. The answer is B.   *(Microbiology)*
A "wheal and flare" (induration and erythema) appears rapidly in individuals with Type I hypersensitivity after a skin prick test, if the appropriate allergen is used. A drop containing the allergen is placed on the skin, which is then pricked lightly with a needle at the center of the drop. This introduces an extremely small amount of the allergen into the epidermis, thus reducing the risk for a systemic anaphylactic reaction. In hypersensitive individuals, the specific allergen binds to the antigen-binding portion of the specific immunoglobulin E (IgE), which is fixed to the surface of cutaneous mast cells. The binding induces degranulation and release of pharmacologically active mediators (e.g., histamine), which produce the "wheal and flare." Recall that histamine increases vessel permeability, thus producing this type of cutaneous response.

Intradermal (ID) testing in IgE-mediated diseases is usually perfomed only when the skin prick test gives negative or 1+ results. Some individuals develop a late-phase reaction that appears 6 to 12 hours after a "wheal and flare." The late-phase reaction is thought to be caused by certain cytokines (e.g., tumor necrosis factor-α, which is preformed and stored in mast cell granules) and other mediators (prostaglandins and leukotrienes) that are synthesized after mast cell degranulation.

A positive response to ID injection of purified protein derivative (PPD) or lepromin is seen at 48 and 72 hours in individuals with cutaneous delayed-type hypersensitivity to *Mycobacterium tuberculosis* or *M. leprae*. It is characterized by induration and erythema at the injection site. The inflammatory infiltrate primarily consists of mononuclear cells. A positive response in one or more skin tests for delayed hypersensitivity indicates that T-dependent immune responses are generally intact.

In some patients, the same test antigen (when injected ID) can induce a "wheal and flare" at 15 to 20 minutes, a late-phase inflammatory response at 6 to 12 hours, and a positive response at 48 to 72 hours.

Patch testing is commonly used to detect cutaneous hypersensitivity (cellular immunity) to substances associated with contact dermatitis (e.g., detergents, nickel). A low concentration of the test substance is applied directly on the skin and covered with a bandage (or "patch") for 48 hours. Erythema and papules or vesicles indicate a positive response. Induration is rare, because the antigen is not injected ID. Patch testing during active contact dermatitis may exacerbate the condition.

The Schick test is a skin test performed to determine the presence of neutralizing antibodies against diphtheria toxin. Currently, it is rarely performed, and is mostly of historical value.

105. The answer is B. *(Behavioral science)*
"What brings you here today?" is the most open-ended question or statement because it is the most useful in obtaining information about the patient and does not close off other important topics. "Have you been to a physician within the last year?" and "Is there a history of heart disease in your family?" are direct questions, requiring only a yes or no answer, and are therefore less likely to elicit information. "Why didn't you come in sooner?" may make the patient defensive and, consequently, is not likely to lead to good rapport, important for eliciting patient information. "Tell me about the pain in your chest" limits the patient's response to one particular body area and does not allow for a completely open-ended response.

106. The answer is D. *(Biochemistry)*
Termination of translation occurs when the ribosome arrives at a nonsense or chain termination codon on the messenger RNA (mRNA) molecule, and this nonsense codon becomes aligned with the A site on the ribosome. No transfer RNA (tRNA) molecule has an anticodon that can bind to a nonsense codon and enter the A site. Release factor is a protein that recognizes this situation and stimulates the ribosome to terminate protein synthesis, release the completed polypeptide chain, and dissociate from the message. Uncharged tRNA is not involved in any stage of translation. AUG is the initiation codon, not a chain-termination codon. Energy for termination of translation is provided by guanosine triphosphate (GTP), not adenosine triphosphate (ATP).

107. The answer is A. *(Behavioral science)*
Both the federal and state governments contribute to the cost of Medicaid. Medicare is funded completely by federal monies. Blue Cross and Blue Shield are part of a nonprofit, private health insurance plan.

108. The answer is D. *(Microbiology)*
Several DNA viruses possess linear genome molecules with ends that have terminal repetitions. Terminal repetitions mean that the two ends of a linear DNA molecule have identical base sequences; all members of the herpesvirus group have this characteristic. These viruses are well known for their ability to produce latent infections, which can be mediated by the insertion of a provirus into a host cell chromosome or by the presence of a plasmid-like (Epstein-Barr virus circular DNA plasmid) molecule. Insertion of the linear molecule requires a circular intermediate. In a circular intermediate, a linear DNA genome has assumed a circular shape and has been stabilized by a ligase enzyme. The intermediate term indicates that the DNA molecule will reassume a linear format once it has been cut and inserted into a host chromosome by an integrase enzyme. Endonuclease activity on single-end strands creates "sticky" ends that match complimentary bases, forming the requisite circle. The provirus can be inserted and ligated into place by enzymes. Such a mechanism may form the basis of a latent infection of host cells.

109. The answer is B. *(Behavioral science)*
Medicare is a federal program designed to provide coverage for the elderly, for people on social security disability, and for patients on chronic dialysis.

110. The answer is E. *(Biochemistry)*
Normally, 95% of the bile acids secreted into the intestine are reabsorbed in the ileum and returned to the liver via the portal circulation. The soluble fibers, such as pectin and oat bran, lower cholesterol levels by binding to the bile acids, thus preventing their reabsorption. Cholestyramine and colestipol, ion exchange resins used pharmaceutically to lower cholesterol levels, act by a similar mechanism.

Vitamin C is a cofactor, rather than an inhibitor, of cholesterol 7 α-hydroxylase. This enzyme catalyzes the rate-limiting step in the synthesis of bile salt from cholesterol.

In general, an increased serum lipoprotein concentration is associated with an increased risk of atherosclerosis. An exception is an increase in high density lipoprotein (HDL), which decreases the risk.

Pharmacological levels of niacin decrease serum cholesterol levels by inhibiting very low density lipoprotein (VLDL) secretion from the liver into the circulation. It does not inhibit 3-hydroxy-3-methylglutaryl-coenzyme A (HMG-CoA) reductase, the rate-limiting step in cholesterol synthesis. Lovastatin and mevastatin are HMG-CoA reductase inhibitors used clinically to reduce serum cholesterol levels.

Primary chylomicronemia, most often caused by a deficiency of lipoprotein lipase, is generally managed by limiting the fat and oil intake, to decrease the amount of circulating chylomicrons, and by restricting caloric intake, to reduce the *de novo* synthesis of fatty acids and their release into the circulation as VLDL.

111. The answer is A. *(Behavioral science)*
The statement "Please continue" will best encourage this man to continue speaking. This statement is an example of the interviewing technique known as facilitation. "How much liquor do you drink per week?" and "Are you a heavy drinker?" are direct questions that will elicit restricted answers. The statement "Many people are upset by situations like this" is an example of validation, which gives credence to the patient's feelings and thus helps to establish rapport. "You should have come in 6 months ago" preaches to the patient and does not encourage rapport or information gathering.

112. The answer is D. *(Microbiology)*
The first exposure to an immunogen results in a relatively weak antibody response that consists primarily of immunoglobulin M (IgM), not immunoglobulin G (IgG), and is of short duration (the exact length of time can vary depending upon the nature and persistence of the inducing antigen). Because B lymphocytes that are specific for a particular epitope are rare, the antigen is processed by low-affinity cells and presented to antigen-specific T-helper lymphocytes (also rare). The T-helper cells then contact and activate the B lymphocytes, which differentiate into plasma cells. The IgM antibodies have low average affinity for the antigen, because many are secreted by B cells, which are incidentally activated by T-helper cell factors. The appearance of IgG usually follows IgM, but the amount produced is highly variable. Long-lived memory cells are generated during this priming event. Upon subsequent encounter with the same immunogen (as in a booster vaccine), a secondary (anamnestic or memory) response ensues that is faster, results in a higher level of antibody (mostly IgG), and persists longer.

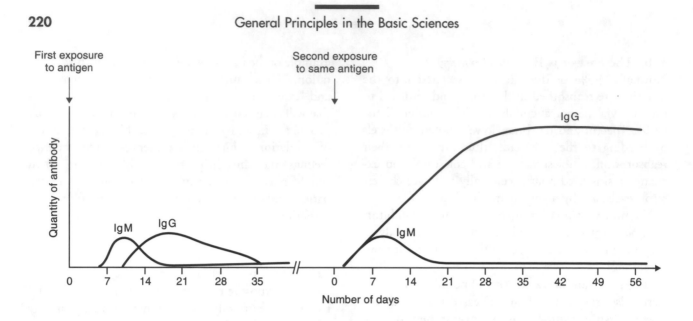

Both primary and secondary responses are characterized by a lag or latent phase (length of time from exposure to detectable antibody level), exponential phase (rapid increase in antibody concentration and number of plasmacytes), steady-state or plateau phase (antibody level remains relatively constant because its secretion and degradation proceed at similar rates), and declining phase (antibody level declines because of decreasing production and demise of plasmacytes).

The rapid kinetics seen during a secondary response are caused by the memory T and B cells generated during a primary response.

Relative Characteristics of Primary and Secondary Antibody Responses

Characteristic	Primary	Secondary
Dose of antigen needed for induction	High	Low
Length of time for induction (lag phase)	Long (7–10 days)	Short (3–5 days)
Major class of antibody	IgM	IgG
Titer of antibody	Low	High
Affinity of antibody	Low	High
Persistence of antibody	Short (A few weeks)	Long (Up to a lifetime)

113. The answer is D. *(Pathology)*
Benign tumors are more likely to retain their ABO antigens on the surface than malignant cells, which often shed their surface antigens.

Lack of a capsule is more likely to represent a malignant tumor. An exception is a leiomyoma of the uterus, which lacks a capsule. An increased nuclear/cytoplasmic ratio is characteristic of a malignant cell. Nuclear chromatin is dense, the nuclear membrane is

irregular, and nucleoli are large and irregular. Malignant cells are immortal in tissue culture. Atypical mitotic spindles (e.g., tetraploid) indicate a malignant cell. A mitosis can appear normal in a benign or a malignant cell.

114. The answer is B. *(Behavioral science)*
Motor vehicle accidents are the most common cause of death between 1 and 4 years of age. Injuries, in

fact, account for the most deaths through the age of 24; automobile accidents are the leading cause, followed closely by burns and drowning. Cancer is the third leading cause of death from 1 to 4 years of age. Sudden infant death syndrome (SIDS) is the most common cause of death from 1 to 12 months of age.

115. The answer is A. *(Pathology)*
Third degree burns primarily differ from first or second degree burns in that they lack sensation, because the nerves are destroyed.

The severity of a burn is dependent on depth, surface area, site of the burn, and whether or not inhalation is a factor. Current emphasis on burn healing has lead to the designation of burns as partial thickness burns, which heal spontaneously, versus full thickness burns, which require skin grafting. First degree burns cause pain, erythema, and edema in the epidermis, with focal necrosis of epidermal cells. They are partial thickness burns that most commonly occur from scalding and sunburn. Healing is uneventful and scarring does not occur. Second degree burns (blisters) involve the entire epidermis, and form blisters within the epidermis. They are considered partial thickness burns and are subdivided into superficial and deep types,

the latter resulting in scarring (grafting is useful in this situation). Healing with scar formation occurs by the regeneration of squamous epithelium from the edge of the wound and from residual adnexal epithelium. Blisters are an example of serous inflammation. Third degree burns are full thickness and have extensive necrosis of the epidermis and adnexa, and involvement of underlying subcutaneous fat and connective tissue. The only potential for reepithelialization is from the margins of the wound; therefore, grafting is frequently required. Dermal scarring is extensive and often associated with keloid formation.

116. The answer is E. *(Biochemistry)*
Melanin synthesis is decreased in phenylketonuria, because the absence of phenylalanine hydroxylase decreases production of tyrosine, which is the key amino acid for melanin synthesis.

Melanin is synthesized in melanocytes, which are located in the epidermis. They are derived from neural crest cells. Melanin is formed when the enzyme, tyrosinase, converts tyrosine to 3,4-dihydroxyphenylalanine (DOPA), which, in turn, is polymerized in the Golgi apparatus into membrane-bound organelles called melanosomes.

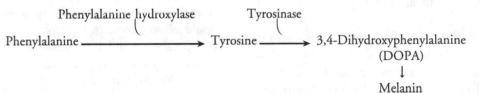

117. The answer is E. *(Pathology)*
A point mutation leading to the formation of a stop codon and premature termination of globin-chain synthesis is operative in β-thalassemia.

Four genes control α–globulin-chain synthesis (two genes on each chromosome 16). In α-thalassemia, there is a deletion in one or more of the four genes responsible for the synthesis of α-chains. In α-thalassemia minor, a one- or two-gene deletion results in mild anemia and a proportional decrease in the synthesis of hemoglobin (Hgb) A (two α- and two β-chains), Hgb A_2 (two α- and two δ-chains) and Hgb F (two α- and two γ-chains). In Hgb H disease, there is a three-gene deletion, resulting in a hemolytic anemia and the formation of tetramers of four β-chains (Hgb H). In hemoglobin Bart disease, there is a four-gene

deletion, which is fatal. Hgb Bart occurs when four γ-chains form a tetramer.

118. The answer is C. *(Anatomy)*
Genes for testicular development reside on the Y chromosome. Genetic sex is determined by the presence or absence of a Y chromosome. Gonadal sex is determined by the histologic appearance of the gonads (testis or ovary). Ductal sex is determined by the presence of derivatives of the Mullerian or Wolffian ducts. Phenotypic or genital sex is determined by the appearance of the external genitalia.

An XY karyotype leads to medullary differentiation of the primitive gonadal tissue into sex cords (seminiferous tubules) and Leydig cells. Females with an XX karyotype preferentially develop the germinal cortex into primordial follicles. By the twelfth week of gestation in a male fetus, testosterone is produced by the Leydig cells, which allows for the development of Wolffian duct structures, rather than Mullerian. In addition, a Mullerian inhibitory factor is produced by Sertoli cells, which further inhibits any development of the Mullerian structures. In the absence of a Y chromosome, the Mullerian duct develops into the uterus, fallopian tubes, and upper third of the vagina. In the male fetus, testosterone is primarily responsible for development of the seminal vesicles, vas deferens, and the epididymis. The more potent dihydrotestosterone derivative of testosterone induces male external genitalia formation including penis, scrotum, and prostate. The enzyme, 5–α-reductase, is responsible for conversion of testosterone to dihydrotestosterone, both of which attach to androgen receptors.

According to the Lyon hypothesis, one of the two X chromosomes in females is randomly inactivated and becomes a Barr body; therefore, approximately 50% of the X chromosomes are of maternal origin and the remainder are of paternal origin. In rare cases, only the maternally derived X chromosome is inactivated. This leads to the possibility of a female having a sex-linked recessive disease if the paternally derived X chromosome has an abnormal gene (e.g., hemophilia A).

A normal female has one Barr body, while a normal male has no Barr bodies. Buccal smears are used to count the number of Barr bodies in the squamous cells. Barr bodies can be identified as projections from the nucleus of a cell.

119. The answer is A.   *(Pathology)*
This patient has fragile X syndrome, which is a sex-linked recessive disease. It is the second most common cause of inheritable mental retardation after Down syndrome. The incidence is 1 out of 1000 males. The mutation is characterized by multiple tandem repeats of three nucleotides, mainly CGG. Patients have the following characteristics:

• mental retardation
• long face with a large mandible
• 80% of post-pubertal males have macro-orchidism (enlarged testicles)
• 30% of carrier females have mental retardation

The diagnosis is confirmed by ordering a fragile X chromosome study.

An XYY karyotype is associated with individuals who are tall, exhibit aggressive behavior, and have acne. Whether or not the aggressive, antisocial behavior is related to the extra Y chromosome is controversial. A single Barr body, representing a randomly inactivated X chromosome, is characteristic of a normal female. A mutation in a mitochondrial gene is unique to females, because ova contain more mitochondria than sperm, after the sperm lose their mitochondria normally located in the base of their tail on penetration of the egg during the fertilization process. The mitochondrial DNA (mtDNA) codes for enzymes in oxidative phosphorylation. The affected female passes the trait on to all of her children, both male and female. Affected males do not transmit the disease. A mutation with insertion of nucleotide bases into DNA is characteristic of Tay-Sachs disease. This insertion produces a frameshift mutation, which codes for a defective hexosaminidase.

120. The answer is B.   *(Biochemistry)*
The Guthrie test is a bacterial growth assay for the presence of an elevated concentration of phenylalanine in the blood. An infant with such phenylalaninemia would be suspected to have phenylketonuria (PKU). The patient should be placed on a diet with a low content of phenylalanine to maintain blood phenylalanine within the normal range. Patients with untreated PKU develop severe mental retardation, whereas infants immediately placed on a low phenylalanine diet retain normal mental function.

121. The answer is B.   *(Microbiology)*
Mycoplasmas are a class of cell wall–free bacteria; any antimicrobial whose mechanism of action targets bacterial cell walls (penicillins, cephalosporins, and bacitracin) have no targets to affect in *Mycoplasma* species. Vancomycin is also ineffective.

Tetracyclines and erythromycin are effective anti-*Mycoplasma* reagents and are the drugs of choice in *Mycoplasma* pneumonias. Some *Ureaplasma* strains are resistant to tetracyclines.

Acyclovir is an antiherpes simplex reagent. Although *Mycoplasma* organisms are small (similar size range as viruses) and obligate intracellular parasites, they are not inhibited by acyclovir. Acyclovir affects the virally coded thymidine kinase and DNA polymerase enzymes.

122. The answer is D. *(Behavioral science)*
Biofeedback aimed at regulating peripheral temperature is most useful in the treatment of Raynaud disease, a condition characterized by poor peripheral blood flow and low temperature in the periphery. Biofeedback using muscle relaxation is most useful in the treatment of tension headache, hypertension, and asthma. Biofeedback aimed at gaining sphincter control is useful in the treatment of anal incontinence.

123. The answer is D. *(Microbiology)*
Many gram-negative bacteria possess rigid surface structures known as pili or fimbriae. They are smaller than flagella and consist of protein subunits called pilins. Ordinary pili play a role in the adherence of bacteria to host cells. Pili in streptococci, the M proteins, associate with lipotechoic acids to help the group A streptococci adhere to epithelial cells. *Neisseria gonorrhoeae* virulent strains possess pili, which assists these organisms to adhere to mucous membrane cells.

Adherence to tissue cells inhibits phagocytic ability of white blood cells to a certain degree, but capsules perform this function directly. Protein A of *Staphylococcus aureus* binds the Fc portion of IgG molecules and prevents complement attachment–activation. Flagella are organs of locomotion and allow bacterial movement toward or away from a chemotactic substance. Plasmids are circular DNA molecules that provide genes for antibiotic resistance.

124. The answer is C. *(Behavioral science)*
Children from single-parent households face a greater likelihood of failure in school than children from intact families. They are also more likely to suffer from depression, drug abuse, and suicidal and criminal behavior, and to be divorced in adulthood.

125. The answer is C. *(Biochemistry)*
Hyperuricemia is least likely to occur in the presence of high doses of salicylate, because at these concentrations, salicylates act as a uricosuric (increase the urine

excretion of uric acid) agent. Uric acid is an end-product of purine metabolism. An abbreviated schematic follows.

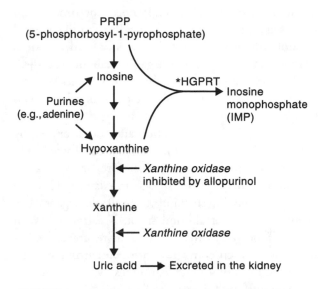

*HGPRT=hypoxanthine-guanine phosphoribosyltransferase

Hyperuricemia is a disorder in uric acid metabolism representing decreased excretion in the kidneys (most common), increased production (decrease in hypoxanthine-quanine phosphoribosyltransferase [HGPRT] or an increase in 5-phosphoribosyl-1-pyrophosphate [PRPP]), or a combination of the two. This may be the result of a primary or secondary disorder that predisposes patients to an increase in purines. These include such diseases as

- polycythemia rubra vera—increased breakdown of hematopoietic cells
- leukemia—increased breakdown of leukemic cells usually associated with chemotherapy
- multiple myeloma—increased breakdown of malignant plasma cells plus renal failure (decreased excretion)
- diuretic therapy—increased reabsorption caused by volume contraction
- treatment of disseminated cancer—increased breakdown of neoplastic cells

Because uric acid crystals precipitate at an acid pH, maintaining an alkaline urine prevents stone formation.

126. The answer is B. *(Pathology)*
Poisoning caused by isopropyl alcohol, or rubbing alcohol, produces deep coma, hyporeflexia, and excessive amounts of acetone in the blood and urine from metabolism of the alcohol. It does not produce an increased anion gap metabolic acidosis, unlike methyl alcohol, which is converted to formic acid and does produce an increased anion gap metabolic acidosis.

Cyanide is a systemic asphyxiant that blocks cytochrome oxidase in the oxidative phosphorylation system in the mitochondria, thus preventing adenosine triphosphate (ATP) production and use of oxygen by the cell. It is released by the combustion of wool, silk, and plastics in upholstery; therefore, it is a factor to consider in cases of smoke inhalation. Cyanide produces hypoxic cell injury in multiple organs. The breath has a bitter almond smell. Treatment is with nitrites, followed by thiosulfate. Nitrites create methemoglobin, which competes with cytochrome oxidase for cyanide. Thiosulfate combines with cyanide to form a nontoxic thiocyanate.

Arsenic is the most common cause of acute heavy metal poisoning, and is associated with garlic breath. Haloperidol is an antipsychotic drug that is associated with severe extrapyramidal side effects (e.g., oculogyric crisis). Strychnine is a powerful central nervous system stimulant that produces tetanic convulsions and death.

127. The answer is A. *(Biochemistry)*
Heme is the most important of the porphyrins in humans. It consists of a ferrous iron (Fe^{2+}) atom combined with protoporphyrin IX. The important proteins containing heme as a prosthetic group include catalase, the cytochromes, hemoglobin, and myoglobin. δ-aminolevulinate synthase contains pyridoxal phosphate as its prosthetic group and is the rate-controlling enzyme in the pathway for heme biosynthesis.

128. The answer is E. *(Microbiology)*
With nonenveloped viruses, the antigenic epitopes that determine serotype are part of the capsid (protein coat) of the virion. Proteins would be easily detected as a basis for serotyping by the immune system of the host. Such components would be easily reached by the antigen processing cells (APCs). Enveloped virions may also have multiple or single serotypes, as determined primarily by glycoproteins found on the envelope. Influenza viruses have multiple serotypes, based

on the hemagglutinin and neuraminidase glycoproteins.

The RNA polymerase contained in many RNA viruses is concerned with messenger RNA (mRNA) synthesis and has no function in determining viral antigenic epitopes.

129. The answer is C. *(Biochemistry)*
Phenylalanine is an essential amino acid and is not synthesized in the human body. The coenzyme tetrahydrobiopterin is required for the activity of the enzymes phenylalanine hydroxylase, tyrosine hydroxylase, and tryptophan hydroxylase. If phenylalanine hydroxylase remains inactive because it lacks tetrahydrobiopterin, tyrosine cannot be synthesized. The accumulation of excess phenylalanine results in a variant form of phenylketonuria. If tyrosine hydroxylase remains inactive, synthesis of the catecholamines (dopamine, epinephrine, and norepinephrine) from tyrosine is inhibited. If typtophan hydroxylase remains inactive, serotonin cannot be synthesized from tryptophan.

130. The answer is B. *(Pathology)*
In burns occupying more than 10% of the body surface, hypovolemia, caused by the isotonic loss of plasma from damaged vessels, occurs rather than hypervolemia. Other complications associated with burns include infection, which is the most common cause of death; *Pseudomonas aeruginosa* is the key offender (*Staphylococcus aureus* is also a common pathogen). Stress ulcers (called curling ulcers—things curl in a fire), adult respiratory distress syndrome, carbon monoxide poisoning, and cyanide poisoning from combustion of wool, silk, and plastic upholstery can also occur.

131. The answer is D. *(Pharmacology)*
Recurrent pulmonary infections in cystic fibrosis patients are often caused by mucoid strains of *Pseudomonas aeruginosa*. All of the choices have antipseudomonal activity except trimethoprim/sulfamethoxazole. A combination of antipseudomonal pencillin and an aminoglycoside is sometimes employed. Oral or parenteral therapy with a fluoroquinolone is a new option for *Pseudomonas* infections.

Not all third generation cephalosporins have antipseudomonal activity. Ceftazidime and cefoperazone are effective against *Pseudomonas aeruginosa*, while ceftriaxone, cefotaxime, and others are not. Aztreonam is a monocyclic β-lactam (monobactam) with excellent activity against gram-negative bacilli, including *Pseudomonas*.

132. The answer is D. *(Microbiology)*
Group A (Lancefield classification) streptococci are beta hemolytic (complete destruction of red blood cells; clear zone) on blood agar plates and cause 95% of human streptococcal infections. Streptococci produce the following six important toxins and enzymes: streptokinase (dissolves fibrin clot), streptodornase (DNAse), hyaluronidase (destroys hyaluronic acid in connective tissue), erythrogenic toxin (scarlet fever), streptolysin S (oxygen stable hemolysin). All of these materials contribute to the development of the typical lesion of streptococci (cellulitis).

Lipoteichoic acids are components of many gram-positive organisms. They are involved in attachment to tissues, allowing organisms to set up an area of colonization. As such, these qualify as virulence factors.

Collagenase is a tissue-degrading enzyme, breaking down collagen. It is a major product of anaerobic organisms, namely *Clostridium* and *Bacteroides*.

133. The answer is E. *(Biochemistry)*
Insulin increases the rate of glucokinase synthesis, which promotes the uptake of glucose in the liver by increasing the concentration gradient. This process helps to lower blood glucose levels after a carbohydrate meal and sets the stage for the synthesis of glycogen and fatty acids by the liver. Insulin also promotes the transport of amino acids and glucose into muscle cells by recruiting an increased number of specific transporter proteins into the membrane. This process also helps to lower blood glucose and promotes anabolic activity in the muscle cell. Conversely, when blood glucose levels and insulin levels are low, muscle is less able to take up glucose, thus conserving it for the brain and red blood cells. These tissues are normally dependent on glucose as an energy source; this dependence is complete for the red blood cell, whereas the brain can utilize ketones for fuel in the starvation state.

The binding of insulin to its receptor activates tyrosine kinase activity on an intracellular domain of the receptor. This autophosphorylates the receptor as well

as other proteins. Induction of a phosphorylation on tyrosine is also characteristic of growth factors. The protein kinases activated by cyclic adenosine monophosphate (cAMP; protein kinase A) or by calcium and diacylglycerol (protein kinase C) differ in that they phosphorylate seryl or threonyl residues; however, in all cases the phosphorylations represent the manner by which the cell responds to the signal carried by the hormones.

Another manifestation of the anabolic activity of insulin is increased transport of potassium along with glucose into cells. This may lead to a serious depletion of serum potassium, potentially resulting in death. Insulin plus glucose is one of the modalities of therapy for hyperkalemia.

134. The answer is D. *(Microbiology)*
Although exotoxin production is essential for pathogenesis, establishment of the organism in the throat must occur. The DNA that codes for the toxin is part of the genome of a temperate bacteriophage. The prophage integrates into the bacterial chromosome, adding the genetic ability to produce the toxin. Diphtheria toxin inhibits protein synthesis by adenosine diphosphate (ADP) ribosylation of elongation factor 2 (EF-2) and affects all eukaryotic cells. The toxin has two fragments or domains. One mediates binding to glycoprotein receptors on the cell membrane and the other possesses enzymatic activity that cleaves nicotinamide from nicotinamide adenine dinucleotide (NAD) and transfers the ADP ribose to EF-2. Myocarditis accompanied by arrhythmias and circulatory collapse is one of the prominent complications.

The preexisting antibody in the serum that is involved in the Schick test (assessment of immune status) blocks the interaction of fragment B with the receptors.

The Schick test is performed by injecting 0.1 ml of purified toxin into the skin of the forearm. A control consists of a similar amount of toxin, heated to 60° C for 30 minutes, injected into the other arm. A positive reaction is a local inflammatory reaction that maximizes in 4 to 7 days and fades. A positive test indicates absence of immunity to diphtheria. A negative test (no inflammation) indicates the presence of antitoxin in the serum, and the individual is considered immune. No reaction should occur on the heated, control-injected arm. The antigen is not generally available.

135. The answer is D. *(Pharmacology)*
Antibiotics that may cause ototoxicity include the aminoglycosides, such as gentamicin, tobramycin, and amikacin. These drugs accumulate and contribute to toxicity in the endolymph/perilymph of the inner ears and in the renal cortex. Hearing loss caused by aminoglycosides may be permanent, whereas that caused by erythromycin is almost always reversible. Dose-dependent eighth cranial nerve damage and deafness are the most serious adverse effects caused by vancomycin. Clindamycin is not associated with ototoxicity.

136. The answer is D. *(Microbiology)*
There are at least three regulatory molecules involved in the complement system: C4 binding protein, factor H, and S protein. Factor I and C1 inhibitor (C1INH) are the two major inhibitors.

C4 binding protein (C4BP) binds to C4b and facilitates its cleavage by factor I, which is a proteolytic enzyme. Thus, C4BP and factor I are both important in the classic complement pathway.

Factor H serves as a cofactor for I-mediated cleavage of C3b and C3(H₂O). Although some breakdown of the latter two components will occur on cell surfaces without factor H, it is critical in the soluble phase. One result of this action is the production of iC3b, a partially degraded C3b, which is inactive in terms of continuing the cascade. However, iC3b can act as an opsonin.

S protein (or vitronectin) binds to the membrane-binding site of C5b67 and prevents its attachment to cell membranes. C8 and C9 can bind to the free-floating S protein-C5b57 complex, but cell lysis is prevented.

Protein	MW	Function
Inhibitors		
C1INH	105,000	Has serine protease activity; dissociates C1rs from C1
Factor I	88,000	Cleaves C4b, C3b, and C3(H₂O) C4BP or factor H act as cofactors
Regulators		
C4BP	560,000	Blocks C3 convertase formation in classic pathway by binding to C4b (so it is more readily cleaved by factor I)
Factor H	150,000	Blocks C3 convertase formation in alternative pathway by acting as cofactor for factor I
S protein	80,000	Blocks cell lysis by binding to C5b57 and preventing insertion into cell membrane
Alternative pathway		
Properdin	53,000	Stabilizes C3bBb convertase by binding to it
Factor B	90,000	Is the Bb subunit of C3bBb, has serine protease activity, activates C3 and C5
Factor D	25,000	Activates factor B, has serine protease activity

137. The answer is D. *(Behavioral science)*
This child's friends, teachers, and group leaders have become more important to him than his family over the last 5 years. A child of this age has the capacity for logical thought and his conscience is formed. Boys of this age identify with their fathers and prefer to play predominantly with other boys.

138. The answer is A. *(Microbiology)*
Live vaccines induce long-term protection against disease. Most live vaccines in use today induce life-long protection, if given appropriately. Whole killed vaccines and portions of an infectious agent induce only short-lived immunity. Boosters are required in order to maintain protection.

Live vaccines multiply within the immunized individual for a period of time and allow ample interaction of foreign antigens with the immune system of the host. When given via the usual route of infection, they induce protective immune responses similar to those seen after a natural infection (i.e., the oral polio vaccine induces both IgG and IgA). They are the most immunogenic of all vaccines.

Immunization that requires the host to produce antibodies or a cell-mediated response is known as active immunization. Passive immunization occurs when preformed antibodies or immunoreactive cells are administered.

Pathogenic infectious agents are usually attenuated by growing in a nonhuman host or in cultured cells (i.e., chick embryo, monkey kidney cells, or human diploid fibroblasts). These agents are unable to cause disease in healthy individuals, but retain sufficient immunogenicity.

Live vaccines can revert to virulence, although the possibility is low. If reversion occurs during production, it can be detected by testing prior to immunization; however, it may also occur during multiplication in the immunized individual. For example, reversion of the attenuated polio virus in the vaccine accounts for most of the rare cases of paralytic polio in the United States.

The processes used to manufacture live vaccines would not be expected to kill any "passenger" agents that might be present as contaminants. The presence of a secondary agent may also be a problem with killed vaccines. For example, several decades ago simian virus 40 (SV40) was found in the killed polio vaccine after many people had already been immunized. SV40 was resistant to the formaldehyde used to inactivate the polio virus. SV40 can cause sarcomas in rodents, but it has not been associated with cancer in humans.

139. The answer is A.   *(Pharmacology)*
β-adrenergic, dopamine D1, and histamine H_2 receptors are linked with G_s to increase adenylyl cyclase activity and cyclic adenosine monophosphate (cAMP) formation. α_2-Adrenergic and dopamine D2 receptors are linked with G_i to decrease adenylyl cyclase activity and cAMP production. Nitric oxide is believed to directly activate cytoplasmic guanylyl cyclase, thereby increasing cyclic guanosine monophosphate (GMP) production and leading to smooth muscle relaxation.

140. The answer is E.   *(Microbiology)*
The vaccine for influenza is inactivated ("killed") with formalin or β-propiolactone, and the viral antigens are isolated from egg proteins. Hemagglutinin is the major antigen present in the final preparation. Administration of the vaccine induces immunoglobulin G (IgG), but not IgA or T-cytotoxic cells. A new vaccine must be prepared nearly every year because of antigenic changes in influenza A and B viruses. The greatest changes are seen in influenza A during "antigenic shift." Immunizations are generally given before November (e.g., before the peak influenza season). The typical influenza vaccine contains two variations of influenza A and one of influenza B.

The influenza vaccine is given primarily to healthy individuals over the age of 65, medical personnel taking care of high-risk patients, and others with chronic pulmonary or cardiovascular diseases.

The measles, mumps, and rubella (MMR) vaccine consists of live viruses. It is usually given to children at approximately 15 months of age and again before entry into school. The vaccine is effective in 95% or more of individuals and induces life-long immunity.

The live (Sabin) polio vaccine is an oral trivalent vaccine that contains virus types I, II, and III. Three doses are generally given, followed by a fourth dose if the third dose was given before the age of 4 years. Because the virus is shed in the stool, it displaces the wild-type virus in the environment and thus decreases the risk of paralytic disease in the nonimmunized. A trivalent inactivated (Salk) polio vaccine is also available for parenteral (intramuscular) immunization of immunocompromised patients. After a full course of 4 to 5 injections, a booster is recommended every 5 years until the age of 18. The live polio vaccine is the one of choice in the United States.

Other live viral vaccines include the vaccines for yellow fever, smallpox, and adenovirus. They are given under special circumstances (e.g., used for military personnel or for those traveling to an endemic country).

The rabies vaccines, including human diploid cell vaccine (HDCV), are killed. The hepatitis B vaccine consists of the major surface antigen of the virus (HBsAg; genetically engineered in yeast).

Vaccines in which the virus is first grown in embryonated eggs (e.g., influenza, measles, mumps, and yellow fever vaccines) may induce a type I hypersensitivity reaction in some persons. Antibiotics and preservatives added to the vaccine may also provoke an allergic response.

141. The answer is E.   *(Behavioral science)*
Personality tests include the Thematic Apperception Test, the Minnesota Multiphasic Personality Inventory (MMPI), Rorschach Test, and Sentence Completion Test. The Wechsler Adult Intelligence Scale-Revised (WAIS-R) is an intelligence test.

142. The answer is A.   *(Microbiology)*
The activation of T-suppressor cells would not be expected to result in a breakdown of tolerance. Tolerance to self-antigens is thought to be maintained by a population of continuously activated T suppressors.

T-helper cells respond to antigen in the context of class II molecules. Induction of class II molecules after exposure to interferon-γ or other cytokines increases the likelihood that T-cell help will be generated. The induced T-cell help may be against an autologous antigen.

Numerous extrinsic agents, especially certain viruses, have antigens with epitopes that are very similar to those found in the body. This phenomenon is sometimes referred to as "molecular mimicry." Infection with one of these agents may induce a cross-reactive response against the host.

Certain tissues of the body (i.e., lens of the eye, central nervous system, and spermatozoa) have little or no interaction with cells of the immune system. If the antigens present in those sites are released into the circulation, as may occur after surgery or accidental trauma, an autoimmune response may be generated.

Polyclonal activation of lymphocytes may be induced by agents such as the Epstein-Barr virus and lipopolysaccharide (endotoxin) found in the walls of gram-negative bacteria. In the case of B cells, antibodies that react with self-antigens may be secreted.

143. The answer is D.   *(Pharmacology)*
Genes conferring bacterial resistance to antibiotics are constituents of both chromosomal and extrachromosomal (plasmid) DNA. Spontaneous chromosomal mutations conferring resistance enable strains to survive antibiotic exposure and become dominant. Plasmid genes conferring resistance are called R-factors, and may be transferred among bacteria by conjugation or transduction. Such genes often confer resistance to multiple drugs; however, there is no evidence that bacterial resistance is dependent upon specific defects in cellular immunity.

144. The answer is C.   *(Microbiology)*
Paramyxoviruses include four important human pathogens: measles, mumps, respiratory syncytial virus, and parainfluenza viruses. They differ from orthomyxoviruses in that their genomes are not segmented, are larger, and have different envelope surface spikes.

The helical nucleocapsid contains the negative sense RNA genome and is inside an outer lipoprotein envelope. Negative sense RNA, by definition, is the opposite of messenger RNA (mRNA), or positive sense RNA, and cannot be translated into a protein at the ribosome. The outer spikes are enzymes (hemagglutinin–neuraminidase on one and a fusion protein on another).

Parvoviruses, picornaviruses, and adenoviruses are icosahedral (cubic) viruses without an envelope, whereas the herpesviruses are icosahedral and possess an outer lipid-containing envelope.

145. The answer is A.   *(Pharmacology)*
Spectinomycin is an aminocyclitol antibiotic that inhibits bacterial protein synthesis. The other drugs all inhibit bacterial cell wall synthesis. Vancomycin and bacitracin inhibit early steps in the biosynthesis of the peptidoglycan component of the cell wall, whereas β-lactams such as aztreonam (a monobactam), penicillins, cephalosporins, and carbapenems inhibit the cross-linking (transpeptidation) of the cell wall peptidoglycan polymers.

146. The answer is C.   *(Microbiology)*
The terms "hapten" and "epitope" are not synonymous. A hapten can have more than one epitope, and it may constitute only a portion of one epitope (the remainder being contributed by the carrier).

Historically, hapten refers to a small (MW of <1000 kD), chemically well-defined substance that is normally not an integral part of a larger molecule and is not immunogenic on its own.

An epitope is that small portion (usually only a few amino acids or sugar moieties) of an antigenic molecule to which antibody binds. One immunogenic molecule can have several different epitopes (also known as antigenic determinants). An epitope can be linear (amino acids or sugar residues that are positioned sequentially) or conformational (amino acids or sugar residues that are brought together in close proximity by the three-dimensional configuration of the molecule).

Haptens can be made to be immunogenic when coupled to a large carrier molecule, such as a protein. The hapten will bind to the appropriate immunoglobulin M (IgM) expressed on the surface of B cells, but antibody production requires T-cell help.

T helpers are triggered by the carrier portion of the complex. Immunization with a hapten-carrier complex results in production of antibodies against the carrier and the hapten.

Injection of the hapten-carrier complex would be required in order to generate a secondary response against a hapten, because injection of only the hapten is not enough.

Most prescription drugs have low molecular weights and are not immunogenic in and of themselves; however, they (or one of their metabolites) may bind to tissue proteins and act as haptens. A good example is penicillin G. Most patients who are allergic to this antibiotic react against the penicilloyl moiety, which is generated by cleavage of the β-lactam ring. Penicillin is known to cause a variety of hypersensitivity reactions including anaphylaxis, cytotoxic hypersensitivity, immune complex disease, and contact dermatitis.

147. The answer is C. *(Behavioral science)*
Adult hormone levels are normal in male homosexuals. Markers on the X chromosome, evidence of decreased prenatal testosterone levels, and difference in size of a sexually-dimorphic hypothalamic nucleus have been implicated recently in the etiology of male homosexuality.

148. The answer is B. *(Microbiology)*
The major histocompatibility complex (MHC) in all mammalian species tested is located on a single chromosome. In humans, it is found on the short arm of

chromosome 6. The human MHC is known as the human leukocyte antigen system, or HLA. Its counterpart in mice is the H-2 complex present on chromosome 17.

The genes within the HLA are classified into three groups: class I, class II, and class III, according to their location, molecular structure of the produced proteins, and their functions. The three genes within the class I region are referred to as the HLA-A, HLA-B, and HLA-C loci, whereas the three genes within the class II area are designated as HLA-DP, HLA-DQ, and HLA-DR. Class III genes are wedged in between class I and class II regions; they code for several complement components (C2, C4, B, and F) and tumor necrosis factor-α and -β.

Class I and II genes are polymorphic; each exists in multiple forms, (i.e., they are not identical in all individuals). HLA-B exhibits the greatest degree of polymorphism. At least 50 different alleles of HLA-B have been identified in the human population. A given copy of chromosome 6 contains only one of the possible allelic forms of each gene. Because humans have two copies of each chromosome, and the HLA class I and II genes are codominant, the cells of one individual can express two HLA-A proteins, plus two HLA-B, proteins plus two HLA-C proteins, and so forth.

The chance of finding a perfect HLA match among siblings is 25% ($\frac{1}{4}$). Parents and 50% of siblings are matched at one haplotype. Cadaveric donors to a random recipient will be genotypically mismatched.

The HLA consists of only approximately 3000 kilobase pairs, and is usually inherited as a unit according to classic Mendelian mechanisms. The likelihood of genetic recombination between parental chromosomes within the MHC is dependent upon size and is approximately 1%.

Class I and II molecules are extremely important in regulating acquired immune responses. CD4 positive T cells react with class II molecules, while CD8 positive T cells react with class I molecules. They are also important in determining the success or failure of organ transplantation. Inheritance of some of the HLA genes has been associated with a predisposition to certain diseases.

Short arm of chromosome 6

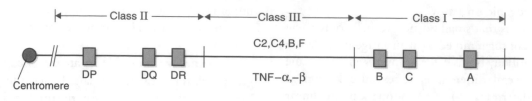

149. The answer is E.   *(Biochemistry)*
In the elongation phase of translation, the ribosome moves along the messenger RNA (mRNA) molecule in the 5′ to 3′ direction, synthesizing the protein specified by that particular message. Peptidyl transferase is the enzymatic activity of the ribosome that forms peptide bonds by covalently linking together the amino acids. Guanosine triphosphate (GTP) provides the energy necessary for the elongation stage of translation. Formylmethionyl-transfer RNA (tRNA) is the initiator tRNA that is used in the initiation phase of translation in bacteria. Methionyl-tRNA, rather than formylmethionyl-tRNA, is used during elongation.

150. The answer is E.   *(Microbiology)*
Infectious agents can avoid immune attack by making frequent changes in the antigenic makeup of their surface molecules. An often-cited example is *Borrelia recurrentis*, the cause of relapsing fever. Antibodies that are initially induced select for one or a few antigenically distinct variants of *Borrelia*, which survive and multiply until another wave of antibody appears. Approximately three to ten recurrences of this phenomenon may occur. *Neisseria gonorrhoeae* has three surface antigens (pili, lipooligosaccharide, and protein II) that very rapidly switch their immunogenic characteristics. Changes in each of these antigens are under the control of different genetic mechanisms. The influenza A virus can undergo antigenic shift—a large antigenic change that results in a new subtype of hemagglutinin or neuraminidase (HA and NA, respectively). This is presumably caused by genetic reassortment. Antigenic drift (accumulation of small point mutations) also occurs. These changes render the population susceptible to reinfection with influenza A.

Many pathogenic bacteria have a hydrophilic polysaccharide capsule that inhibits phagocytosis. A capsule can also mask cell surface antigens, including lipopolysaccharide, and prevent immune recognition. A capsule may also interfere with the lytic activity of complement. If free soluble capsular material is present, it can form immune complexes with antibodies and prevent opsonization of the microorgansim itself. Examples of bacteria with a capsule include *Streptococcus pyogenes* (group A), *Staphylococcus aureus, Haemophilus influenzae, Neisseria meningitidis, Escherichia coli,* and *Klebsiella pneumoniae.*

Some bacteria, most notably *Neisseria meningitidis, Neisseria gonorrhoeae, Haemophilus influenzae,* and *Streptococcus pneumoniae,* produce proteases that are specific for the immunoglubulin A (IgA) class of antibody (i.e., IgA1 proteases). The enzymes split IgA1 in the hinge region and inactivate it. The IgA2 subclass has a different amino acid sequence in the hinge region and is not affected by the proteases. IgA is the secretory antibody and is important in local protection of mucous membranes of the genitourinary and respiratory tracts.

Some antigens of microorganisms are virtually identical to those of the normal individual (antigenic mimicry). For example, the hyaluronic acid that makes up the capsule of *Streptococcus pyogenes* is also present in human connective tissue. Thus, the host does not recognize the capsule as foreign material.

In addition, mechanisms by which pathogens evade host defenses include the absorption of normal host products. For example, *Staphylococcus aureus* has a protein A on its surface that binds strongly to the Fc′ portion of immunoglobulin G (IgG), thus rendering the antibody ineffective. Some bacteria, such as *Mycobacterium tuberculosis, Brucella,* and *Legionella,* survive well within macrophages and neutrophils. They may be resistant to lysosomal enzymes, prevent phagosome–lysosome fusion, or may avoid entry into phagolysosomes.

151. The answer is C. *(Biochemistry)*
The steroid ring structure of cholesterol cannot be degraded.

The decrease in blood glucose levels enhances the release of glucagon and catecholamine and inhibits insulin release. The increase in catecholamines and glucagon increases the activity of the hormone sensitive lipase, causing the degradation of stored triacylglycerols. The fasting state constrains the formation of chylomicrons and very low density lipoproteins (VLDL), and results in decreased lipoprotein lipase activity, which is normally enhanced by insulin.

Elevated levels of glucagon activate the transcription of phospho*enol*pyruvate carboxykinase, thereby increasing its activity, promoting gluconeogenesis, and inducing the phosphorylation of pyruvate kinase, which inhibits its activity, preventing a futile cycle at one of the irreversible steps in glycolysis.

Alanine–α-ketoglutarate transaminase activity of muscle and liver increases as muscle protein is broken down and the amino groups are transported as alanine to the liver, where the alanine is again transaminated and the carbons used for gluconeogenesis. Although the breakdown of muscle protein to provide carbons for gluconeogenesis increases ammonia formation in the liver, enhancing the activity of mitochondrial carbamoyl phosphate synthetase I and urea synthesis, the absence of dietary protein results in a net decrease in these processes. Prolonged fasting is almost always accompanied by decreased levels of urea and total nitrogen excretion.

152. The answer is C. *(Microbiology)*
Clonal deletion of potentially self-reactive T-cell clones takes place in the fetal thymus; it does not accelerate with age. The process occurs after rearrangement of the gene segments for the T-cell antigen receptor (TCR) and after the lymphocytes simultaneously express CD4 and CD8 molecules on their surface.

The presentation of self-antigens to double-positive (CD4$^+$CD8$^+$) thymocytes with TCR that recognizes autoantigen induces apoptosis (programmed cell death). Apoptosis is a form of induced suicide that is under genetic control. The lymphocyte degrades its own DNA, blebs appear in the cytoplasmic and nuclear membranes, and the cell breaks itself down into small globules that can be readily phagocytized.

Apoptosis may partly account for the fact that more than 95% of developing thymocytes die in the thymus.

Clonal deletion is an important mechanism, but not the only one, by which an autoimmune response is controlled. This mechanism is also known as negative selection.

Much less is known about deletion of self-reactive B lymphocytes. Evidence shows that it probably occurs in the bone marrow among early B cells. When surface immunoglobulin makes contact with self-antigen, the early B lymphocytes either die or cease further development into mature immunocompetent cells.

153. The answer is A. *(Pathology)*
Germ cell tumors are totipotential tumors that have the capability of differentiating in any direction. They are most commonly located in the testes, ovaries, mediastinum, and the pineal gland. An acute leukemia derives from stem cells in the bone marrow that are committed to differentiating into a specific line of hematopoietic cells. Acute lymphoblastic leukemia most commonly derives from a B-cell precursor. Acute myelogenous leukemia most commonly develops from a myeloid stem cell.

The female counterpart of a seminoma in the testicle is a dysgerminoma of the ovary. Both ovaries and testes can have cystic teratomas and yolk sac (endodermal sinus) tumors. Struma ovarii refers to the presence of thyroid tissue in a cystic teratoma.

154. The answer is A. *(Microbiology)*
Class I molecules consist of two noncovalently linked polypeptide chains; however, only the α chain is encoded within the HLA region found on chromosome 6. More specifically, it is encoded by the genes within the HLA-A, -B, and -C loci. The α chain is large and polymorphic. The other chain is β_2-microglobulin. It is smaller, nonpolymorphic, and is encoded by a gene on chromosome 15.

The α chain and the β_2-microglobulin are globular molecules, but only the C-terminal of the α chain is embedded in the cytoplasmic membrane. The α chain has three globular domains (α_1, α_2, and α_3), whereas β_2-microglobulin has only one. β_2-microglobulin is not directly involved in antigen presentation, but probably serves to stabilize the α chain and to facilitate its transport through the cell after it is synthesized. Cells that do not synthesize β_2-microglobulin (e.g., Daudi tumor cells) are unable to express the α chain on the cytoplasmic membrane. In addition, recent studies suggest that the association of β_2-microglobulin with the α chain is needed for optimal peptide ligand binding. β_2-microglobulin is also found free in body fluids. It has greater than 20% homology with virtually all constant domains of every immunoglobulin.

Antigens are processed and presented to T-cytotoxic cells by antigen-presenting cells (APCs) in the context of the class I molecule. Presented peptides are bound noncovalently within a groove consisting of the α_1 and α_2 domains of the α chain.

Major histocompatibility complex (MHC) class I molecules are found on virtually all nucleated cells. They are known as the classic transplantation antigens. In contrast, MHC class II molecules are much more restricted in their distribution and are found primarily on cells involved in immune responses.

	CD4$^+$ T cells (helpers)	CD8$^+$ T cells (cytotoxic)	Macrophages and other APCs
Class I	–	+	+
Class II	+	–	+

155. The answer is A.   (Biochemistry)

Enzymes catalyze reactions without being consumed themselves. The velocity of the reaction increases with an increase in enzyme concentration, substrate, temperature (up to a point), and varies with different pHs. In the following schematic, the product (P) exerts a negative feedback on enzyme E_1; therefore, if E_3 is deficient, P is decreased and you would expect activation of the enzyme E_1 with a subsequent decrease in substrate (S) as it is converted into intermediates (I_1 and I_2), which increase in concentration behind the E_3 enzyme block.

$$\uparrow E_1 \quad \uparrow E_2 \quad \downarrow E_3$$
$$\downarrow S \rightarrow \uparrow I_1 \rightarrow \uparrow I_2 \rightarrow \downarrow P$$

156. The answer is C.   (Microbiology)

The major histocompatibility complex (MHC) class II (and class I) molecules are not highly specific, as is the case for antibodies. One cell can bind and display many different peptide fragments from a wide range of pathogens, as well as inanimate materials.

MHC class II molecules consist of two polypeptide chains, α and β. They are encoded by polymorphic genes within the HLA-DP, HLA-DQ, and HLA-DR loci of the MHC.

The distribution of class II molecules is restricted to only a few cell types, unlike class I molecules, which are found on virtually all nucleated cells in the body.

Class II molecules are found primarily on B lymphocytes and macrophages; however, they also appear on CD4$^+$ T-helper lymphocytes after they are activated.

Processed peptide fragments are presented by antigen-presenting cells (APCs) to CD4$^+$ T-helper cells in a cleft or groove made up of the α_1 and β_1 domains of a class II molecule. The basic structural characteristics of the peptide-binding site is very similar to that of MHC class I molecules.

All human cells with a nucleus are diploid (i.e., they carry one complete chromosome set from each parent; the only exceptions are sperm and egg, which are haploid). Thus, each individual has two chromosome 6s and three class II genes (one each for the HLA-DP, -DQ, -DR) per chromosome (2 chromosomes × 3 class II genes/chromosome = 6 class II proteins). This is also true for the MHC class I molecules.

157. The answer is D.   (Behavioral science)

The social smile (i.e., smiling in response to a human face) appears in normal infants between 1 and 2 months of age. Visual tracking, turning away from a noxious odor, the rooting reflex, and the stepping reflex are all seen in normal infants at birth.

158. The answer is E.   (Microbiology)

The intracellular processing pathways of proteins before presentation to lymphocytes are different.

Peptide fragments from endogenously synthesized proteins (such as a viral proteins in infected cells) are processed in large proteasome complexes within the cytoplasm, and then pumped into the lumen of the rough endoplasmic reticulum (RER) by peptide transportation proteins (TAP-1 and TAP-2). The endogenously synthesized peptides will associate with the major histocompatibility complex (MHC) class I molecules while they are both still in the RER. The binding of the peptide to the class I α chain promotes the association of β_2-microglobulin, which facilitates transport of the entire complex to the cell surface.

In contrast, peptide fragments derived from exogenous proteins (i.e., proteins in the medium that have been internalized by antigen-presenting cells) associate with MHC class II molecules in an endosomal compartment after the class II molecule has left the RER.

The end result of these different processing pathways can be summarized as follows:

- Cells with intracellular infectious agents are attacked by MHC class I-restricted T-cytotoxic cells. For example, a herpes simplex virus-infected cell presents a viral peptide in the groove of its class I molecule to a cytotoxic T-lymphocyte, which kills the infected cell.
- Exogenous protein fragments are presented by antigen-presenting cells (APCs) to MHC class II-restricted T-helper cells. For example, purified proteins of *Mycobacterium tuberculosis*, which are injected intradermally (PPD skin test), are processed into peptides and presented together with a class II molecule on the surface of an APC to a T-helper lymphocyte. The activated T cell responds by secreting lymphokines.

Presentation of peptides in the context of MHC class I could, at least theoretically, be performed by many different cell types, because all nucleated cells express class I molecules. Presentation of peptides in the context of MHC class II can be done by relatively few cell types, because only a few cell types have class II molecules.

159. The answer is A.   (Pathology)

Mixed connective tissue disease (MCTD) presents with a constellation of findings that include mixtures of systemic lupus erythematosus, progressive systemic sclerosis, and polymyositis. Unlike many of the other autoimmune diseases, MCTD usually spares the kidneys. Anti-ribonucleoprotein (RNP) antibodies are a characteristic finding.

Regarding the other distracters in the question:

- Multiple myeloma, a malignant plasma cell disorder producing a monoclonal gammopathy, commonly involves the kidney. Problems range from a tubulointerstitial reaction against Bence Jones protein (light chains) to nephrocalcinosis (metastatic calcification of the tubular basement membranes from hypercalcemia) to actual infiltration of the kidney by myeloma cells.
- Amyloidosis, particularly those variants associated with light chains (primary type) and the serum-associated amyloid protein (secondary, or reactive type), commonly involves the kidneys. It produces a nephrotic syndrome. Renal disease is the most common cause of death in systemic amyloidosis.
- Polyarteritis nodosa, an immune vasculitis involving medium sized arteries, commonly involves the kidneys. It produces renal infarctions. Renal disease is the most common cause of death.
- Sjögren syndrome is commonly involved with tubulointerstitial disease, producing renal tubular acidosis.

160. The answer is E.   (Behavioral science)

The dream censor works primarily on an unconscious level. The dream censor, which integrates the latent dream (the unconscious meaning of the dream) with events that happened during the day (the day residue), is less active in naive individuals, disguises the latent dream, and operates according to the rules of primary process.

161. The answer is D.   (Microbiology)

Poxviruses are the largest (400 × 230 nanometers) viruses and have a complicated structure. It is neither icosahedral nor helical. The outer lipoprotein, or envelope, encloses a core and two structures of unknown function called lateral bodies. The core contains a large genome of double-stranded DNA. The viruses contain more than 100 structural polypeptides and a multiplicity of enzymes. These viruses are necessary because the entire growth cycle of poxviruses occurs in the cytoplasm of the host cell.

Adenoviruses, papovaviruses, and parvoviruses are all "naked" viruses, indicating that none have an envelope of any kind. The surface antigen of hepadnaviruses has been termed an envelope (although not of lipid structure), and should be referred to as the surface antigen layer. The surface antigen of hepatitis B virus (HBV) is protein and is usually compared with the HBV core antigen (also protein) when structure is discussed.

Herpesviruses have a lipid envelope that is derived from the nuclear membrane of the host cell.

162-163. The answers are: 162-E, 163-A. *(Biochemistry)*
Stercobilin, the compound responsible for the brown color of stools, is formed as a by-product of heme degradation. Heme is first degraded to form the green pigment biliverdin and then the red-orange pigment bilirubin. Bilirubin travels to the liver bound to albumin and is then conjugated to two molecules of glucuronic acid to increase its solubility. The bilirubin diglucuronide is excreted into bile. Bacteria in the intestine convert bilirubin diglucuronide to colorless urobilinogen and then to brown stercobilin.

Some of the colorless urobilinogen is reabsorbed from the intestine and travels to the kidney. Here the urobilinogen is converted to the yellow urobilin and excreted in the urine.

164-168. The answers are: 164-E, 165-F, 166-A, 167-G, 168-B. *(Biochemistry)*
Two of the most important hormonal or drug-signaling mechanisms are the cyclic nucleotide and phosphoinositide pathways. Many receptors are linked with guanine nucleotide-binding proteins (G proteins) that either stimulate (G_s) or inhibit (G_i) adenylyl cyclase to increase or decrease cyclic adenosine monophosphate (cAMP) production. cAMP activates protein kinases that phosphorylate proteins leading to specific effects in different types of cells. The phosphoinositide pathway begins with stimulation of phospholipase C activity that hydrolyzes a membrane phospholipid to release inositol triphosphate (IP_3) and diacylglycerol. IP_3 releases calcium from the sarcoplasmic reticulum and eventually leads to muscle contraction and other responses. Diacylglycerol (DAG) activates protein kinase C, leading to substrate phosphorylation and cellular

effects. Nitric oxide diffuses through cell membranes, to activate a cytoplasmic guanylyl cyclase to form cyclic guanosine monophosphate (GMP), which leads to smooth muscle relaxation.

169-171. The answers are: 169-C, 170-A, 171-B. *(Biochemistry)*
The isoelectric point is the pH at which a compound is electrically neutral. The amino acid alanine has two dissociable hydrogens, one from the carboxyl group and one from the amino group. Region C lies midway between the pKs for these two groups. At this point, the carboxyl group is dissociated and is negatively charged, and the amino group is protonated and positively charged. The net charge on the compound is zero.

Full protonation of a compound occurs at the lowest pH of a titration curve. At this point, the amino group is protonated and is positively charged, and the protonated carboxyl group is uncharged.

The pK of a dissociable group is the pH at which that group is half dissociated. The carboxyl group is the first to dissociate of any of the amino acids; thus, the carboxyl group will be half dissociated at point B, when one-half equivalent of NaOH has been added. A compound acts as a buffer when the pH is near the pK, because the solution resists change in pH following the addition of acid or base.

172-176. The answers are: 172-E, 173-G, 174-C, 175-I, 176-H. *(Pharmacology)*
Most drugs bind reversibly to receptors. Receptor affinity for a drug determines its potency, which is the dose or concentration required to produce a defined response. The maximal response obtained with a drug is an indication of its efficacy. Full agonists produce 100% of the maximal response, whereas partial agonists produce less than 100%. Competitive or surmountable antagonists increase the median effective dose (ED_{50}) of an agonist but do not change its maximal response, whereas noncompetitive antagonists reduce the maximal response. Tolerance occurs when increasing doses are required to elicit a specified response. It may be caused by down-regulation of receptors, in which the number of receptors declines over a relatively long period of drug exposure, or by desensitization, which is an acute response that occurs during

a short period of drug exposure. Both down-regulation and desensitization may lead to tolerance, whereas the up-regulation of receptors may cause supersensitivity.

177-180. The answers are: 177-A, 178-C, 179-B, 180-A. *(Biochemistry)*
The DNA base sequences are written in terms of the antitemplate strand. In messenger RNA (mRNA), U would substitute for the T's in DNA. In mutant #1, codon #6 is mutated from the glutamate codon GAG to a valine codon, GUG. In the protein molecule, the negatively charged glutamate would be replaced by the neutral valine. Because the protein is less negatively charged, it would move more slowly toward the positive electrode. Such a single amino acid substitution would be called a missense mutation. This particular mutation causes sickle cell disease.

In mutant #3, codon #4 is mutated from ACT to ACG. Because these are both threonine codons, there would be no effect on the final protein molecule. This is called a silent mutation.

In mutant #2, codon #8 is changed from AAG (lysine) to UAG (stop). The ribosome would prematurely terminate protein synthesis at this point. Such a mutation is called a nonsense mutation.

This restriction enzyme cleavage site is found at codons 5, 6, and 7 in the normal β-globin gene. It remains intact in all mutants except mutant #1. The mutation causing sickle cell disease thus brings about a change in the restriction fragments produced in this region by MstII, and serves as the basis for prenatal diagnosis and carrier detection for this disease.

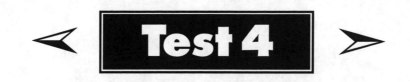

Test 4

DIRECTIONS:

Each of the numbered items or incomplete statements in this section is followed by answers or by completions of the statement. Select the ONE lettered answer or completion that is BEST in each case.

1. Over the past 10 years, the percentage of adults who have been hospitalized on at least one occasion is

(A) 10%
(B) 25%
(C) 35%
(D) 75%
(E) 90%

2. Endotoxin is a component part of the

(A) gram-positive bacterial cytoplasmic membrane
(B) gram-positive bacterial cell wall
(C) gram-negative bacterial outer membrane
(D) gram-negative bacterial peptidoglycan
(E) peptidoglycan techoic acid residues

3. The creatinine content of urine would be expected to be lower than normal in a patient with

(A) hepatitis
(B) muscular dystrophy
(C) Alzheimer's disease
(D) lead poisoning
(E) malaria

4. The genus Candida reproduces by

(A) arthrospore formation
(B) blastospore formation
(C) sexual spores
(D) ascospore formation
(E) sporangiospore formation

5. Study the following human leukocyte antigen (HLA) makeups (represented in groups on one chromosome), ABO groups, and Rh antigen typing of the following family. The woman and her present husband, the brother of her former husband, are represented in the chart. Which child is the product of the woman's first marriage?

	A1	B8	Dw3	A3	B7	Dw2	A2	B12	Dw2	A9	B5	Dw1	ABO group	D antigen
Mother	+	+	+	+	+	+	−	−	−	−	−	−	O	+
Present Husband	−	−	−	−	−	−	+	+	+	+	+	+	AB	+
(A)	+	+	+	−	−	−	−	−		+	+	+	B	+
(B)	−	−	−	+	+	+	+	+	+	−	−	−	A	−
(C)	+	+	+	−	−	−	+	+	I	−	−	−	A	−
(D)	−	−	−	+	+	+	−	−	−	+	+	+	O	−
(E)	+	+	+	−	−	−	+	+	+	−	−	−	B	+

6. Several chemical agents inhibit bacterial growth. Detergents' mode of antibacterial action is explained by which one of the following mechanisms?

(A) Damage to DNA
(B) Protein denaturation
(C) Disruption of cell membrane or wall
(D) Removal of suflhydral groups
(E) Chemical analogue antagonism

7. The catecholamines are synthesized from which amino acid?

(A) Tyrosine
(B) Tryptophan
(C) Histidine
(D) Glutamate
(E) Proline

8. Which one of the following organisms is endemic to the central San Juaquin Valley in California?

(A) *Histoplasma capsulatum*
(B) *Coccidioides immitis*
(C) *Blastomyces dermatitidis*
(D) *Cryptococcus neoformans*
(E) *Paracoccidioides braciliensis*

9. Which statement concerning viral carcinogenesis is correct?

(A) DNA oncogenic viruses are able to both integrate and replicate themselves in the host cell
(B) Acute, transforming retroviruses carry oncogenes that must be activated in the host cell
(C) Retroviruses insert their DNA directly into the host genome without the aid of enzymes
(D) Oncogenic viruses usually activate oncogenes by gene amplification, inactivation of suppressor genes, or inducing translocations
(E) Tumors evoked by a specific oncogenic retrovirus tend to have different tumor-specific antigens

10. Serotonin is synthesized from which amino acid?

(A) Cysteine
(B) Histidine
(C) Serine
(D) Tryptophan
(E) Tyrosine

11. A 9-month-old infant has a small fishlike mouth, low-set notched ears, cardiac insufficiency, hypocalcemia, and lymphopenia. The patient already has had several episodes of viral pneumonia, a fungal infection of the oral mucosa, and fever blisters caused by herpes simplex virus. The infant is diagnosed as having an immunodeficiency disease. Which of the following disorders is the most likely diagnosis?

(A) X-linked hypogammaglobulinemia
(B) Hereditary angioedema
(C) Ataxia-telangiectasia
(D) Severe combined immunodeficiency disease
(E) DiGeorge syndrome

12. Arrange the following into the proper sequence of glucagon stimulation of glycogenolysis.

1. Increased protein kinase activity
2. Increased phosphorylase A
3. Increased phosphorylase kinase
4. Activation of adenylate cyclase

(A) 1-4-2-3
(B) 4-1-3-2
(C) 1-4-3-2
(D) 4-2-1-3
(E) 1-2-3-4

13. A patient with eczema, thrombocytopenia, and recurrent infections is best characterized by which disorder?

(A) Deficiency of reduced nicotinamide adenine dinucleotide phosphate oxidase
(B) Defect in microtubule polymerization
(C) Combined B-cell and T-cell immunodeficiency
(D) Chromosomal instability syndrome
(E) Deficiency of adenosine deaminase

14. Vanillylmandelic acid (VMA) and homovanillic acid are metabolic products derived from the degradation of

(A) folic acid
(B) histamine
(C) serotonin
(D) heme
(E) catecholamines

15. A woman whose Rh haplotype is cde has an infant. The woman's infant would most likely have hemolytic disease of the newborn if he had which of the following Rh haplotypes?

(A) cdE
(B) CdE
(C) Cde
(D) cDe
(E) cde

16. Suppose that the radioactive amino acid ^{14}C-cysteine is charged onto its proper tRNA and then treated chemically so that the ^{14}C-cysteine residue is converted to ^{14}C-alanine. What is most likely to happen if this ^{14}C-ala-tRNA^{cys} is added to a protein synthesizing system?

(A) Radioactivity will be incorporated into protein only in response to cysteine codons in the mRNA
(B) Radioactivity will be incorporated into protein only in response to alanine codons in the mRNA
(C) Radioactivity will be incorporated into protein in response to both cysteine and alanine codons in the mRNA
(D) Radioactivity will be incorporated into random positions in the protein
(E) Protein synthesis will terminate prematurely

17. Which mechanism of tissue destruction is predominant in type III hypersensitivity reactions? The activation of

(A) natural killer cells with direct tissue destruction in areas of immune-complex deposition
(B) macrophages by immune complexes with the release of cytokines, which damage the tissue
(C) the complement system with the release of histamine and chemotactic agents that directly result in tissue damage
(D) the complement system and subsequent chemotaxis of neutrophils to areas of immune-complex deposition
(E) CD8 cytotoxic T cells with subsequent release of cytokines, which directly damage tissue

18. An emergency medical worker rescuing individuals trapped in a collapsed building finds a man with a beam across his right thigh. Signs of stasis are evident in the victim's right leg. The best course of action is to

(A) remove the beam immediately
(B) tourniquet and amputate the leg
(C) administer an intravenous drip of bicarbonate and insulin in a 5% dextrose solution, then remove the beam
(D) administer an intravenous drip of sodium lactate and insulin in a 5% dextrose solution, then remove the beam
(E) administer an intravenous drip of sodium lactate, 2 mmol potassium, and insulin in a 5% dextrose solution, then remove the beam

19. Which of the following diseases has a type of hypersensitivity reaction that the other diseases listed do not?

(A) Goodpasture syndrome
(B) ABO incompatibility
(C) Febrile transfusion reaction
(D) Graves disease
(E) Farmer's lung

20. Which one of the following amino acids would serve as the best buffer at physiologic pH?

(A) Glycine
(B) Aspartic acid
(C) Serine
(D) Lysine
(E) Histidine

21. A live bacterial vaccine is available for which of the following diseases?

(A) Whooping cough
(B) Tuberculosis
(C) Diphtheria
(D) Tetanus
(E) Meningitis

22. In the diagram below, curve 1 shows the oxygen dissociation for hemoglobin under normal conditions.

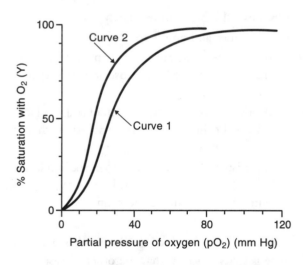

Curve 2 would most likely result from

(A) a decrease in pH
(B) an increase in the concentration of carbon dioxide
(C) an increase in the concentration of 2,3-bisphosphoglycerate
(D) stabilization of the deoxyhemoglobin
(E) an increase in pH

23. Three formulations of a drug (A, B, and C) were administered orally to human subjects, and the resulting pharmacokinetic values are shown in the following table.

Formulation	C_{max}	T_{max}	AUC[1]
A	50 mg/l	1 hour	250 mg/l × hours
B	25 mg/l	1 hour	125 mg/l × hours
C	35 mg/l	2 hours	250 mg/l × hours

[1] Area under the plasma drug concentration versus time curve.

The above data show that

(A) A is absorbed more rapidly than the other formulations
(B) A is absorbed more completely than the other formulations
(C) B is absorbed at the same rate as A but less completely
(D) C is absorbed slower and less completely than A
(E) B and C are absorbed slower and less completely than A

24. A postpartum woman with galactosemia is able to synthesize lactose in her breast milk due to the presence of

(A) galactose 1-phosphate uridyltransferase
(B) galactokinase
(C) β-galactosidase
(D) epimerase
(E) glucose-6-phosphatase

25. Which rickettsial diseases are transmitted to humans by *Pediculus*, the body louse?

(A) *Rickettsia rickettsii* and *Ehrlichia canis*
(B) *Rickettsia prowazekii* and *Rickettsia typhi*
(C) *Rickettsia rickettsii* and *Coxiella burnetii*
(D) *Rochalimaea quintana* and *Ehrlichia canis*
(E) *Rochalimaea quintana* and *Rickettsia prowazekii*

26. Which of the following is an imino acid?

(A) Glycine
(B) Histidine
(C) Arginine
(D) Proline
(E) Tryptophan

27. A woman is allergic to dogs. Within minutes after being in a room with a dog, she begins sneezing. The dog is best described as the

(A) unconditioned stimulus
(B) conditioned stimulus
(C) unconditioned response
(D) conditioned response
(E) discriminative status

Questions 28-29

An individual inherits a gene from his father that codes for a defective enzyme that normally would add a stretch of 20 to 80 amino acids to the NH_2 terminus of a protein synthesized on a "free" ribosome (i.e., a ribosome that is not attached to the endoplasmic reticulum). This added amino acid sequence forms an amphipathic α-helix, which is nonpolar on one side and positively charged on the other.

28. Normally, the final destination of the protein to which this amphipathic α-helix is added is the

(A) nucleus
(B) cytosol
(C) mitochondria
(D) cell membrane
(E) lysosome

29. Provided the gene coded is not sex-linked and that a normal allele is inherited from the proband's mother, the clinical manifestation of the defective gene inherited from the proband's father would be an observable defect in

(A) oxidative phosphorylation
(B) secretion of a specific circulating protein such as a hormone
(C) cytoskeletal structural elements
(D) spindle formation
(E) there should be no clinical effect

30. Both tetracycline and chloramphenicol are described by which of the following functions? They both

(A) cause a dose-dependent microcytic anemia
(B) are metabolized by glucuronide conjugation
(C) form a complex with divalent and trivalent cations
(D) may deposit in growing teeth and bones
(E) are effective in the treatment of rickettsial infections

31. The following pedigree involves a family with individuals who have developed a progressive loss of central vision.

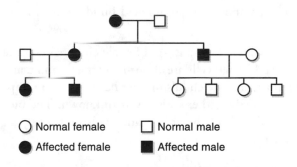

○ Normal female   □ Normal male
● Affected female   ■ Affected male

This family pedigree exhibits which of the following inheritance patterns?

(A) Multifactorial inheritance
(B) Mitochondrial genetic defect
(C) Autosomal dominant inheritance
(D) Sex-linked dominant inheritance
(E) Autosomal recessive inheritance

32. Which method is the most effective in teaching a dog to jump through a flaming hoop?

(A) Classical conditioning
(B) Operant conditioning
(C) Stimulus generalization
(D) Extinction
(E) Respondent conditioning

33. Which of the following is a high-energy compound that can donate a phosphate group to adenosine diphosphate (ADP) to form adenosine triphosphate (ATP)?

(A) Adenosine monophosphate (AMP)
(B) Creatine phosphate
(C) Glucose 6-phosphate
(D) Glycerol 3-phosphate
(E) Phosphatidic acid

34. The *Bacillus anthracis* capsule is unusual because it

(A) does not impede phagocytosis
(B) stains blue in the Gram stain procedure
(C) stains red in the Gram stain procedure
(D) is composed of short-chained polysaccharides
(E) is composed of amino acid building blocks

35. A white, 32-month-old female child has chronic anemia. Her red cells are abnormally fragile and many are spherical. The child's mother has no similar symptoms, and the father's history is unknown. The biochemical basis of the child's anemia is most likely an abnormal

(A) glucose 6-phosphatase
(B) pyruvate kinase
(C) spectrin
(D) ankyrin
(E) intrinsic factor

36. On which method is biofeedback based?

(A) Classical conditioning
(B) Operant conditioning
(C) Stimulus generalization
(D) Extinction
(E) Respondent conditioning

37. A man with chronic alcoholism has just been admitted to a veterans hospital. The patient is hallucinating and has an unsteady gait, uncoordinated eye movements, and a lack of fine motor coordination. Laboratory results show that he is acidotic because of a high concentration of lactate in his serum. His symptoms diminish almost immediately after the intravenous injection of a multivitamin mixture. The molecular basis of this patient's symptoms is most likely due to an inhibition of

(A) pyruvate kinase
(B) pyruvate dehydrogenase
(C) lactate dehydrogenase
(D) isocitrate dehydrogenase
(E) pyruvate carboxylase

Questions 38-39

A nine-year-old boy gets an injection during a visit to his physician. That night, he dreams that a cartoon character shoots him in the arm.

38. Which term best describes the boy's actual dream?

(A) Latent dream
(B) Dream censor
(C) Day residue
(D) Manifest dream
(E) Dream work

39. The injection that the boy received at the doctor's office is the

(A) latent dream
(B) dream censor
(C) day residue
(D) manifest dream
(E) dream work

40. The half-lives for the mRNAs of C-fos and β-globin are about 30 minutes and 10 hours, respectively. Which of the following conclusions can most logically be deduced from this observation?

(A) Normally, more C-fos than β-globin is synthesized
(B) The half-life of C-fos is greater than that of β-globin
(C) Each molecule of C-fos mRNA will direct the synthesis of more protein molecules than will each β-globin mRNA molecule
(D) It is more important for the cell to regulate C-fos levels than β-globin levels
(E) No particular significance can be attached to the relative half-lives of mRNAs

41. The ideal method to protect a population from tetanus is

(A) immunization with the toxin
(B) immunization with the toxoid
(C) immunization with the antitoxin
(D) immunization with γ-globulin
(E) use of the antibiotic prophylactically

42. In a patient with systemic lupus erythematosus, which one of the following functions would most likely be directly affected by this disease?

(A) 5'mRNA capping
(B) Addition of a poly-A tail to mRNA
(C) Removal of introns from mRNA
(D) Methylation of specific adenylate residues of mRNA
(E) Degradation of the poly-A tail of mRNA

43. In order to estimate the expected body weight of a one-year-old child, multiply his birth weight by

(A) 1.5
(B) 2.0
(C) 2.5
(D) 3.0
(E) 4.0

44. Which of the following statements describes both metronidazole and cefoperazone? They

(A) are active against a wide range of aerobic gram-negative bacilli
(B) may cause adverse effects when administered with ethanol
(C) are effective in the treatment of giardiasis
(D) may cause the urine to be dark or reddish-brown
(E) inhibit bacterial cell wall synthesis

45. A baby who usually smiles at everyone begins to cry when strangers pick her up. The age of this child is most likely

(A) one month
(B) two months
(C) four months
(D) five months
(E) seven months

46. In an inner-city clinic that is seriously underfunded, testing for *Chlamydia* would be economically impractical in

(A) male patients with urethritis and no intracellular gram-negative diplococci
(B) female patients using nonbarrier contraceptives
(C) female patients presenting with cervicitis and admission of multiple sex partners
(D) neonatal patients with inclusion conjunctivitis and/or pneumonia
(E) patients with a history of sexually transmitted diseases

47. A 4-year-old girl insists on bandaging even the smallest insect bite or injury. This behavior is

(A) an early sign of obsessive-compulsive disorder
(B) an indication of an adjustment disorder
(C) an early sign of depression
(D) an early sign of passive-aggressive behavior
(E) normal for this age

48. Which virus is associated with hemorrhagic cystitis?

(A) Parvovirus
(B) Echovirus
(C) Varicella-zoster virus
(D) Adenovirus
(E) Parainfluenza virus

49. A patient with tuberculosis is most likely to develop peripheral neuritis and paresthesia as a result of taking

(A) pyrazinamide
(B) rifampin
(C) ethambutol
(D) isoniazid
(E) streptomycin

50. A 12-year-old girl develops a diffuse maculopapular rash, a tender posterior cervical, auricular and occipital nodes, a mild sore throat, and a low-grade fever. During the next 24 hours, the girl develops conjunctivitis and her wrists swell. The rash subsides three days after the onset of her illness. The most likely diagnosis is

(A) varicella
(B) rubeola
(C) erythema infectiosum
(D) roseola
(E) rubella

51. A pediatric resident is having a birthday party for his daughter and overhears one of the little girls being taunted for being too dumb to eat her ice cream and cake. By talking to the girl, the resident learns that the child has an older sister who is retarded and has very poor sight. The little girl's mother warned her that she too would become retarded and blind if she consumes any product containing large quantities of milk. The symptoms suggested by the little girl's mother indicate an

(A) accumulation of a disaccharide in the lens and neural tissues
(B) accumulation of galactitol (dulcitol) in the lens and neural tissues
(C) accumulation of fructose 1-phosphate in the lens and neural tissues
(D) autoimmune reaction initiated by an immune reaction to cow's milk lactalbumin initiated in early infancy
(E) autoimmune reaction initiated by an immune reaction to cow's milk casein initiated in early infancy

52. Acyclovir and azidothymidine interfere with virus growth by affecting which of the following functions?

(A) Cell wall synthesis
(B) Cell membrane metabolism
(C) Nucleic acid metabolism
(D) Protein synthesis
(E) Receptor attachment

53. In a catheterized patient, a lower urinary tract infection caused by *Pseudomonas aeruginosa* may be treated with

(A) trimethoprim with sulfamethoxazole
(B) amoxicillin
(C) doxycycline
(D) nitrofurantoin
(E) ofloxacin

54. Live, attenuated vaccines exist for which viral disease?

(A) Hepatitis B and poliovirus
(B) Influenza and measles viruses
(C) Rubella and mumps viruses
(D) Rabies and measles viruses
(E) Poliovirus and influenza viruses

55. An 83-year-old woman's husband died 6 months ago. Which of the following reactions is considered normal bereavement for this woman?

(A) A suicide attempt
(B) Intense feelings of worthlessness
(C) Problems with sleep
(D) Grief lasting 4 years after the death
(E) Feelings of hopelessness

56. Which structure describes the respiratory syncytial virus?

(A) DNA-dependent RNA polymerase
(B) DNA-dependent DNA polymerase
(C) Double-stranded RNA-dependent RNA polymerase
(D) RNA-dependent DNA polymerase
(E) Single-stranded RNA-dependent RNA polymerase

57. A researcher has prepared a human complementary DNA (cDNA) library using an expression vector. She wants to identify the specific bacterial colonies producing human hypoxanthine phosphoribosyltransferase (HPRT) protein. Which of the following would be the best way to identify these specific colonies?

(A) Bacterial growth medium containing ampicillin
(B) Bacterial growth medium containing tetracycline
(C) Radioactive messenger RNA (mRNA) coding for HPRT
(D) Radioactive antibody specific to HPRT
(E) Radioactive nucleic acid probe complementary to HPRT introns

58. A middle-aged man, who has been an avid bicyclist and tennis player, is hospitalized for heart failure. The next day he is found doing push-ups on the floor of his hospital room. This is an example of which defense mechanism?

(A) Regression
(B) Dissociation
(C) Displacement
(D) Intellectualization
(E) Denial

59. Which drug is correctly matched with the seroto-nin, or 5-hydroxytryptamine (5-HT), receptor subtype to mediate the drug's effects?

(A) Buspirone—5-HT$_4$
(B) Cisapride—5-HT$_3$
(C) Metoclopramide—5-HT$_4$
(D) Sumatriptan—5-HT$_{1D}$
(E) Ondansetron—5-HT$_2$

60. A 26-year-old woman exhibits different personal-ities at different times. These actions are examples of which defense mechanism?

(A) Regression
(B) Dissociation
(C) Displacement
(D) Intellectualization
(E) Denial

61. The product of the v-*src* gene is a

(A) protein tyrosine kinase
(B) G protein
(C) growth factor
(D) growth factor receptor
(E) DNA-binding protein

62. A 15-month-old child placed in an orphanage will most likely experience which one of the following?

(A) Severe developmental retardation
(B) Generally good health
(C) Inadequate physical care
(D) Few problems as an adult
(E) Normal social relationships in childhood

63. Gluconeogenesis provides most of the fuel for the brain when fasting for

(A) 2 to 6 hours
(B) 8 to 12 hours
(C) 20 to 24 hours
(D) 10 to 20 days
(E) 30 to 40 days

64. Which of the following factors is associated with patient noncompliance?

(A) Extended waiting room time
(B) Older age of the physician
(C) Simple treatment regimen
(D) Increased time the physician spends with the patient
(E) Patient knowledge of how the medication will help the illness

65. Which of the following statements is true of a human genome?

(A) Genes that encode related enzymes are usually organized into operons
(B) Normal cells contain proto-oncogenes
(C) Transcriptionally-active chromatin is usually highly condensed
(D) Most of the DNA codes for protein sequences
(E) Each chromosome has a single origin of repli-cation

66. A surgeon argues with his son in the morning, then he takes his anger out on his residents by answer-ing their questions abruptly. The surgeon is exhibiting which defense mechanism?

(A) Regression
(B) Displacement
(C) Sublimation
(D) Denial
(E) Dissociation

67. The loss or inactivation of an anti-oncogene causes

(A) sickle cell anemia
(B) β-thalassemia
(C) the color pattern of a calico cat
(D) Burkitt lymphoma
(E) retinoblastoma

68. While hospitalized for treatment of pneumonia, a young lawyer does not shave, watches cartoons on television, and reads *Mad* magazine. These actions illustrate which defense mechanism?

(A) Regression
(B) Dissociation
(C) Displacement
(D) Intellectualization
(E) Denial

69. In eukaryotes, the TATA sequence functions as

(A) an indication of the starting point for replication
(B) a part of the binding site for a transcription factor and RNA polymerase
(C) a common part of the messenger RNA (mRNA) molecule
(D) a termination signal for transcription
(E) an indication of the starting point for translation

70. Patients with chronic pain who receive psycho-therapy and behavior therapy exhibit which sign?

(A) Need more pain medication
(B) Show excessive dependence on the therapist
(C) Become less mobile
(D) Show fewer attempts to get back to their preillness lifestyle
(E) Spend less time in the hospital

71. A young child has a liver that appears normal upon palpitation. She has a history consistent with hypoglycemia that is relieved by eating, and she metabolizes fat normally (i.e., there is no ketosis). Although alanine fails to increase her blood glucose levels, fructose or glycerol administration restores the patient's blood glucose to normal. Enzyme assays of liver tissue are pending, but you expect that she has a deficiency of active

(A) glucose-6-phosphatase
(B) fructose-1,6-bisphosphatase
(C) glycogen phosphorylase
(D) phospho*enol*pyruvate-carboxykinase
(E) aldolase B

72. Which statement describes both amphotericin B and fluconazole? They

(A) are orally effective
(B) often cause chills, fever, and nephrotoxicity
(C) inhibit fungal cell membrane ergosterol synthesis
(D) are effective in treating cryptococcal meningitis
(E) inhibit cytochrome P-450 enzymes

73. If an individual exercises strenuously before eating breakfast, the exercise will increase the levels of

(A) high density lipoprotein (HDL)
(B) very low density lipoprotein (VLDL)
(C) triacylglycerol micelles
(D) chylomicrons
(E) albumin-bound free fatty acids

Questions 74-75

Six medical students received test scores of 20, 20, 40, 50, 100, and 30.

74. The median of this group of scores is

(A) 20.0
(B) 30.0
(C) 35.0
(D) 40.0
(E) 43.3

75. The distribution of this group of scores is

(A) normal
(B) Gaussian
(C) skewed to the left
(D) skewed to the right
(E) bimodal

76. A young woman, who is very conscious of her weight, complains that she is fatigued and has even fainted in the late afternoon. A physical examination finds no abnormalities. The doctor learns that the patient's breakfast consists of a small glass of orange juice, a bagel, and a cup of coffee with cream, while her lunch is usually a garden salad, hamburger, and small glass of milk. The doctor suspects that the patient is hypoglycemic and recommends that she self-measure her blood glucose levels at hourly intervals. The results show that her blood glucose level is 80 mg/dl at about 2 P.M., and by 4 P.M., this level has dropped to 40 mg/dl. The doctor finds that if the patient eats a carbohydrate-rich meal at noon, she maintains a normal blood glucose level until at least 8 P.M. However, when she eats a protein-rich, carbohydrate-poor meal, her blood glucose level drops. The extreme nature of the woman's levels indicates that there is a metabolic aberration in addition to her insufficient diet. During follow-up, oral administration of neither fructose, glycerol, nor alanine results in an increase in blood sugar levels. The young woman probably has a defect in

(A) glycogenolysis
(B) β-oxidation of fatty acids
(C) glycolysis
(D) gluconeogenesis
(E) pentose phosphate shunt function

77. Which statement describes mycoplasmas? They

(A) are sensitive to penicillin
(B) lack peptidoglycan cell walls in all stages of growth
(C) cannot divide by binary fission
(D) require low salt concentration to maintain cellular integrity
(E) are sensitive to cephalosporins

78. The most serious cause of stress for children and adolescents is

(A) school transfer
(B) trouble with law enforcement authorities
(C) sexual abuse
(D) divorce of parents
(E) suspension from school

79. One of two reactions in which vitamin B_{12} acts as a cofactor is the isomerization of methylmalonyl coenzyme A (CoA) to succinyl CoA by methylmalonyl CoA mutase. With this reaction, a vitamin B_{12} deficiency causes

(A) a secondary functional folate deficiency
(B) a decrease in energy because of a lack of succinate as a substrate for oxidative phosphorylation
(C) an accumulation of branched-chain amino acids
(D) an accumulation of fatty acids having an odd number of carbon atoms
(E) a deficiency of fumarate in the tricarboxylic acid cycle

80. An overweight, diabetic woman asks a doctor for help in dieting. The physician prepares a diet for her and spends 45 minutes discussing it with her. One month later, the patient has not lost weight and tells the doctor that she has not had a chance to buy the required food. This behavior is characteristic of which of the following personality types?

(A) Schizoid
(B) Passive-aggressive
(C) Paranoid
(D) Histrionic
(E) Dependent

81. A 6-month-old infant presents with a history of one-day periods of nasal congestion, sneezing, and coughing. Other members of the family have had similar symptoms. The child now presents with dyspnea, nasal flaring, hyperexpansion of the chest, and inspiratory and expiratory wheezes in both lung fields. Which infection best explains these symptoms?

(A) Epstein-Barr virus infection with bronchiolitis

(B) Cytomegalovirus infection with acute epiglottitis

(C) Parainfluenza virus infection with croup

(D) Respiratory syncytial virus infection with bronchiolitis

(E) Adenovirus infection with interstitial pneumonia

82. Which viral disease can be managed, in part, by using passive immunity techniques?

(A) Hepatitis A infections

(B) Rubella infections

(C) Rotavirus infections

(D) Poliovirus infections

(E) Influenza A virus infections

83. What happens when the lipid envelope of an orthomyxovirus is destroyed by ether?

(A) The virus will not attach to a host cell

(B) Infectious RNA will be produced

(C) The virus will multiply without the benefit of a host cell

(D) The genome of the virus will also be destroyed

(E) The virus may be successfully treated by amantadine

84. The renal threshold for a solute denotes the

(A) maximun filtration rate

(B) maximum reabsorption rate

(C) plasma concentration at which a solute begins to appear in the urine

(D) maximum secretion rate

(E) maximum tubular secretory capacity (Ts)

85. A 1-year-old child with a history of hypoglycemia and hepatomegaly is referred to a pediatrician. The patient's previous doctor has stabilized conditions by prescribing small high-protein meals every 2 to 3 hours. However, the child's parents are anxious to obtain a diagnosis. After running a series of tests, the pediatrician determines that the patient has a glucose-6-phosphatase deficiency. Which of the following observation sets is consistent with this diagnosis?

Liver Glycogen on Liver Biopsy	Blood Glucose Post Fructose Infusion	Fructose Levels in Urine
(A) Normal Amount but unbranched	Increased	Normal
(B) Normal Amount Normal Structure	No Increase	Increased
(C) Increased Amount Normal Structure	No Increase	Normal
(D) Increased Amount Normal Structure	Increased	Normal
(E) Increased Amount Normal Structure	No Increase	Increased

86. The ED_{50}s (median effective doses) for cardiac stimulation and bronchial muscle relaxation of a new adrenergic agonist and isoproterenol are shown below.

Drug	Cardiac ED_{50}	Bronchial Muscle ED_{50}
Isoproterenol	30	30
New Agonist	160	40

One can conclude that the new agonist is a

(A) selective α_1 agonist

(B) selective α_2 agonist

(C) selective β_1 agonist

(D) selective β_2 agonist

(E) nonselective β_1 and β_2 agonist

87. In this figure, the cell in the center with secretory granules (SG) oriented away from the lumen side is

(A) a goblet cell
(B) an acinar cell
(C) an absorptive cell
(D) a Paneth cell
(E) an enteroendocrine cell

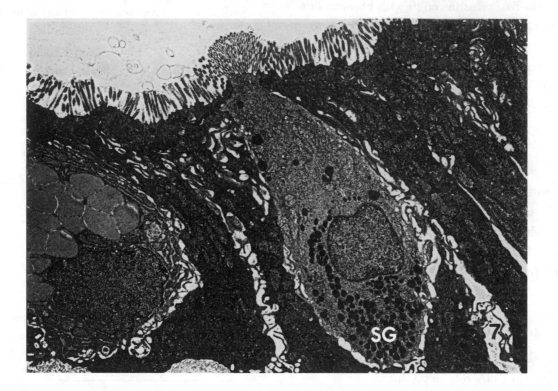

88. Neutrophils and monocytes use both oxygen-dependent and oxygen-independent mechanisms to kill engulfed bacterium. Normally, the oxygen-dependent mechanism is due to a macrophage enzyme that converts molecular oxygen to superoxide (a free radical). An inborn error of metabolism causes chronic granulomatosis, which is characterized by severe and persistent pyogenic infections. Patients suffering from chronic granulomatosis lack a macrophage enzyme called

(A) reduced nicotinamide adenine dinucleotide phosphate (NADPH) oxidase
(B) superoxide dismutase
(C) myeloperoxidase
(D) catalase
(E) glutathione peroxidase

89. For coronary artery disease, the standard for a positive stress electrocardiogram is a 1-mm ST depression. If the criteria for a positive test is changed to 2 mm, this change would

(A) increase the sensitivity of the test
(B) decrease the number of false negatives (FNs)
(C) increase the number of false positives (FPs)
(D) increase the specificity of the test
(E) have no effect on the sensitivity or specificity of the test

90. Which of the following statements best characterizes toxoids? Toxoids are

(A) toxins that are degraded to haptens
(B) nonimmunogenic because the epitopes are missing
(C) toxins that have been treated with neutralizing antibodies
(D) immunogenic but not harmful to the host
(E) immunogenic and toxic to the host

91. A restriction map of bacteriophage λ-DNA is shown below. What size fragments would be produced by cutting λ-DNA with a combination of Apa I and Xba I?

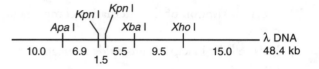

(A) 5.5 and 10.0 kb
(B) 10.0 and 38.4 kb
(C) 10.0, 13.9, and 24.5 kb
(D) 5.5, 6.9, 9.5, and 10.0 kb
(E) 1.5, 5.5, 6.9, 9.5, 10.0, and 15.0 kb

92. Which of the following immune globulins is most likely to be given to a hospital employee who is accidentally stuck with a hypodermic needle?

(A) Varicella-zoster
(B) Tetanus
(C) Rabies
(D) Hepatitis B
(E) Vaccinia

93. A pharmaceutical company develops an anticancer agent. When the company completes the first phase III trial (Experiment A) in five different centers, it reports that the patients who received the agent lived significantly longer than the patients who received the placebo. Further phase III testing (Experiment B) uses the same number of patients, and all of these patients are in one center. Experiment B reveals that the drug is ineffective in increasing the survival time of cancer patients. The best conclusion is that a

(A) type I error was committed in Experiment A
(B) type I error was committed in Experiment B
(C) type II error was committed in Experiment A
(D) type II error was committed in Experiment B
(E) type III error was committed in both Experiments A and B

94. Which statement best describes a function of the lipopolysaccharide that is present in the cell wall of gram-negative bacteria?

(A) Inhibits the release of interleukin-1 and other cytokines
(B) Blocks activation of the alternative complement cascade
(C) Kills cells by inactivating peptide elongation factor EF-2
(D) Induces disseminated intravascular coagulation
(E) Enables the organisms to survive within phagocytes

95. A 75-year-old woman, who lives with her daughter, is brought to the emergency room with a fractured forearm, bruises on both wrists, and bilateral contusions on her face. When you question the elderly patient about her injuries, she says that she "fell." Your first course of action is to

(A) tell the daughter that you believe the mother is being abused
(B) contact a social service agency
(C) contact the police
(D) send the mother home with instructions to come back in one week
(E) instruct the daughter on how to reduce her own stress to better take care of her mother

96. Ten months after surgery for colon cancer and radiation treatments, a 70-year-old male patient is informed that the concentration of a tumor marker in his serum has increased substantially. The tumor marker is most likely to be

(A) antibody light chains
(B) α-fetoprotein
(C) human chorionic gonadotropin
(D) carcinoembryonic antigen
(E) prostate-specific antigen

97. In bacteria, all enzymes of a given metabolic pathway are often coordinately expressed because

(A) all enzymes in bacteria are expressed constitutively
(B) the enzymes are all the same size
(C) the enzymes all require the same cofactors
(D) the pathway is regulated by feedback inhibition
(E) the enzymes are all produced from one polycistronic message

98. Which of the following choices is most likely to serve as a substrate for the enzyme ribonucleotide reductase?

(A) Adenosine monophosphate
(B) Uridine diphosphate
(C) Guanosine triphosphate
(D) Adenine
(E) Inosine

99. Which of the following agents is known to enhance immune responsiveness?

(A) Cyclophosphamide
(B) Methotrexate
(C) Levamisole
(D) Prednisone
(E) Total lymphoid irradiation

100. A midstream, "clean-catch" urine culture from an asymptomatic 24-year-old pregnant woman yields numerous bacteria that are lactose positive, motile, and susceptible to many common antibiotics. Which organism is most likely causing the infection?

(A) *Serratia marcescens*
(B) *Escherichia coli*
(C) *Klebsiella pneumoniae*
(D) *Pseudomonas aeruginosa*
(E) *Proteus vulgaris*

101. Which of the following *Escherichia coli* types produces a disease similar in pathogenesis to cholera?

(A) Enteropathogenic *E. coli*
(B) Enterotoxigenic *E. coli*
(C) Enterohemorrhagic *E. coli*
(D) Enteroinvasive *E. coli*
(E) Nephropathogenic *E. coli*

102. In mitochondria, oxygen will be used at the fastest rate with added

(A) 2,4-dinitrophenol
(B) adenosine diphosphate (ADP)
(C) succinate
(D) succinate, plus ADP
(E) succinate, plus 2,4-dinitrophenol

103. HIV type 1 binds to which of the following receptors?

(A) Human leukocyte antigen (HLA) class I molecules
(B) HLA class II molecules
(C) T-cell antigen receptor
(D) CD4 molecule
(E) CD8 molecule

104. A 29-year-old female is addicted to drugs and is diagnosed with AIDS. The woman delivers an infant who fails to thrive. The best evidence that the newborn is infected with HIV type 1 is

(A) identification of HIV type 1 (HIV-1) genome in cells
(B) high titer of HIV-1 immunoglobulin
(C) low birth weight
(D) high titer of immunoglobulin G against HIV-1
(E) low response to bacterial polysaccharides

105. The antigens on erythrocytes that determine ABO blood groups are

(A) proteins
(B) lipids
(C) glycoproteins
(D) carbohydrates
(E) lipoproteins

106. Which statement describes a function of the genetic mechanisms of erythrocyte ABO group antigens?

(A) Involve genes that code for carbohydrates
(B) Provide information in paternity disputes
(C) Involve genes that code for enzymes
(D) Are suppressed in all other cell types
(E) Are the same as those for the Rh system

Questions 107-108

A 6-month-old infant was admitted to the hospital with an upper respiratory infection, which was found to be caused by bacteria. Although he responded well to antibiotics, the infant was admitted again one month later for severe otitis media. After two more episodes of infection and a diagnosis of *Haemophilus influenzae* pneumonia, the infant had an extremely low serum antibody titer and was diagnosed as having an immunodeficiency disease.

107. The infant is most likely to have which of the following diseases?

(A) Selective immunoglobulin A deficiency
(B) X-linked hypogammaglobulinemia
(C) Thymic aplasia
(D) Ataxia-telangiectasia
(E) Wiskott-Aldrich syndrome

108. The best therapy for this infant is

(A) immunoglobulin G from pooled random donors
(B) a thymus transplant
(C) a blood transfusion
(D) immunization with attenuated vaccines
(E) antifungal agents

109. An 8-month-old infant has a history of chronic diarrhea, several episodes of pneumonia, and otitis media. He also has had oral candidiasis (thrush) and infections with herpes simplex virus. He has no detectable thymus upon radiograph, and B lymphocytes are absent. A rash was evident at birth. The most likely diagnosis is

(A) ataxia-telangiectasia
(B) hereditary angioedema
(C) severe combined immunodeficiency disease
(D) chronic granulomatous disease
(E) Chédiak-Higashi syndrome

110. An example of a malignant tumor of mesenchymal origin is

(A) mesothelioma
(B) hemangioma
(C) chondroma
(D) rhabdomyoma
(E) meningioma

111. If a blood group A patient inadvertently receives a blood group B donor heart, which reaction would be expected?

(A) Intimal thickening of vessels in the donor heart with rejection in the next 3 months
(B) A predominantly CD8 T lymphocyte infiltrate in the donor coronary artery vessels with subsequent vessel thrombosis and rejection of the heart
(C) Acute necrotizing vasculitis with vessel thrombosis in the donor heart with rejection in the first 24 hours
(D) A combination of humoral and cellular immune reactions against the donor heart with destruction after 3 months
(E) A predominantly humoral reaction after 3 to 4 months with dense intimal fibrosis of vessels producing ischemia

112. A newborn boy with DiGeorge syndrome inadvertently received crossmatch compatible blood that was not irradiated prior to transfusion. The infant developed a fever, diarrhea, liver abnormalities, a skin rash, and lost weight. Which disorder is most likely responsible for the infant's condition?

(A) A cytomegalovirus infection
(B) A graft versus host reaction
(C) An anaphylactic reaction to donor leukocytes
(D) A febrile transfusion reaction
(E) A hemolytic transfusion reaction

113. A 20-year-old woman has a history of chronic sinopulmonary infections and allergies. Her 2-year-old boy developed hepatitis A in a nursery. When given a shot of γ-globulin, the woman had an anaphylactic reaction requiring resuscitation in the doctor's office. The woman most likely has which of the following disorders?

(A) Wiskott-Aldrich syndrome
(B) Immunoglobulin A deficiency
(C) Common variable immunodeficiency
(D) C1 esterase inhibitor deficiency
(E) Immunoglobulin G subset deficiency

114. A 26-year-old man has recurrent attacks of facial swelling and inspiratory stridor that last up to 24 hours, often requiring hospitalization because of airway obstruction. There is no family history of allergies, and preliminary tests reveal a low C4 complement level. This patient most likely has which of the following disorders?

(A) A low complement C3 level
(B) A normal complement C2 level
(C) A decrease in C1 esterase inhibitor
(D) An increase in serum immunoglobulin E
(E) The presence of autoantibodies against the C3 complement component

115. A newborn boy with truncus arteriosus has carpopedal spasm and absence of the mediastinal shadow on a chest radiograph. The newborn most likely has which of the following disorders?

(A) Severe combined immunodeficiency syndrome
(B) Ataxia-telangiectasia
(C) Bruton agammaglobulinemia
(D) DiGeorge syndrome
(E) Sex-linked lymphoproliferative syndrome

116. Which of the following conditions would be expected in a patient with a pure B-cell deficiency state?

(A) Anergy to skin testing with common antigens
(B) Abnormal phytohemagglutinin mitogen assay
(C) Plasma cells in lymph nodes
(D) Antibody response to routine immunizations
(E) Absence of isohemagglutinins in the serum

117. Which of the following reactions most closely resembles the hypersensitivity reaction associated with poison ivy?

(A) Scratch testing
(B) Skin testing for penicillin allergy
(C) Skin reaction to nickel
(D) Arthus reaction
(E) Shwartzman reaction

118. A stimulus for insulin release would be expected with

(A) hyperkalemia
(B) increased glucagon
(C) increased somatostatin
(D) hypercortisolism
(E) dawn effect

Questions 119-120

The following questions refer to the process of generating adenosine triphosphate (ATP) from one molecule of glucose.

119. What is the total set number of ATPs generated per molecule of glucose from pyruvate through the tricarboxylic acid cycle (TCA cycle)?

(A) 22
(B) 24
(C) 26
(D) 28
(E) 30

120. What is the net number of ATPs that can be generated from one molecule of glucose without using oxidative phosphorylation?

(A) 2
(B) 4
(C) 6
(D) 8
(E) 12

121. When bacterial cells are fractionated, the major components of the electron transport system are found in

(A) cell walls
(B) membrane fragments
(C) ribosomes
(D) capsule or glycocalyx
(E) the supernatant from high speed centrifugation

DIRECTIONS:

Each of the numbered items or incomplete statements in this section is negatively phrased, as indicated by a capitalized word such as NOT, LEAST, or EXCEPT. Select the ONE lettered answer or completion that is BEST in each case.

122. All of the following are common reasons for noncompliance with medical advice EXCEPT

(A) oral rather than written dosage instructions
(B) deliberate misuse of medication
(C) failure to understand the instructions for taking the medication
(D) dislike of the physician
(E) an illness that has few or no symptoms

123. Bacteria that produce IgA proteases, which helps to allow efficient colonization of mucosal surfaces, include all the following EXCEPT

(A) *Neisseria gonorrhea*
(B) *Neisseria meningitidis*
(C) *Staphylococcus aureus*
(D) *Streptococcus pneumoniae*
(E) *Haemophilus influenzae*

124. Which one of the following amino acids is NOT optically active?

(A) Glycine
(B) Alanine
(C) Tyrosine
(D) Glutamic acid
(E) Asparagine

125. The following combinations each represent secondary descriptor paired with a cancer location. In which combination does the secondary descriptor NOT apply to the usual morphology of one of the primary cancers in that location?

(A) Papillary–bladder cancer
(B) Medullary–breast cancer
(C) Mucinous–ovarian cancer
(D) Comedo–breast cancer
(E) Scirrhous–central nervous system cancer

126. Tumor cells can escape immune defenses by all of the following mechanisms EXCEPT

(A) immunoselection
(B) induction of low-dose tolerance
(C) activation of cytotoxic T lymphocytes
(D) immunologic blinding
(E) formation of soluble immune complexes

127. Which test would be LEAST useful in the evaluation of a patient with expiratory wheezes in all lung fields, particularly during the early Spring?

(A) Scratch test
(B) Radioimmunosorbent test
(C) Radioallergosorbent test
(D) Complete blood cell count
(E) Patch test

128. Patients with a viral meningitis have all of the following conditions EXCEPT

(A) normal cerebrospinal fluid glucose
(B) normal cerebrospinal fluid protein
(C) lymphocyte predominant cell count and differential
(D) negative Gram stain on spun sediment
(E) spinal fluid glucose level lower than the blood glucose level

129. Which response is NOT an expected cellular immune response leading to eventual destruction of a renal transplant?

(A) Antigen-presenting cells in the graft interact with host CD8 cytotoxic T cells through their class I antigen recognition sites
(B) Antigen-presenting cells in the graft interact with host CD4 T-helper cells through their class II antigen recognition sites
(C) CD4 T-helper cells in the host are activated and release interleukin-2, stimulating further proliferation of host T cells and stimulating B cells to synthesize antibodies
(D) Antigen-presenting cells in the graft release interleukin-1, increasing the host's proliferation of CD4 T-helper cells
(E) Host CD8 cytotoxic T cells, using an antibody-dependent cell-mediated cytotoxicity, interact with class I antigens on donor cells and destroy them

130. Tetracyclines, such as doxycycline, treat all of the following infections EXCEPT

(A) syphilis in patients allergic to penicillin
(B) chlamydial urethritis
(C) legionnaires disease
(D) cholera due to *Vibrio* genus
(E) brucellosis

131. All of the following statements are true about families in the United States EXCEPT

(A) most of the population marries at some time
(B) approximately half of the marriages will end in divorce
(C) 10% to 15% of couples are childless
(D) the nuclear family commonly includes parents and their dependent children
(E) approximately 10% of children live in families in which both parents work

132. The following descriptions of *Streptococcus pneumoniae* are all true EXCEPT that it

(A) is bile soluble
(B) is catalase positive
(C) is optochin sensitive
(D) causes sinusitis in children
(E) contains polysaccharide capsules

133. All of the following statements are true about hypnosis EXCEPT that

(A) less intelligent people are easier to hypnotize than more intelligent people
(B) people with a hypnotic capability of five are easy to hypnotize
(C) the effects of hypnosis are commonly short term
(D) hypnotic capability can be increased only marginally with training
(E) the subject under hypnosis can disregard suggestions made by the hypnotist

Questions 134-135

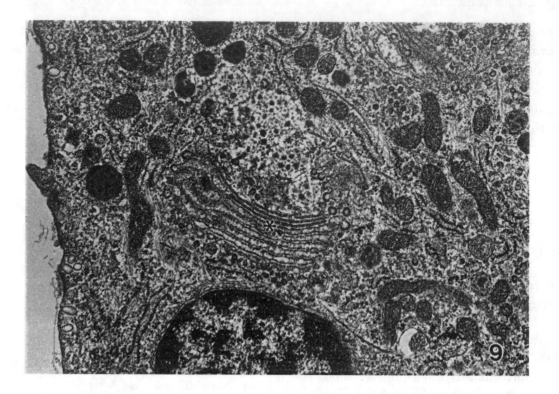

134. Identify the organelle at the asterisk in this figure. The nucleus is in the lower portion of the figure.

(A) Microtubules
(B) Golgi complex
(C) Annulate lamellae
(D) Rough endoplasmic reticulum
(E) Smooth endoplasmic reticulum

135. The organelle in this figure serves all of the following functions EXCEPT

(A) sulfating
(B) packaging
(C) glycosylation
(D) concentration
(E) detoxification

136. When a middle-aged couple tried to have intercourse, the husband could not maintain an erection. Which of the following is LEAST likely to have caused this problem?

(A) Antihypertensive medication
(B) Alcohol
(C) Diabetes
(D) Illegal diet pills (amphetamines)
(E) Antidepressant medication

137. All of the following statements are correct regarding tumor-associated antigens EXCEPT that

(A) they may be products of reactivated fetal genes
(B) they are not capable of inducing tumor rejection
(C) virus-associated tumor antigens are cross-reactive
(D) radiation-induced tumor antigens are unique
(E) chemically-induced tumor antigens are unique

138. All of these statements regarding immune defense against tumors are correct EXCEPT that

(A) antibodies against tumor antigens are of major importance
(B) natural killer cells are involved in immune surveillance
(C) cytotoxic T lymphocytes can kill tumor cells
(D) T-helper lymphocytes augment antitumor defense mechanisms
(E) activated macrophages preferentially kill tumor cells

139. Which of the following choices is LEAST likely to be involved in regulation of gene expression in eukaryotes?

(A) Gene rearrangement
(B) Messenger RNA stability
(C) Attenuation
(D) Increased rate of transcription
(E) Decreased rate of translation

140. All of the following statements are correct regarding adoptive immunotherapy for cancer EXCEPT that

(A) peripheral blood mononuclear cells are activated
(B) interleukin-2 is used for cell activation
(C) lymphokine-activated killer cells are generated
(D) the procedure is in clinical trials
(E) specific antitumor immunoglobulin is administered

141. Which of the following attributes is NOT a characteristic of transfer RNA?

(A) It can be covalently attached to an amino acid
(B) It contains many modified bases
(C) It contains an anticodon
(D) It binds messenger RNA during protein synthesis
(E) A given transfer RNA molecule can carry any of the 20 amino acids

142. A patient with AIDS would be expected to have all of these findings EXCEPT

(A) lymphopenia
(B) a great variety of immunoglobulin specificities
(C) high $CD4^+:CD8^+$ cell ratio
(D) decreased or absent delayed-type hypersensitivity in advanced cases
(E) decreased interleukin-2 and interferon-γ production

143. The HIV type 1 virus avoids the immune system by all of these mechanisms EXCEPT

(A) antigenic variation
(B) induction of neutralizing antibodies
(C) latent infection
(D) decreased cytotoxic T-cell activity
(E) destruction of lymph nodes

144. Which of the following country—most common cancers relationships is NOT correctly matched?

(A) China—nasopharyngeal carcinoma, esophageal cancer
(B) Russia—hepatocellular carcinoma, esophageal cancer
(C) Egypt—squamous cell carcinoma of the bladder
(D) Japan—T-cell lymphoma, stomach cancer
(E) Africa—Burkitt lymphoma, Kaposi sarcoma

145. In diabetes mellitus, nonenzymatic glycosylation is primarily operative in all of the following processes EXCEPT

(A) hyaline arteriolosclerosis
(B) formation of hemoglobin A$_{1c}$
(C) generation of oxidized low density lipoprotein (LDL)
(D) increased vessel permeability
(E) peripheral neuropathy

146. None of the following organisms stain well in the Gram staining procedure EXCEPT

(A) *Mycobacterium tuberculosis*
(B) *Mycoplasma pneumoniae*
(C) *Chlamydia trachomatis*
(D) *Treponema pallidum*
(E) *Actinomyces israelii*

DIRECTIONS:

Each set of matching questions in this section consists of a list of four to twenty-six lettered options (some of which may be in figures) followed by several numbered items. For each numbered item, select the ONE lettered option that is most closely associated with it. To avoid spending too much time on matching sets with a large number of options, it is generally advisable to begin each set by reading the list of options. Then for each item in the set, try to generate the correct answer and locate it in the option list, rather than evaluating each option individually. Each lettered option may be selected once, more than once, or not at all.

Questions 147-151

Select the drug of choice for each infection.

(A) Pentamidine
(B) Metronidazole
(C) Mefloquine
(D) Mebendazole
(E) Praziquantel

147. Treatment of drug-resistant malaria

148. *Pneumocystis carinii* pneumonia

149. Schistosomiasis

150. Vaginal trichomoniasis

151. *Trichuris trichiura* (whipworm) infection

Questions 152-153

For each set of characteristics, select the most likely organism.

(A) *Escherichia coli*
(B) *Enterobacter*
(C) *Klebsiella*
(D) *Proteus*
(E) *Pseudomonas*

152. A motile, gram-negative rod that ferments lactose with the production of acid and gas, forms indole from tryptophan, and is a common cause of septicemia in hospitalized patients

153. Has a large gelatinous capsule and is found in the respiratory and intestinal tracts of healthy humans

Questions 154-158

For each numbered example, choose the decision statement on doctrine with which it is most closely associated.

(A) Tarasoff decision
(B) Good Samaritan statute
(C) Doctrine of *parens patriae*
(D) *O'Connor* v. *Donaldson*
(E) *Rouse* v. *Cameron*

154. Patients who are judged to be mentally ill but are not dangerous to themselves or to others cannot be held against their will without treatment.

155. If a patient issues significant threats, the therapist must warn the intended victims of those threats.

156. The state can make decisions for persons who cannot take care of themselves or who may harm themselves (i.e., mentally ill persons or minors).

157. Patients who are hospitalized involuntarily have a right to treatment.

158. Limitation of liability for physicians who provide emergency medical care outside of their usual practice.

Questions 159-163

Select the correct term for each of the following descriptions of drug regulation and evaluation.

(A) Phase I clinical study
(B) Phase II clinical study
(C) Phase III clinical study
(D) Abbreviated New Drug Application (ANDA)
(E) Investigational New Drug (IND) Application
(F) New Drug Application (NDA)
(G) Orphan drug
(H) Generic drug
(I) Schedule I drug
(J) Schedule II drug
(K) Schedule IV drug

159. A drug for the treatment of patients with rare diseases

160. Contains the results of a bioequivalence study comparing an approved brand-name product with a generic formulation

161. A drug that has high abuse potential and no approved medical use in the United States

162. A study of the safety and pharmacokinetics of a new drug in normal human volunteers

163. Contains a summary of preclinical drug tests and protocols for studies in human subjects

Questions 164-165

For each set of findings, select the most likely causal organism.

(A) *Vibrio cholerae*
(B) *Vibrio parahaemolyticus*
(C) *Campylobacter jejuni*
(D) *Campylobacter fetus*
(E) *Helicobacter pylori*

164. A 45-year-old tourist returned from a trip to South America and abruptly began having cramps and diarrhea. The watery bowel movements came rapidly one after another and contained small bits of grayish-white stool. The man was sweaty and nauseated. Upon admission to the hospital, 2 liters of fluid were administered intravenously, which was supplemented by oral fluid. The patient was discharged 48 hours after admission. A gram-negative rod with the O1 antigen was isolated.

165. Histologic examination of a duodenal biopsy specimen from a 59-year-old executive reveals active inflammation within the epithelium and lamina propria. A silver stain shows the presence of comma-shaped organisms in the mucous layer.

Questions 166-170

Select the drug that is associated most frequently with the adverse effect.

(A) Erythromycin
(B) Moxalactam
(C) Ampicillin
(D) Gentamicin
(E) Tetracycline

166. Maculopapular rash during viral infections

167. Cholestatic jaundice

168. Discoloration of teeth

169. Permanent deafness

170. Platelet dysfunction and bleeding

Questions 171-175

Match each description with the appropriate heading.

(A) Pepsin
(B) Pinocytic absorption of proteins
(C) Enteropeptidase
(D) Carboxypeptidases
(E) Aminopeptidase
(F) Amino acid transport
(G) Chymotrypsin
(H) Trypsinogen
(I) Rennin

171. Defect associated with Hartnup disease

172. Initiation of zymogen activation

173. Involved in establishing food allergies

174. Has the most acidic pH optima

175. Of primary significance in an infant's digestion of milk

Questions 176-180

Select the pair of receptors that mediates each physiologic effect.

(A) α_1-Adrenergic—serotonergic $5HT_{1D}$
(B) β_2-Adrenergic—cholinergic muscarinic
(C) Serotonergic $5HT_4$—cholinergic muscarinic
(D) Histamine H_2—β_1-adrenergic
(E) α_1-Adrenergic—cholinergic nicotinic
(F) Histamine H_2—serotonergic $5HT_3$
(G) Histamine H_1—cholinergic muscarinic

176. Positive cardiac inotropic effect

177. Vasodilation in skeletal muscle

178. Bronchoconstriction

179. Vasoconstriction

180. Increased gastrointestinal motility

ANSWER KEY

1. D	31. B	61. A	91. C	121. B	151. D
2. C	32. B	62. A	92. D	122. B	152. A
3. B	33. B	63. C	93. A	123. C	153. C
4. B	34. E	64. A	94. D	124. A	154. D
5. D	35. C	65. B	95. B	125. E	155. A
6. C	36. B	66. B	96. D	126. C	156. C
7. A	37. B	67. E	97. E	127. E	157. E
8. B	38. D	68. A	98. B	128. B	158. B
9. D	39. C	69. B	99. C	129. E	159. G
10. D	40. D	70. E	100. B	130. C	160. D
11. E	41. B	71. D	101. B	131. E	161. I
12. B	42. C	72. D	102. E	132. B	162. A
13. E	43. D	73. E	103. D	133. A	163. E
14. E	44. B	74. C	104. A	134. B	164. A
15. D	45. E	75. D	105. D	135. E	165. E
16. A	46. B	76. D	106. C	136. D	166. C
17. D	47. E	77. B	107. B	137. B	167. A
18. C	48. D	78. C	108. A	138. A	168. E
19. E	49. D	79. D	109. C	139. C	169. D
20. E	50. E	80. B	110. A	140. E	170. B
21. B	51. B	81. D	111. C	141. E	171. F
22. E	52. C	82. A	112. B	142. C	172. C
23. C	53. E	83. A	113. B	143. B	173. B
24. D	54. C	84. C	114. C	144. B	174. A
25. E	55. C	85. C	115. D	145. E	175. I
26. D	56. E	86. D	116. E	146. E	176. D
27. A	57. D	87. E	117. C	147. C	177. B
28. C	58. E	88. A	118. A	148. A	178. G
29. E	59. D	89. D	119. B	149. E	179. A
30. E	60. B	90. D	120. B	150. B	180. C

ANSWERS AND EXPLANATIONS

1. The answer is D. *(Behavioral science)*
Over the past 10 years, 75% of adults have been hospitalized on at least one occasion. Hospitalized patients are more likely to be elderly women. Although the average hospital stay is approximately 6 days, the length of hospital stays is decreasing.

2. The answer is C. *(Microbiology)*
Gram-negative cell walls are composed of three components that lie outside the peptidoglycan layer: lipoprotein, outer membrane, and lipopolysaccharide (LPS). Lipoprotein cross-links the outer membrane and peptidoglycan layers. Its function is to stabilize the outer membrane.

The outer membrane is a bilayered structure, somewhat like the cytoplasmic membrane, where the phospholipids of the outer part are replaced by LPS molecules. The outer membrane excludes hydrophobic molecules and protects the gram-negative cells from materials such as bile salts. Protein molecules, called porins, permit the passive diffusion of low–molecular-weight compounds and ions.

Lipid A, phosphorylate glucosamine disaccharide units, makes up the LPS layer. When LPS is split into lipid A and polysaccharide, the toxicity is associated with the former. LPS, also called endotoxin, is released only when cells are lysed. Endotoxin is heat stable and can cause hemorrhagic tissue necrosis, disseminated intervascular coagulation, fever (via interleukin 1), and activation of complement via the alternative pathway.

Gram-positive cells do not contain endotoxin. The gram-positive cell wall consists of a thick layer of peptidoglycan. Techoic acid or lipotechoic acid residues are attached to gram-positive cell walls, which are antigenic and aid in the adherence of gram-positive organisms to tissue. The gram-positive bacterial cytoplasmic membrane also does not contain endotoxin.

3. The answer is B. *(Biochemistry)*
Creatine and creatine phosphate from muscle are spontaneously converted to creatinine, which is excreted in the urine. Measurement of creatinine production can be used to estimate muscle mass. Creatinine excretion in a patient with muscular dystrophy would be lower than normal, because muscular dystrophy leads to a loss of muscle. None of the other diseases mentioned has a major effect on muscle mass.

4. The answer is B. *(Microbiology)*
Candida albicans is an oval, budding yeast that produces pseudohyphae in culture, tissues, and exudates. It is a member of the normal human flora and an efficient opportunist. Candida produce a pseudomycelium by the formation of elongate buds, which fail to detach. Buds are developed that serve as spores at the nodules of pseudohyphae.

Coccidioides immitis produces spores as part of its aerial hyphae. The aerial hyphae contain alternating arthroconidia (arthrospores) and empty cells. When released into the air, the arthroconidia are highly infectious.

Ascospores consist of four to eight spores that form in a specialized cell called an ascus, following meiosis. This represents a sexual fusion process and occurs in the genera *Tricophyton* and *Microsporum*. *Rhizopus* species develop sporangioconidia (sporangiospores) and are opportunists.

Fungi are classified on the basis of their sexual reproduction. The sexual stages are usually difficult to induce in the laboratory and are rarely observed in clinical specimens. Most fungi reproduce by forming conidia through mitosis (asexual reproduction), during which the chromosome number remains the same.

5. The answer is D. *(Pathology)*
Determining the parentage of a child is facilitated by using human leukocyte antigen (HLA) typing of the parents and child along with ABO, Rh, and other blood group antigens. An individual inherits one HLA haplotype from each parent in codominant fashion (both haplotypes are able to express themselves), and when combined, this becomes the HLA genotype of the individual. There is at least a 25% chance that two offspring will have identical haplotypes, a 50% chance of at least one haplotype match, and a 25% chance of no haplotype match. Identical haplotype match is rarely achieved because of crossovers between the loci during fertilization and possibly other HLA loci that have not yet been characterized.

In the chart, child D has compatible HLA haplotypes with the mother and present husband (the brother of the previous husband), but the AB blood group does not match. Blood group O and AB parents cannot have an AB child.

	A	B
O	AO	BO
O	AO	BO

It is possible for two heterozygote D-antigen parents to have an Rh-negative child (dd).

	D	d
D	DD	Dd
d	Dd	dd

Regarding children a, b, c, and e, their HLA, ABO, and Rh findings are compatible with the present parents.

6. The answer is C. *(Microbiology)*

Compounds that have the property of concentrating at interfaces are called detergents or surface-acting agents. The interface between the lipid-containing membrane of a bacterial cell and the surrounding aqueous medium attracts these anionic (negative charge) and cationic (positive charge) detergents. Detergents act by disrupting the normal function of the cell membrane, leading to cell death.

Alcohols and phenols denature proteins, and oxidizing agents (e.g., hydrogen peroxide, hypochlorite) inactivate cells by affecting free sulfhydral groups. Dyes such as crystal violet (Gram stain reagent) attach to nucleic acids and interfere with normal function. Sulfa drugs are analogues of para-aminobenzoic acid, a component of the tetrahydrofolate coenzyme. The coenzyme will not be produced by the microorganism as long as the sulfa drug is present. Once it is removed, normal folate metabolism can occur.

7. The answer is A. *(Biochemistry)*

The catecholamines—dopamine, norepinephrine, and epinephrine—are synthesized from the amino acid tyrosine. The first step in the pathway, which is also the rate-limiting step, is the hydroxylation of tyrosine to form dopamine. Tyrosine is catalyzed by the enzyme tyrosine hydroxylase in a tetrahydrobiopterin-requiring reaction. Dopa is then converted to dopamine by the enzyme dopa decarboxylase. Dopamine is hydroxylated to form norepinephrine. Finally, donation of a methyl group from *S*-adenosylmethionine converts norepinephrine to epinephrine.

8. The answer is B. *(Microbiology)*

Coccidioides immitis, which causes coccidioidomycosis, is endemic in the arid regions of the southwestern United States. It exists in the central San Juaquin Valley in California and in Arizona and New Mexico. It is spread by dust and inhaled into the respiratory tract.

Aerial hyphae form alternating arthrospores (arthroconidia) and empty cells. Hyphae fragment easily and release the conidia. The arthroconidia are light, float in the air, and are highly infectious. When inhaled, the conidia develop into tissue spherules. Most infections are subclinical, and about 15% of individuals develop a symptom complex called valley fever (rash, rheumatism), which is self-limited. Fewer than 1% of infected persons develop the disseminated, often lethal, form.

Histoplasma capsulatum exists in the Ohio and Mississippi River valleys, whereas blastomycosis occurs mainly in the northern midwest United States and Canada. *Paracoccidioides brasiliensis* is in Central and South America. *Cryptococcus* infections are associated with bird droppings.

9. The answer is D. *(Microbiology)*

Oncogenic viruses can activate oncogenes by gene amplification, inactivation of suppressor genes, or inducing translocations. Some of these viruses activate proto-oncogenes (normally functioning oncogenes) in the host cell by inserting their genome above or below a proto-oncogene causing them to overexpress their gene product (gene amplification).

10. The answer is D. *(Biochemistry)*

Serotonin (5-hydroxytryptamine) is synthesized from the amino acid tryptophan. The first step in the pathway is the hydroxylation of tryptophan to produce 5-hydroxytryptophan, catalyzed by the enzyme tryptophan hydroxylase in a tetrahydrobiopterin-requiring reaction. Decarboxylation of 5-hydroxytryptophan yields serotonin.

11. The answer is E.   *(Pathology)*

DiGeorge syndrome (congenital thymic aplasia) is the most important of the primary T-cell deficiencies. This deficiency is caused by an interference of some sort in the development of the third and fourth pharyngeal pouches at approximately 12 weeks gestation. The parathyroid also is affected because it develops from these same pouches. Facial abnormalities may or may not be present, and congenital heart disease may include various types of abnormalities (e.g., truncus arteriosus). Tetany is the most common initial presentation.

In DiGeorge syndrome, symptoms are seen immediately after birth, unlike in the great majority of other primary immunodeficiencies. The lymphocyte count is usually low and T-lymphocyte responsiveness to antigens or mitogens is missing at birth. Immunoglobulin levels may or may not be normal. T-lymphocyte deficiencies are often associated with viral, fungal, and protozoal infections.

X-linked hypogammaglobulinemia is a B-cell deficiency that is characterized by a total lack of B lymphocytes and plasma cells.

Hereditary angioedema is a deficiency of the C1 esterase inhibitor, which controls the classic complement pathway. The disease is characterized by recurrent attacks of subcutaneous and mucosal swelling. There is no increase in infections.

Severe combined immunodeficiency disease encompasses a variety of disorders, all of which involve defective T-lymphocyte and B-lymphocyte immunity.

12. The answer is B.   *(Biochemistry)*

The correct sequence is:

- 4. Activation of adenylate cyclase
- 1. Increased protein kinase activity
- 3. Increased phosphorylase kinase
- 2. Increased phosphorylase A

Glycogenolysis occurs primarily in the fasting state when glucose is necessary for fuel. It normally begins 2 to 3 hours after eating, and stores are usually depleted by 30 hours. Glucagon only stimulates glycogenolysis in the liver, whereas epinephrine stimulates glycogenolysis in both the liver and muscle. Glucose derived from the liver is used primarily to maintain the blood glucose levels in the fasting state, whereas glucose released from muscle glycogen stores is only used by the muscle for energy. Glucagon in liver and epinephrine in muscle have a similar mode of action, as illustrated by the figure.

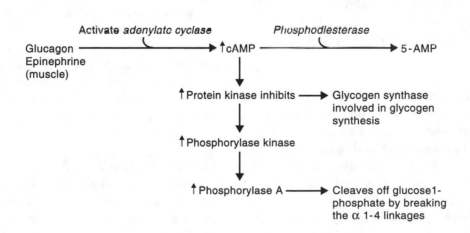

Note that both glucagon and epinephrine activate adenylate cyclase to produce cyclic adenosine monophosphate (cAMP). cAMP activates protein kinase, which inhibits glycogen synthetase and activates phosphorylase kinase. Phosphorylase kinase phosphorylates inactive phosphorylase B forming active phosphorylase A, which cleaves α1-4 bonds to release glucose 1-phosphate up to four glucose residues from a branching point. A 4:4 debrancher enzyme moves three of the four remaining glucose residues on the residual branch and attaches these to the main glycogen core with an α1-4 linkage, thus making them amenable to further breakdown by phosphorylase A. The remaining single glucose molecule with an α1-6 linkage attached to the main glycogen core is acted upon by an α1-6 debranching enzyme, which releases free glucose. Normally, there is approximately an 8:1 glucose 1-phosphate:free glucose ratio.

13. The answer is E. *(Pathology)*
The Wiskott-Aldrich syndrome is a sex-linked recessive disease with a characteristic triad of thrombocytopenia, eczema, and recurrent infections.

Additional clinical findings include bloody diarrhea, cerebral hemorrhage, septicemia, severe infections by encapsulated bacteria, and an increased propensity for malignant lymphomas.

Laboratory findings include low lymphocyte counts as the T cells decrease with subsequent impairment in cellular immunity, low immunoglobulin M levels, and increased levels of immunoglobulin G, immunoglobulin A, and particularly immunoglobulin E.

14. The answer is E. *(Biochemistry)*
The catecholamines—dopamine, norepinephrine, and epinephrine—are inactivated in two steps catalyzed by monoamine oxidase (MAO) and catechol *O*-methyltransferase (COMT). MAO catalyzes an oxidative deamination reaction, whereas COMT catalyzes an *O*-methylation reaction. The two steps can occur in either order. The end-product of epinephrine and norepinephrine degradation is vanillylmandelic acid (VMA). The end-product of dopamine degradation is homovanillic acid. MAO inhibitors block degradation of these catecholamine neurotransmitters.

15. The answer is D. *(Pathology)*
According to the Fisher-Race nomenclature, presence of the D antigen classifies the individual as being Rh positive. The D antigen is the most immunogenic antigen in the Rh system. More than 90% of cases of hemolytic disease of the newborn (erythroblastosis fetalis) are due to the D antigen. The small d represents the lack of a D antigen.

The disease may develop if the mother is Rh negative and the infant is Rh positive. In response to Rh-positive fetal erythrocytes, which may enter maternal circulation, the mother produces Rh antibodies of the immunoglobulin G (IgG) class. In subsequent pregnancies where the fetus is D-antigen positive, the antibody crosses the placenta, binds to the fetal erythrocytes, and this complex is removed by macrophages through their Fc receptors for IgG (extravascular hemolytic anemia). The infant develops anemia, jaundice reticulocytosis, and erythroblastosis.

According to the Fisher-Race terminology, D, C, c, E, and e are the most commonly expressed Rh-system antigens.

CDe			Cde	
CDE	Rh positive		CdE	Rh negative
cDe			cde	
cDE			cdE	

Hemolytic disease of the newborn also may occur when there is an ABO blood group incompatibility between the mother and fetus. Maternal IgG against the A and B antigens may cross the placenta. Most cases are seen when the mother is blood group O and the fetus is group A. However, serious problems are rare because soluble A or B substances in the fetus can neutralize the maternal antibodies before these antibodies cause damage to the erythrocytes.

16. The answer is A. *(Biochemistry)*
Once an amino acid has been charged onto a tRNA molecule, the specificity for incorporation of that amino acid lies entirely with the anticodon of the tRNA. The amino acid is not involved in codon selection. In this example the anticodon of the tRNA would still recognize and bind to cysteine codons, although it is carrying a different amino acid. Radioactive amino

acid would be incorporated into newly synthesized protein molecules only in response to cysteine codons.

17. The answer is D. *(Pathology)*
Type III hypersensitivity is an immune-complex disease involving the deposition of immune complexes in a target tissue, complement activation, production of chemotactic factors (C5a), and subsequent destruction of tissue by neutrophils and macrophages. Immune-complex disease may be localized (e.g., Arthus reaction) or systemic (e.g., serum sickness). Factors that determine if immune-complex formation will produce disease include the size and solubility of the complexes and whether or not macrophages are able to remove the complexes from the circulation.

Only complement-fixing antibodies (immunoglobulins M and G) are involved in immune-complex disease. The first exposure to an antigen results in the formation of antibodies. The second exposure results in antigen/antibody complexes, which attract complement and deposit in tissue. Complement is activated and chemotactic agents attract neutrophils and macrophages to the tissue causing their destruction.

The Arthus reaction is localized immune-complex disease. Localized vasculitis with thrombosis and ischemic damage to tissue are key in the Arthus reaction. Serum sickness is the prototype of systemic type III hypersensitivity. Clinical manifestations include urticaria, fever, edema, generalized lymphadenopathy, arthritis, glomerulonephritis, and vasculitis.

18. The answer is C. *(Biochemistry)*
Blocked circulation causes oxygen deprivation to the muscle cells in the limb. The cells survive for a while through anaerobic glycolysis, which produces lactic acid as a by-product. Because of the inefficient production of adenosine triphosphate (ATP) [net gain of only 2 ATPs per glucose used], the ATP-dependent Na^+/ K^+ pump is not fully operative, causing K^+ to leak from the cell and Na^+ to enter. If the beam is raised without initial preparation, the accumulated lactate and K^+ is added to the systemic circulation causing a generalized lactic acidosis and hyperkalemia. Pretreatment with bicarbonate neutralizes the acidosis, while insulin in the presence of glucose will cause a rapid influx of K^+ into the cells and Na^+ out of the cells. Adding more lactate or K^+ would insult the system further.

19. The answer is E. *(Pathology)*
Initially, farmer's lung is a type III hypersensitivity, but later, it invokes type IV hypersensitivity to form granulomas. The other conditions listed are all type II hypersensitivity reactions.

Farmer's lung is a classic example of an Arthus reaction. The farmer is exposed to thermophilic actinomycetes in the air and then develops antibodies against the antigen. Re-exposure to the antigen produces local immune-complex formation of the antigen, and the antibodies in the interstitium of the lung produce hypersensitivity interstitial pneumonitis, a type of restrictive lung disease. Later in the disease, granulomas develop in the interstitium, which illustrates type IV hypersensitivity.

Type II hypersensitivity reactions refer to cytotoxic reactions involving immunoglobulins G or M antibodies, which are deposited on target tissue and cause damage to the tissue or lysis of cells.

20. The answer is E. *(Biochemistry)*
Histidine can serve as a buffer at physiologic pH of between 5 and 7 because its side chain has a pK of about 6.0. The side chain of aspartic acid contains a carboxyl group, which would give it buffering properties at low pH. The side chain of lysine contains an amino group, which would give it buffering properties at high pH. Glycine and serine do not contain dissociable side chains. All the amino acids serve as buffers at high pH owing to their amino groups and at low pH owing to their carboxyl groups.

21. The answer is B. *(Microbiology)*
Bacillus Calmette-Guérin (BCG), a live attenuated strain of *Mycobacterium bovis*, is used in some countries for immunization against tuberculosis. The vaccine induces conversion to a positive purified protein derivative (PPD) skin test. The vaccine's degree of efficacy in preventing tuberculosis remains somewhat controversial. BCG is not used routinely in the United States, but it is available for high-risk groups or PPD-negative contacts of active cases.

The diptheria-tetanus-pertussis (DTP) vaccine consists of *Corynebacterium diphtheriae* toxoid, *Clostridium tetani* toxoid, and killed *Bordetella pertussis* (whooping cough). After an initial course of 4 to 5 doses, booster injections are needed every 10 years in order to maintain protection. Occasionally, seizures, encephalitis, and other neurological problems have been associated with the pertussis portion of the DTP vaccine. Now, an acellular vaccine, containing at least two antigens of *B. pertussis* but not the whole organism, is available.

The *Haemophilus influenzae* type b (HIB) vaccine is administered to young children (starting at 2 months old) for prevention of meningitis due to *H. influenzae.* HIB consists of type b capsular polysaccharide. This vaccine has been only modestly effective because children under the age of 2 years generally do not produce large amounts of antibodies against polysaccharide antigens. There are three conjugated HIB vaccines available, but the polysaccharide–protein conjugate is the most immunogenic.

22. The answer is E.   *(Biochemistry)*
A shift to the left from curve 1 to curve 2 indicates an increase in the affinity of hemoglobin for oxygen.

An increase in the concentration of hydrogen ions (lower pH), carbon dioxide, and 2,3-bisphosphoglycerate all stabilize the deoxyhemoglobin and would shift the curve to the right. A higher pH (lower hydrogen ion concentration) would tend to stabilize oxyhemoglobin, increase the affinity of hemoglobin for oxygen, and shift the curve to the left.

23. The answer is C.   *(Pharmacology)*
Formulation A is rapidly absorbed because T_{max} is 1 hour and C_{max} and AUC are high. Formulation B is absorbed as rapidly as A, but its absorption is not as complete because C_{max} and AUC are low.

Formulation C is absorbed as completely as A but at a lower rate because its T_{max} is greater.

24. The answer is D.   *(Biochemistry)*
Galactosemia is an autosomal-recessive disease usually characterized by a total lack of galactose 1-phosphate uridyltransferase (GALT). A schematic of galactose metabolism is as follows:

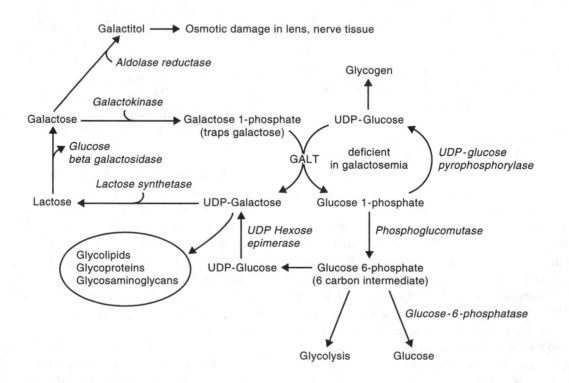

Note that a deficiency of GALT results in the build-up of galactose 1-phosphate behind the block. Galactose 1-phosphate is toxic and damages tissue resulting in jaundice at birth caused by a fatty liver eventually leading to scarring and liver failure, damage to the central nervous system leading to mental retardation, and damage to the kidneys resulting in aminoaciduria.

There is also an accumulation of galactose, which can be converted into the polyol (sugar alcohol), galactitol. Galactitol is osmotically active and produces osmotic damage in the lens of the eye (cataracts), nerves, and other tissues.

Because galactose is a reducing substance, when it is spilled into the urine, it can be detected with a Clinitest tablet, which has chemicals that combine with the galactose to produce a color reaction. This underscores the use of Clinitest tablets in screening the urine of newborns for inborn errors of metabolism, which in this case is galactosemia.

Most complications can be prevented by removing lactose (source of galactose) from the diet for the first two years. Women with galactosemia who have children can still make lactose in their milk by the uridine diphosphate (UDP) hexose epimerase reaction. This reaction converts UDP-glucose into UDP-galactose, which is then converted by lactose synthetase into lactose.

25. The answer is E.   (Microbiology)
Trench fever (caused by *Rochalimaea quintana*) and epidemic typhus (caused by *Rickettsia prowazekii*) are transmitted to humans by the bite of the body louse, *Pediculus*.

Other rickettsial diseases are also transmitted by insect vectors. Rocky mountain spotted fever (caused by *Rickettsia rickettsii*) is spread by tick bites, and endemic typhus (caused by *Rickettsia typhi*) is transmitted by lice. Rickettsial pox (*Rickettsia akari*) and scrub typhus (caused by *Rickettsia tsutsugamushi*) are transmitted by mites.

The only rickettsia not spread by an arthropod vector is Q fever (caused by *Coxiella burnetii*). It is transmitted to humans by inhalation of aerosols.

26. The answer is D.   (Biochemistry)
The side chain of proline forms the ring with an α-amino group. Thus, proline contain an imino group.

All the other common amino acids contain an α-amino group in addition to an α-carboxyl group and a distinctive side chain.

27. The answer is A.   (Behavioral science)
The dog in the example is best described as the unconditioned stimulus because the dog automatically or naturally produces the unconditioned response (sneezing).

28–29. The answers are: 28-C, 29-E.   (Biochemistry)
All proteins, except the 13 mitochondrial ones that are coded for by mitochondrial DNA, are coded by nuclear DNA and are synthesized on cytoplasmic ribosomes. These ribosomes may either be "free" or complexed with the endoplasmic reticulum (ER). The complex between endoplasmic reticulum and a multitude of ribosomes is known as the rough endoplasmic reticulum (RER), because of its appearance on electron microscopy.

Free and ER-bound ribosomes are identical in structure; both are reconstituted from the same pool of small and large ribosomal subunits when translation is initiated. However, whether they remain free or become part of the RER is important because this is the initial determinant of the final location of the protein product. Proteins synthesized on the RER have a different destiny than do proteins synthesized on free ribosomes. Whether a given ribosome functions on the ER or remains free is determined by the presence or absence of a unique "leader sequence." (This is different from the amphipathic leader referred to in the question.) Ribosomes that form a translation initiation complex with an mRNA coding for this leader sequence become ER bound; those that do not remain free.

This leader sequence on the nascent protein directs the ribosome to the RER via a two-step mechanism. The leader sequence is recognized by a large protein complex called the signal recognition particle (SRP). The binding of the nascent peptide–ribosomal complex with the SRP causes translational arrest. Translation restarts when the SRP–ribosomal complex interacts with a protein in the ER membrane called the docking protein. Now, however, the newly synthesized protein is pushed through the membrane of the ER as it is synthesized. Proteins synthesized on the ER membrane are destined to become part of the ER itself or are modified in the lumen of the ER and shipped to the Golgi apparatus. Once in the Golgi apparatus, the proteins undergo further modifications that determine if they become part of the Golgi apparatus or if they are shipped to the lysosomes, become part of the plasma membrane or are shipped externally to be circulated in the blood system.

Ribosomes that form translational complexes with mRNAs lacking the code for this leader sequence that attracts the SRP do not become part of the RER. Such "free" (they are in actuality associated with other elements of the cytoskeleton) ribosomes synthesize proteins destined for the cytosol, mitochondria, nucleus, and peroxisomes. All elucidated mechanisms indicate that there are specific sequences added to either end or incorporated within the amino acid sequence that determines the final destination of these proteins. An amphipathic α-helix on the N-terminus of some of these proteins serves as the signal that directs them into the mitochondria, where they will bind to a signal receptor on the outer mitochondrial membrane.

The whole complex then moves laterally across the outer membrane until it reaches a site at which the outer and inner mitochondrial membranes are joined. The complex crosses both membranes at this site. The receptor and signal peptide are removed; the protein is directed to its functional site and unfolded, ready to go to work.

Some of the more salient features concerning regulations of protein trafficking are summarized in the table.

Type of Ribosome	Destination of the Protein Product	Signalling Mechanism
ER Bound	ER	Alternating start and stop signals that "sew" the protein into the membrane as it is translated
ER Bound	Cell surface (as part of the membrane or secreted)	None; this is the "default fate"
ER Bound	Regulated secretion (e.g., a hormone regulated by a trophic hormone)	Concentration into clathrin-coated vesicles that release their contents when signalled to do so
ER Bound	Lysosomes	For at least the acid hydrolases, mannose 6-phosphate; in I cell disease this mannose 6-phosphate cannot be formed, and the acid hydrolases follow the default pathway and are secreted
"Free"	Cytosol	Default
"Free"	Peroxisomes	Unknown
"Free"	Nucleus	Receptors on the nuclear pores that recognize a divergent number of signalling sequences
"Free"	Mitochondria	Amphipathic α-helix added to the N-terminus

ER = endoplasmic reticulum.

Enzymes are generally synthesized at levels that are at least an order of magnitude higher than that required for normal function. Therefore, if only half the normal amount of an enzyme were synthesized that would still meet the cell's requirements. This is what happens in most recessive diseases. One genetic allele is aberrant and its enzyme product is defective, often nonfunctional. However, since the other allele codes for a normal product, sufficient enzyme remains and the genetic error has no clinical consequence. Of course, if the proband received two defective alleles, the result would most likely be disastrous.

30. The answer is E.   *(Pharmacology)*
Tetracycline is usually the drug of choice for rickettsial infections; chloramphenicol is an alternative drug. Only chloramphenicol causes dose-dependent anemia (and idiosyncratic aplastic anemia), and only chloramphenicol is metabolized by glucuronide conjugation. Only tetracycline forms a complex with cations and may deposit in growing teeth, bones, and other tissues (e.g., neoplastic tissues).

31. The answer is B.   *(Pathology)*
This pedigree exhibits a mitochondrial DNA (mtDNA) genetic defect. A mutation in a mitochondrial gene is unique to females because ova contain more mitochondria than sperm, which lose the mitochondria in their tail after the sperm penetrates the egg in fertilization. The mtDNA codes for enzymes in oxidative phosphorylation. The affected female passes the trait on to all of her children, both males and females, but males do not transmit the disease. Note that the female proband transmitted the disease to her daughter and her son. The daughter, in turn, transmitted it to her children. However, her son did not transmit the disease to any of his four children. The progressive loss of central vision in this case is called Leber hereditary optic neuropathy.

Multifactorial inheritance refers to the combination of genetic mutations plus the effect of the environment and would not be expected to produce this kind of pattern. Autosomal dominant inheritance is not likely because the affected son did not transmit the disease to any of his children (normally, a 50% chance). In sex-linked dominant inheritance, the affected female transmits the disease to 50% of her sons and daughters, whereas an affected male transmits the disease to 100% of his daughters. An autosomal recessive inheritance requires two parents with the abnormal gene in order for them to have an affected child.

32. The answer is B.   *(Behavioral science)*
The most effective way to teach a dog to jump through a flaming hoop is by operant conditioning. In operant conditioning, a behavior that is not the organism's natural response can be learned through reward or punishment. In classical conditioning, only a natural or reflex behavior can be elicited in response to a stimulus. Extinction in operant conditioning is the disappearance of a learned behavior when the reward is withheld. Stimulus generalization is seen in classical conditioning when a new stimulus that resembles a conditioned stimulus results in the conditioned or learned response.

33. The answer is B.   *(Biochemistry)*
Compounds such as creatine phosphate, phosphoenolpyruvate, and 1,3-bisphosphoglycerate contain phosphate with a standard free energy of hydrolysis higher than that for adenosine triphosphate (ATP). Such compounds can donate their phosphate to adenosine diphosphate (ADP) to form ATP in an energetically favorable reaction. Creatine phosphate donates its phosphate group to ADP to maintain adequate ATP levels for a short period of time during muscle contraction. Transfer of phosphates to ADP by low-energy compounds such as adenosine monophosphate (AMP), glucose 6-phosphate, glycerol 3-phosphate, and phosphatidic acid is energetically unfavorable.

34. The answer is E.   *(Microbiology)*
Bacillus anthracis causes anthrax, an accidental infection in humans related to contact with spore-contaminated animal products. An important reason for pathogenicity of this organism is the presence of a well-defined capsule, which resists phagocytosis. The capsule is composed of D-glutamate, which is unusual because most bacterial capsules are made of polysaccharide residues.

Capsules do not take up a stain color in the Gram stain procedure. A negative staining technique involving India ink can be used to visualize the capsules.

35. The answer is C. *(Biochemistry)*
The patient suffers from hereditary spherocytosis, a dominant trait most commonly observed in whites. In this disorder the red cells are spherical and fragile. The molecular basis of this disease is the presence of an aberrant spectrin molecule in the red cell membrane.

Spectrin is an important component of the skeletal structure of cell membranes, found in different isoforms in various cell types. In red cells, the membranous support structure is particularly flexible, and the skeleton is composed of erythrocyte spectrin coupled to four other proteins: ankyrin, actin, protein 4.1, and "band 3." The flexibility of this structure allows the membrane to accept its normal biconcave shape and to assume different forms as it squeezes through small sinusoids and capillaries.

Patients with spherocytosis have spectrins that are not malleable and force the cell into a spherical shape. (The situation is analogous to a patient with ankylosing spondylitis, in which the spine has lost its flexibility and the patient is forced to assume a 45-degree stance rather than an upright one.) The rigid spherical cells tend to be destroyed in the spleen. Splenectomy is used to treat this condition.

Hereditary elliptocytosis is a similar disease in which the red cells are elliptical in shape. The molecular difference between the two diseases is the site on the spectrin that is affected: the one mutation causing a rigid sphere, the other a rigid ellipse. Both elliptocytosis and spherocytosis are autosomal dominant diseases. The latter is a reflection of the fact that spectrin is a structural protein.

The other potential answers are all associated with anemias. Red cell pyruvate kinase deficiency hemolytic anemia is the most common autosomal recessive disease found in whites. Glucose 6-phosphate dehydrogenase deficiency hemolytic anemia is a sex-linked disease found with high frequency among Africans and other peoples in the malaria zones around the Mediterranean. A problem arises when the red cell is exposed to an oxidizing agent and the activity of the enzyme is insufficient to protect the cell from the oxidative effects. Intrinsic factor is a carbohydrate-rich protein synthesized in the gastric mucosa that is required for absorption of vitamin B_{12}. The absence of intrinsic factor causes pernicious anemia.

36. The answer is B. *(Behavioral science)*
Biofeedback is a behavioral treatment technique based on operant conditioning. In biofeedback, an individual learns to gain control over physiologic parameters. Biofeedback is used to treat hypertension, asthma, peptic ulcer disease, Raynaud disease, temporomandibular joint (TMJ) pain, and migraine and tension headaches.

37. The answer is B. *(Biochemistry)*
The patient is suffering from Wernicke-Korsakoff syndrome, an acute deficiency of thiamine (vitamin B_1). This syndrome is characterized by confusion, ataxia, and nystagmus. The body requires thiamine for three reactions in carbohydrate metabolism: oxidative decarboxylation of pyruvate to form acetyl CoA, oxidative decarboxylation of α-ketoglutarate to form succinyl CoA, and transketolase of the pentose phosphate pathway. The increases in serum pyruvate and lactate acidosis result from failed pyruvate dehydrogenase activity due to a lack of thiamine, a required cofactor. Because pyruvate cannot be converted to acetyl CoA, it is converted into lactate, which induces the metabolic acidosis. The increase in cytoplasmic NADH levels associated with ethanol metabolism will enhance the conversion of pyruvate to lactate. After an intravenous thiamine injection, the symptoms of Wernicke-Korsakoff syndrome often diminish within hours.

38-39. The answers are: 38-D, 39-C. *(Behavioral science)*
In this example, the dream about the cartoon character is a manifest dream. The manifest dream involves the actual content of the dream including events that happen during the preceding day (day residue). The content of a latent dream involves the unconscious thoughts and desires represented in the dream. Dream work is the means by which latent dream content is changed into the manifest dream. The dream censor monitors the dream so that disturbing material is transformed into nondisturbing material so that the dreamer is not awakened.

The injection that the boy received is the day residue, an event from the previous day that is incorporated into a dream.

40. The answer is D. *(Biochemistry)*
Initiation of transcription of a specific mRNA by a specific initiation event starts a chain of reactions that culminate in expression of that gene as its particular protein gene product. If either the mRNA product of transcription or the protein of translation has a relatively long half-life, the effects of the initial initiating event will be long lived. That is, the cell would have been set on a course of action that could not be altered for a long time. This is generally the case for "housekeeping" proteins, such as β-globin, which you would expect the cell (or organisms) to want to keep around for a long time. Regulatory proteins, such as C-fos, however, often need to be fine tuned. They start or stop the cell on a course of action that may not need to be continued. To permit such fine regulation, these protein products and their mRNAs have relatively short half-lives.

The half-lives say nothing about the amount made per mRNA molecule. Since the half-life of C-fos mRNA is less, each molecule will have less not more time to synthesize more protein molecules.

41. The answer is B. *(Microbiology)*
Active immunity (toxoid immunization) is the ideal method to produce a long-term population protection against tetanus. A toxoid is produced by treating the toxin chemically so that pathogenicity is destroyed, while antigenicity is retained. The toxoid is injected and produces crossreading antibodies that neutralize unaltered toxin. The tetanus toxin (tetanospasmin) is an exotoxin produced by vegetative cells at the wound site. The activity of the toxin is in the central nervous system.

Antitoxin and γ-globulin represent short-lived, passive immunization rationales. In a patient with tetanus, antibiotics are administered to destroy the toxin-producing bacteria. Passive immunity (immune globulin) and antibiotics would be appropriate only for management of the acute disease.

42. The answer is C. *(Biochemistry)*
In prokaryotes, translation starts before transcription stops. The mRNA is used as transcribed without further modification. This is not true in eukaryotic cells. The primary transcript of RNA polymerase II, called heterogenous nuclear RNA (hnRNA), is extensively modified after transcription. There are four major steps in this modification: 5′ capping, polyadenylation of the 3′-end, removal of introns, and methylation of specific adenyl groups.

The removal of introns is particularly complex. Introns are sequences in the primary mRNA transcript that must be removed. Therefore, two cuts have to be made, one at the beginning and one at the end of the intron sequence. Then, the two ends of the remaining mRNA ("exons") have to be precisely spliced. If one extra base pair is removed or retained, the remainder of the message, from that point on, will have been altered. Whereas a few mammalian mRNAs have no introns, others, such as collagen, have 50 or more.

To obtain the precision required, the now capped and tailed hnRNA molecule forms a complex with other riboproteins. The total complex is called a splicosome. Included in this splicosome are very abundant small nuclear RNA particles, generally called snRNAs (an older name used less often is U1 RNA).

Patients with systemic lupus erythematosus have antibodies against their own snRNAs. It follows that it is very likely that these patients have problems with intron excision.

43. The answer is D. *(Behavioral science)*
In order to estimate the expected body weight of a one-year-old child, multiply his birth weight by 3.0.

44. The answer is B. *(Pharmacology)*
Certain cephalosporins, including cefoperazone in addition to metronidazole and the hypoglycemic sulfonylureas, may cause disulfiram-like effects (e.g., nausea and vomiting) when administered with ethanol. Cefoperazone is active against aerobic bacteria, whereas metronidazole is active against anaerobes and certain parasitic protozoa, such as *Giardia lamblia* and *Entamoeba histolytica*. Only metronidazole may darken the urine, and only cefoperazone inhibits bacterial cell wall synthesis by blocking transpeptidation of peptidoglycan chains.

45. The answer is E. *(Behavioral science)*
A normal baby who usually smiles at everyone and begins to cry when strangers pick her up is probably

seven months old. This characteristic behavior of normal infants is called stranger anxiety and signals the infant's specific attachment to the mother or primary care giver. Stranger anxiety demonstrates that the child has the ability to identify familiar people.

46. The answer is B. *(Microbiology)*
Under the described conditions, females who use non-barrier contraceptives but have no disease or risk history may be excluded from *Chlamydia* testing.

All methods of *Chlamydia* testing are time and cost intensive. The diagnostic test for *Chlamydia* infections used to be growth of the organism on McCoy cell culture. Now, the preferred methods are fluorescent antibody and enzyme-linked immunosorbent assay (ELISA) tests. In the underfunded clinic, decisions on test limitations are expected. Therefore, the presenting patient condition and history are the most significant factors in making a decision about which patients are tested.

Men with nongonococcal urethritis, women with cervicitis, and patients with a history of sexually transmitted diseases represent high risk populations. Neonates presenting with conjunctivitis may have been infected during passage through the birth canal.

47. The answer is E. *(Behavioral science)*
Children $2\frac{1}{2}$ to 6 years old (preschoolers) are often overly concerned about illness and injury (the "Band-Aid" phase). In a child of this age, such behavior is normal and is not a sign of depression, passive-aggressive behavior, obsessive-compulsive disorder, or an adjustment disorder.

48. The answer is D. *(Microbiology)*
Adenoviruses cause a variety of respiratory tract diseases, including hemorrhagic cystitis, pharyngitis, conjunctivitis (pink eye), and pneumonia.

There are 41 known types of adenoviruses. They can be spread by aerosol droplet, orally, and by direct inoculation. Types 11 and 21 cause hemorrhagic cystitis.

Parvoviruses can cause aplastic crises in sickle cell anemia patients, erythema infectiosum, spontaneous abortions, and arthritis. Parainfluenza viruses produce upper respiratory infections in young children (e.g., croup). Echoviruses cause a variety of diseases (e.g.,

aseptic meningitis, upper respiratory tract infection, infantile diarrhea, and hemorrhagic conjunctivitis). The varicella-zoster virus (chickenpox shingles) causes vascular lesions on the skin that occur at different stages of development. This virus is rarely associated with pneumonia or encephalitis.

49. The answer is D. *(Pharmacology)*
Isoniazid forms a chemical complex with pyridoxal that leads to pyridoxal deficiency and peripheral neuritis. This condition can be prevented and treated by pyridoxine (vitamin B_6) supplementation.

None of the other antitubercular drugs is associated with this adverse effect. Ethambutol may produce optic neuritis with blurred vision and loss of red-green color discrimination. Both isoniazid and rifampin are associated with hepatotoxicity and jaundice.

50. The answer is E. *(Microbiology)*
Rubella (German measles) is a milder, shorter disease than rubeola (measles). Symptoms for German measles include a prodromal fever and malaise, followed by a maculopapular rash. This rash, which typically lasts for three days, starts on the face and progresses downward to the extremities. In adults, especially women, German measles often causes polyarthritis due to immune complexes even before the rash begins.

Varicella (chicken pox) lesions are vesicular in nature. Erythema infectiosum (fifth disease), caused by parvoviruses, is most common in children. Its rash has a typical "slapped cheek" appearance. In the occasional adult case, the hand and knee joints are frequently affected.

Roseola (infantum) is caused by human herpesvirus 6. This disease is common in infants and is characterized by a high fever, which subsides and is followed by a transient rash.

51. The answer is B. *(Biochemistry)*
Mental retardation and cataracts are byproducts of galactosemia, an autosomal recessive disease characterized by the inability to convert galactose (a product of lactose) to glucose. Galactosemia may be due to a deficiency of either galactokinase or galactose 1-phosphate uridylyltransferase. Neither deficiency is benign, unlike fructokinase, which is benign. However,

a nonfunctional galactose 1-phosphate uridylyltransferase causes more severe symptoms than does a deficiency of galactokinase. The molecular basis for the symptomatology associated with the circulation of free galactose lies in the sorbitol pathway. Normally, this pathway, which is active during early development, converts glucose to sorbitol by aldose reductase and then converts sorbitol to fructose by sorbitol dehydrogenase. In adult males, this pathway is most active in the seminal vesicle where fructose is used as the primary fuel for sperm. There is residual activity in other tissues, including the lens. Galactose is converted to galactitol by the aldose reductase, but the sorbitol dehydrogenase does not use galactitol as a substrate. The galactitol, an osmotically active substance, accumulates in the lens and increases movement of water into the lens. This water movement causes proteins to precipitate, resulting in cataracts. Although literature concerning possible mental retardation associated with galactokinase deficiency is contradictory, mental retardation associated with untreated galactose 1-phosphate uridylyltransferase deficiency is inevitable.

When galactose 1-phosphate uridylyltransferase is deficient there is also an accumulation of galactose 1-phosphate in the liver. Unless galactose is removed from the diet the accumulation of hepatic galactose 1-phosphate will lead to death.

An effect analogous to that induced by the accumulation of galactitol is thought to induce the peripheral neuropathy, cataracts, and retinopathy associated with diabetes. In this disease, high glucose levels activate the aldose reductase abnormally and inhibit the sorbitol dehydrogenase by glycosylation. Consequently, sorbitol accumulates and damages the Schwann cells responsible for myelin production, which results in a peripheral neuropathy. In addition, osmotic damage to pericytes in the retinal vessels leads to microaneurysm causing retinopathy.

52. The answer is C. *(Microbiology)*
Acyclovir is a nucleoside analogue with a 3-carbon fragment in place of the normal ribose sugar. It is incorporated preferentially into the infected cells of herpes simplex virus types 1 or 2 and varicella-zoster virus. The virus-coded thymidine kinase (TK) phosphorylates acyclovir more efficiently than the cellular TK. The acyclovir monophosphate is phosphorylated to the triphosphate form and incorporated into the growing herpes virus DNA chain by the virus-coded DNA polymerase. Chain elongation stops and virus growth is terminated.

Azidothymidine (AZT) is a nucleoside analogue that causes chain termination during RNA-dependent DNA synthesis. It has an azide ($-N=N-N-$) group in place of the hydroxyl group on the ribose and is especially efficient in inhibiting DNA synthesis in HIV-infected cells. AZT is a virostatic compound, and, once removed, HIV growth can continue.

53. The answer is E. *(Pharmacology)*
Fluoroquinolones (e.g., ofloxacin, norfloxacin, and ciprofloxacin) are active against a wide range of gram-positive and gram-negative bacteria, including *Pseudomonas* and *Neisseria*. They are useful in treating several infections including genitourinary infections (e.g., sexually transmitted diseases) and bronchitis.

Amoxicillin, nitrofurantoin, and trimethoprim with sulfamethoxazole are useful in treating urinary tract infections caused by *Escherichia coli* and other organisms but not *Pseudomonas*. Tetracyclines, such as doxycycline, are no longer considered the drugs of choice for urinary tract infections.

54. The answer is C. *(Microbiology)*
Rubella, measles, mumps, and polioviruses have live, attenuated viral vaccines. Such vaccines are generally preferred because they lack virulence but allow the virus to complete a normal growth cycle in the human host. A more complete immune response, utilizing both cell-mediated immunity and humoral immunity (antibodies), is activated. Such immunization is long lasting, often imparting life-long protection.

Hepatitis B vaccine consists of surface antigen (HB_sAg), usually derived from yeast containing the HB_sAg gene (recombinant DNA). Influenza and rabies vaccines contain killed viruses. These viruses are grown to high titers, purified, and inactivated by chemical treatment. These vaccines produce an immunity that is less complete and less enduring than the live, attenuated varieties.

55. The answer is C. *(Behavioral science)*
Problems with sleep are common in normal bereavement. Threats of suicide, feelings of worthlessness, grief lasting 4 years after the death, and feelings of

hopelessness are signs of depression, not a normal grief reaction.

56. The answer is E.   *(Microbiology)*
Paramyxoviruses have a negative-sense [opposite base sequence of positive-sense RNA or messenger RNA (mRNA)], linear, single-stranded RNA molecule as the genome. Therefore, in order for respiratory syncytial virus, measles, mumps, and parainfluenza viruses to grow within a host cell, the virus must contain a single-stranded RNA-dependent RNA polymerase or transcriptase. When the virus is uncoated, the growth cycle can begin only when virus-specific mRNA is produced.

For comparison, other viruses also contain polymerases. Retroviruses contain single-stranded RNA-dependent DNA polymerase, and hepatitis B virus contains a DNA-dependent DNA polymerase. Rotaviruses (reoviruses) contain a double-stranded RNA-dependent RNA polymerase.

57. The answer is D.   *(Biochemistry)*
The researcher must use a probe that specifically detects the HPRT protein. A labelled antibody directed against hypoxanthine phosphoribosyltransferase (HPRT) would be the logical choice. Growth media containing antibiotics such as ampicillin or tetracycline are sometimes used to identify bacterial colonies carrying recombinant plasmids, but they do not specify any individual gene. Radioactive messenger RNA (mRNA) could be used as a probe to identify clones carrying the HPRT gene, but this method would not detect the expression of a protein product from that gene. A probe complementary to HPRT introns would not be useful for screening a complementary DNA (cDNA) library because the cDNA produced from mRNA would contain no introns.

58. The answer is E.   *(Behavioral science)*
This patient refuses to believe that he is ill and is using denial to deal with the difficult news of this illness.

59. The answer is D.   *(Pharmacology)*
Serotonin (5-HT) receptors are found primarily in nervous systems and smooth muscle. Buspirone acts as a partial agonist at the 5-HT_{1A} receptors, which are involved in central nervous system (CNS) transmission. In the periphery, 5-HT_{1D} receptors mediate vascular smooth-muscle contraction and vasoconstriction. The antimigraine drug, sumatriptan, is an agonist at these receptors.

The 5-HT_2 receptors are involved in CNS neurotransmission and act peripherally to cause the contraction of gastrointestinal, bronchial, and uterine smooth muscle. These receptors are involved in the pathophysiologic effects of carcinoid syndrome and mediate platelet aggregation. The 5-HT_2 receptors are antagonized by ketanserin and ritanserin.

The 5-HT_3 receptors are found in the chemoreceptor trigger zone (CTZ) of the CNS and peripherally in the enteric nervous system involved in gastrointestinal motility. Ondansetron acts as an antagonist at these receptors and thereby exerts a potent antiemetic effect. Metoclopramide is a weaker antagonist at these receptors.

The 5-HT_4 receptors comprise a new subgroup that is found in the enteric nervous system, where they mediate increased gastrointestinal motility. Cisapride, a prokinetic drug, acts as an agonist at these receptors.

60. The answer is B.   *(Behavioral science)*
This patient's personality is separated into different facets using the defense mechanism of dissociation. Dissociation is often seen in individuals who have been physically or sexually abused as children.

61. The answer is A.   *(Biochemistry)*
Oncogene products fall into five classes of proteins, all of which are involved in some form of growth regulation. The product of the v-*src* gene is a protein tyrosine kinase, an enzyme that phosphorylates tyrosine residues on certain target proteins. Examples of oncogenes for each of the other classes are: G proteins (*ras*), growth factors (*sis*), growth factor receptors (*erb B*), and DNA-binding proteins (*myc*).

62. The answer is A.   *(Behavioral science)*
Despite adequate physical care, children in orphanages show severe developmental retardation. Such children generally have poor health, high death rates, and show severe social problems as adults. There are no orphanages for young children in the United States.

63. The answer is C. *(Biochemistry)*
For 2 to 6 hours after a meal, the brain uses glucose as its major fuel. During this time, glucose is derived from digestion and/or liver glycogen. For 8 to 12 hours after a meal, glucose is derived primarily from liver glycogen. After eight hours, three things occur: 1. The rate of glucose production from liver glycogenolysis slows, ceasing almost entirely within 24 hours. 2. Glucose production from gluconeogenesis increases and reaches its peak at about 30 hours. 3. Ketone body formation from excess acetyl CoA (derived from β-oxidation of fatty acids in the liver) also increases. Therefore, glucose produced by gluconeogenesis is still the main fuel available to the brain between 20 to 24 hours after a meal. Within 10 days, ketone bodies become an important fuel for the brain, replacing its complete glucose dependency. Red blood cells continue to use glucose as their sole fuel, while muscles primarily use fatty acids.

64. The answer is A. *(Behavioral science)*
Increased compliance is associated with decreased waiting room time; patients made to wait for an extended period become angry and may not comply with treatment. Compliance is associated also with older physician age, a simple rather than complex treatment regimen, increased time spent with the patient, and patient knowledge of how the medication treats the illness.

65. The answer is B. *(Biochemistry)*
Cells of higher organisms carry genes called protooncogenes, which are normal growth-regulating genes. Mutation of these genes can lead to cancer.

Operons are groups of organized genes used in bacteria. Related genes in higher organisms are usually scattered, not grouped. Transcriptionally active chromatin usually has a loose structure, while inactive chromatin is generally condensed. Only a small fraction of eukaryotic DNA actually codes for protein structure. Although the bacterial chromosome has a single origin of replication, eukaryotic chromosomes have many such origins.

66. The answer is B. *(Behavioral science)*
The surgeon is using the defense mechanism of displacement; he expresses his repressed anger at his son toward the residents. Using regression, he would exhibit childlike behavior, whereas using denial, he would not express any emotion. If sublimation were used, the surgeon would take out his anger at his son in a more mature way (e.g., by playing a hard game of raquetball). Using dissociation as a defense mechanism, the surgeon separates himself from aspects of his personality.

67. The answer is E. *(Biochemistry)*
Retinoblastoma is cancer of the retina caused by mutation of the *Rb* gene, an anti-oncogene or tumor-suppressor gene. Anti-oncogene products restrain uncontrolled cell growth. When such a gene is lost, cell growth is no longer held back, and cancer may result. Sickle cell anemia is caused by a missense in the β-globin gene. Mutations that lead to decreased synthesis of β-globin cause β-thalassemia. The color pattern of a calico cat results from X chromosome inactivation in females. Burkitt lymphoma is a type of cancer caused by a chromosomal translocation that activates the *myc* oncogene.

68. The answer is A. *(Behavioral science)*
The young lawyer is using the defense mechanism of regression; he is exhibiting childlike behavior under the pressure of his stressful illness.

69. The answer is B. *(Biochemistry)*
The TATA sequence, in both prokaryotes and eukaryotes, is part of the promoter region of a gene (i.e., the binding site for RNA polymerase). In eukaryotes, the TATA sequence must be bound by transcription factor IID before RNA polymerase II can bind. The promoter serves as an initiation signal for transcription, not replication. The promoter region is usually not transcribed and does not appear in the messenger RNA product.

70. The answer is E. *(Behavioral science)*
Patients with chronic pain who receive psychotherapy and behavior therapy spend less time in the hospital. These patients also need less pain medication, become more mobile and show increased attempts to get back to their preillness lifestyle. Patients with chronic pain who receive psychotherapy and behavior therapy do not show excessive dependence on the therapist.

71. The answer is D. *(Biochemistry)*
Phospho*enol*pyruvate-carboxykinase deficiency prevents pyruvate from being converted to phospho*enol*-pyruvate. This deficiency interferes with gluconeogenesis from three carbon precursors, such as alanine, that enter the gluconeogenic pathway at or below the pyruvate level. Because this patient forms glucose from fructose and glycerol, the lesion is not above dihydroxyacetone phosphate (DHAP), which eliminates choices A (glucose-6-phosphatase), B (fructose-1,6-bisphosphatase), and E (aldolase B). There is no sign of excess glycogen storage, and the liver is a normal size, so choice C (glycogen phosphorylase) is also excluded.

Glucose-6-phosphatase, the last enzymatic reaction in gluconeogenesis, converts glucose 6-phosphate to glucose plus inorganic phosphate.

Fructose-1,6-bisphosphatase converts fructose 1,6-bisphosphate to fructose 6-phosphate plus inorganic phosphate. During gluconeogenesis, the enzyme catalyzes the formation of fructose 6-phosphate from fructose 1,6-bisphosphate and avoids the irreversible phosphofructokinase step of glycolysis.

Glycogen phosphorylase, the rate regulating enzyme of glycogenolysis, removes glucose moieties from glycogen as glucose 1-phosphate.

Aldolase B converts fructose 1-phosphate to DHAP and glyceraldehyde 3-phosphate. This reaction is unique to the catabolism of fructose.

72. The answer is D. *(Pharmacology)*
Both amphotericin B and fluconazole may be used in treating cryptococcal meningitis. Fluconazole has the advantage of oral effectiveness and good penetration of the cerebrospinal fluid (CSF). However, amphotericin B must be injected, does not enter the CSF well, and sometimes must be given intrathecally. Amphotericin frequently causes chills, fever, and nephrotoxicity, whereas the azoles (e.g., fluconazole and ketoconazole) may cause hepatic impairment. Azoles also inhibit cytochrome P-450, which increases the serum levels of drugs, such as phenytoin, terfenadine, anticoagulants, and hypoglycemic agents. By inhibiting P-450, azoles also inhibit membrane ergosterol synthesis, whereas amphotericin B binds to fungal membranes and increases their permeability.

73. The answer is E. *(Biochemistry)*
Strenuous exercise activates an adipocyte hormone-sensitive lipase through a cyclic adenosine monophosphate (cAMP)-dependent phosphorylation, which is mediated primarily by catecholamines. The free fatty acids that are released from the adipocyte bind to serum albumin and are transported to tissues where they are used as fuel via β-oxidation.

HDLs carry excess cholesterol from tissues back to the liver. HDLs also carry and add apoproteins to both VLDL and chylomicrons, which transforms these apoproteins from nascent to mature. VLDLs carry triacylglycerol synthesized in the liver to peripheral tissue. While fasting, neither HDL nor VLDL serum levels are immediately affected by exercise. In the long term, however, exercise increases HDL levels and decreases VLDL levels.

Triacylglycerol micelles occur in the intestine as emulsified-triacylglycerol droplets.

Chylomicrons are lipoproteins that carry hydrophobic molecules (mainly triacylglycerol) from the gut to tissues. These lipoproteins are removed primarily by the liver where they are processed and exported as VLDL. Chylomicron levels are increased when an individual eats a breakfast with saturated fats (e.g., bacon and eggs).

74-75. The answers are: 74-C, 75-D. *(Behavioral science)*
The median is the middle number in a sequentially ordered group of numbers. Therefore, the median of this group of scores is 35. The mean or average of this group of scores is 43.3, and the mode or number occurring most often is 20.

The distribution of scores in the question is skewed to the right. In a positively skewed distribution (skewed to the right), the scores cluster toward the low end, the tail is toward the right side, and the modal peak is toward the left side. In a negatively skewed distribution (skewed to the left), the scores cluster toward the high end, the tail is toward the left side, and the modal peak is toward the right side. In a normal or Gaussian distribution, the mean, median, and mode are equal.

76. The answer is D. *(Biochemistry)*
The young woman does not have a glycogen storage disease. This conclusion is based on her maintaining

a normal blood sugar level for at least 8 hours after eating a carbohydrate-rich meal. This observation indicates that carbohydrate is stored as liver glycogen and becomes available postprandially. In addition, she does not have an enlarged liver.

However, the patient does seem to have a problem with gluconeogenesis. Because her usual breakfasts and lunches are too small to build up much liver glycogen, she cannot draw on these meals as sources to maintain her blood glucose levels. Yet, even with insufficient meals, gluconeogenesis should carry the normal individual to at least dinner time, when glycogen stores are usually replenished. This suspicion is confirmed when none of the three gluconeogenic substrates (fructose, glucose, or alanine) are converted to glucose.

If a catabolic process, glycolysis, or β-oxidation were deficient, the patient would have consistent neuro-muscular symptoms that would not be related to postprandial time.

77. The answer is B. (Microbiology)

Mycoplasmas are the smallest free-living organisms. These organisms completely lack a peptidogylcan cell wall. As bacteria, mycoplasmas divide by binary fission. The organisms can be grown in the laboratory on artificial media, but this media must contain complex nutritional materials needed by mycoplasmas. With no cell wall protection, media with a high salt content provide resistance to osmotic lysis needed for organism survival. The organisms may require several days to grow, and the colonies develop a characteristic "fried-egg" shape.

In the presence of penicillin, gram-positive bacteria that exist without cell walls are called an L-form. Removal of the penicillin will allow cell wall production to resume. Mycoplasmas are resistant to antibiotics that inhibit cell wall synthesis (e.g., penicillin and cephalosporin).

78. The answer is C. (Behavioral science)

According to the DSM-IIIR, sexual and physical abuse are considered extreme psychosocial stressors in children and adolescents. School transfer is considered a mild stressor, suspension from school is a moderate stressor, and trouble with law enforcement authorities and divorce of parents are considered severe stressors in children and adolescents.

79. The answer is D. (Biochemistry)

A deficiency of vitamin B_{12} causes small amounts of propionyl coenzyme A (CoA) to accumulate. Because of the cyclic nature of fatty acid synthesis, the propionyl CoA causes significant amounts of fatty acids with an odd number of carbons to accumulate. These fatty acids, which are incorporated into myelin and other membranes, are considered responsible for the neuropathy that accompanies vitamin B_{12} deficiency.

Vitamin B_{12} deficiency causes a functional folate deficiency only when acting as a cofactor in a second reaction. In the absence of vitamin B_{12}, methyltetrahydrofolate cannot transfer its methyl groups to homocysteine to form methionine. Also, much of the tetrahydrofolate is trapped as the methyl derivative, leaving the other forms of folate deficient.

Because of aberrations in this pathway, branched-chain amino acids, or their immediate degradation products, do not accumulate as they do in maple syrup urine disease. In fact, degradations of the branched-chain amino acids are the primary source of the odd-numbered fatty acids.

The reactions involving propionate are not significant enough to influence energy metabolism or the accumulation of tricarboxylic acid cycle intermediates.

80. The answer is B. (Behavioral science)

This behavior is characteristic of the passive-aggressive personality type; an underlying unexpressed anger at the physician results in noncompliance with medical advice. The schizoid personality type becomes anxious and withdrawn with illness, the paranoid type blames the doctor for the illness, the histrionic personality is dramatic and acts inappropriately toward the physician, and the dependent type is afraid of being helpless and needs increased attention during illness.

81. The answer is D. (Microbiology)

Respiratory syncytial virus (RSV) is the most important cause of pneumonia and bronchiolitis in infants. Outbreaks occur in the population every year. RSV infection in infants is more severe and more often involves the lower respiratory tract than in older children and adults. Infection is localized to the respiratory tract.

Severe infant disease appears to have an immunopathogenic mechanism. Immune complexes, such as immunoglobulin G–virus (type III hypersensitivity) and immunoglobulin E–histamine (type I hypersensitivity), may be involved. Multiple infections are common, indicating that protective immunity is incomplete.

Treatment consists of hospitalization to assist respiration and deliver aerosolized ribavirin.

Although the Epstein-Barr virus is widespread and causes a spectrum of diseases, most infections are self-limited illnesses in adolescents and young adults. Similarly, most cytomegalovirus infections are subclinical. Acute epiglottitis is most often bacterial in origin (e.g., *Haemophilus influenzae*), although parainfluenza viruses may cause inflammation of the glottic and tracheal surfaces. Parainfluenza virus infections often manifest as croup (acute laryngotracheitis) but occur in children more than 2 years old. In adenovirus infection with interstitial pneumonia, the pathologic changes are thought to be due to direct tissue damage caused by virus replication within susceptible cells. Severe pneumonia may occur in infants 3–18 months old, and the symptoms include high fever, cough, respiratory distress, rales, vomiting, and lethargy.

82. The answer is A. *(Microbiology)*

Hepatitis A virus (HAV) is one of five known viruses capable of infecting liver cells and causing organ dysfunction. HAV is endemic in many populations and is spread by fecal contamination and usually contracted through a community water source. Children are most frequently affected.

Passive immunity with immune serum globulin (γ-globulin) before infection or early in the incubation period can prevent or mitigate the disease. No direct antiviral therapy against HAV is available. The killed (inactivated) vaccine is now available. No chronic carrier state exists. The diagnosis is based on measuring HAV-specific immunoglobulin M (IgM) in a patient's serum.

None of the other viral diseases listed can be managed by use of passive immunity.

83. The answer is A. *(Microbiology)*

Influenza viruses (groups A, B, and C) are surrounded by a lipid envelope, which is derived from the cytoplasmic membrane of the host cell in the budding-off process. These envelopes contain hemagglutinin, which is the receptor molecule for the virion. If the envelope is destroyed by ether treatment, the virus

cannot accomplish the first requisite step in its growth cycle, which is attachment. On host cells, the virus attaches to sialic acid receptors, but without attachment, there is no viral entry into the cell and no viral growth.

Because orthomyxoviruses have negative-sense RNA (opposite base sequence to positive-sense RNA or messenger RNA), no infectious RNA can be produced. The virus remains an obligate intracellular parasite. The RNA genome would not be destroyed by the ether treatment.

Treatment with amantadine is useless because it inhibits uncoating of the virus within the cytoplasm. The virus does not reach this area because it cannot attach to receptors.

84. The answer is C. *(Physiology)*

The renal threshold for a substance denotes the plasma concentration at which the solute begins to appear in the urine. It is not the plasma concentration that completely saturates the transport mechanism for either reabsorption or secretion. When the plasma concentration of a solute exceeds the renal threshold, the amount of that solute transported through the nephron exceeds the tubular transport maximum (Tm), and the solute appears in the urine in increasing amounts. The filtered load is the amount of a substance entering the tubule by filtration per unit time.

85. The answer is C. *(Biochemistry)*

Von Gierke disease is an autosomal-recessive glycogenosis characterized by a deficiency of glucose-6-phosphatase, a gluconeogenic enzyme. This enzyme converts glucose 6-phosphate to glucose. Because neither phosphorylated sugars nor polysaccharides can escape from the liver cell without this gluconeogenic enzyme, sugars undergoing metabolism can only escape from the cell as lactate, pyruvate, or by conversion to fatty acids.

An increase in glucose 6-phosphate stimulates excess synthesis and storage of structurally normal glycogen in the liver and the kidney. Both of these organs are gluconeogenic and normally produce glucose-6-phosphatase. Because the enzymes of fructose metabolism are normal, fructose is phosphorylated and trapped (not spilled into the urine).

An oral fructose challenge determines if the 3-carbon intermediates derived from fructose (dihydroxyacetone-phosphate and glyceraldehyde 3-phosphate) will be converted to glucose by gluconeogenesis. Because glucose-6-phosphatase is not present, the blood glucose levels are not increased. Similar results occur with a glucagon challenge.

In fructokinase deficiency, fructose is not converted to glucose, and liver glycogen has normal structure. However, fructose is spilled into the urine.

86. The answer is D.   *(Pharmacology)*
Selective adrenergic β_2-receptor agonists relax smooth muscle, but these agonists have little effect on heart rate or contractility. Therefore, cardiac stimulation requires a higher dose than bronchial muscle relaxation.

In contrast, nonselective β_1 and β_2 agonists, such as isoproterenol, produce equivalent effects on heart and smooth muscle. Alpha agonists cause smooth muscle contraction, but these agonists have less effect on the heart than the β agonists.

87. The answer is E.   *(Anatomy)*
In the small intestine, secretory granules are seen at the basal aspect of this enteroendocrine cell. These granules will fuse with the basal membrane and expel their contents across the basal lamina into capillaries. The apical cell membrane, which faces the intestinal lumen, has microvilli as a border modification.

Goblet cells contain mucous granules in the apical cytoplasm. These granules usually appear clear or gray using transmission electron microscopy.

Acinar cells have large granules in the apical cytoplasm. Such cells could be in a gland, such as the pancreatic acinar cell.

Absorptive cells do not contain secretory granules. In the figure, these cells are dark and surround the enteroendocrine cell.

Paneth cells have large granules that are oriented in the apical cytoplasm. These cells are two to three times larger than enteroendocrine cell granules.

88. The answer is A.   *(Biochemistry)*
A deficiency of reduced nicotinamide adenine dinucleotide phosphate (NADPH) oxidase greatly compromises the host's defense mechanism. This enzyme is responsible for chronic granulomatosis because free radicals cannot be formed within the macrophage. Normally, these free radicals are used to kill the engulfed bacterium.

The other four enzymes also operate in this oxygen-dependent defense mechanism. The superoxide formed by NADPH oxidase is converted to H_2O_2 by superoxide dismutase. Myeloperoxidase causes H_2O_2 to react with chloride ion producing hypochlorous acid (bleach), which actually kills the bacterium.

Catalase and glutathione peroxidase destroy excess peroxide. Glutathione peroxidase is unique because it requires selenium as a cofactor. Only trace quantities of selenium are needed in the diet to enable this reaction. In greater-than-optimal concentrations, selenium is toxic.

The reaction sequences are illustrated below.

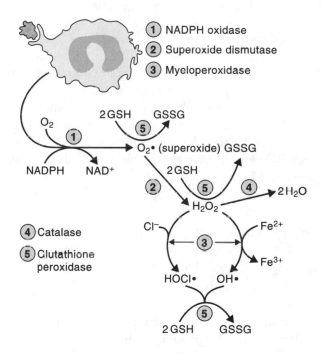

89. The answer is D.   *(Pathology)*
A stress electrocardiogram evaluates patients with suspected ischemic heart disease (angina). Classic angina with exertion is characterized by subendocardial ischemia, which produces sinus tachycardia (ST) depression. Most clinicians use 1 mm or greater ST depression to define a positive test. Therefore, increasing the criteria from 1 mm to 2 mm ST depression increases the chance that a positive test indicates that the patient

has ischemic heart disease by decreasing the number of false positive (FP) test results (normal people misclassified as having disease).

To comprehend this concept, the sensitivity and specificity of a test must be understood. The sensitivity of a test refers to how often the test returns positive in disease. The formula is:

$$\text{Sensitivity} = \frac{\text{true positive (TP)}}{\text{TP + false negative (FN)}} \times 100$$

A test with 100% sensitivity has no FNs. Therefore, when a test result returns negative, it must be a true negative (TN) rather than an FN. If it returns positive, it can be either a true positive (TP) or an FP.

The specificity of a test refers to how often a test is negative (normal) in a patient without disease. The formula is:

$$\text{Specificity} = \frac{\text{TN}}{\text{TN + FP}} \times 100$$

A test with 100% specificity has no FPs. Therefore, a positive test result must be a TP rather than an FP.

By increasing the cutoff for a positive stress test to 2 mm, the specificity of the test is increased, which reduces the number of FPs. A positive test result using this new criteria must be a TP rather than a FP. The problem with this cutoff is that there would be people with ischemic heart disease with an ST depression between 1 mm and 2 mm who would be considered normal.

90. The answer is D.   *(Microbiology)*

Toxoids are toxins that have been chemically altered with agents, such as formaldehyde, so they are no longer toxic to the host but still retain their immunogenicity.

Toxoids can be used for active immunization. Antibodies generated against a toxoid are cross-reactive with the toxin, and, thus, they are protective. Preparation of toxoids for immunization is carefully monitored in order to achieve detoxification with minimal alteration of its epitopes. An epitope is the small portion of a molecule to which a particular immunoglobulin or T-cell antigen receptor binds.

Toxins of bacteria and the venom of snakes and insects are proteins that induce the production of antibodies in vivo. If the antibody binds to the active site of the toxin, it will be neutralized. The formation of antigen–antibody complexes also promotes phagocytosis of the toxin by macrophages and other phagocytes. However, toxins often act rapidly, and there is no time to wait for the individual to produce neutralizing antibodies.

Preformed antibodies against toxins are used therapeutically and prophylactically. Specific immunoglobulin preparations are available for diphtheria, tetanus, botulism, black widow spider venom, and snake venom. These toxins confer passive immunization.

91. The answer is C.   *(Biochemistry)*

The horizontal line in the restriction map represents the bacteriophage λ-DNA molecule, which is shown to be 48.4 kilobase pairs long. The vertical lines show the cleavage sites for the indicated restriction endonucleases. The numbers under the horizontal line show the distance in kilobase pairs between each of the restriction sites. Treatments of λ-DNA with both Apa I and Xba I would cut the molecule in two places, producing three fragments. The sizes of the fragments are determined by adding up the distances shown in the restriction map.

92. The answer is D.   *(Microbiology)*

Hepatitis B virus, the cause of serum hepatitis, is readily transmitted by blood; thus, hepatitis B immune globulin would most likely be administered. Depending on the employee's immunization status, active immunization may also be indicated.

Immune globulin is prepared as whole serum or as fractionated and concentrated antibodies obtained from humans or animals. For specific diseases, the donors are either recovering from the illness or have been immunized with the infectious agent. The antibodies provide immediate, but relatively short-lived, protection for individuals who do not have those specific antibodies or who may be immunocompromised. Immune globulin contains primarily immunoglobulin G (IgG).

As for the other choices, the majority of people in the United States already have antibodies against the varicella-zoster (chickenpox) virus. *Clostridium tetani* is found in the soil and in the feces of horses and other animals. Rabies is usually transmitted by the bite of an animal (there is no viremia). Because smallpox has been eradicated from the world, vaccinia immune globulin is no longer of practical importance.

93. The answer is A. *(Pathology)*

The best conclusion is that a type I error was committed in Experiment A. A type I error occurs when the null hypothesis is rejected even though it is true (i.e., the drug does not increase survival time). A type II error occurs when the null hypothesis is not rejected even though it is false (i.e., the drug really does increase survival time). Because Experiment A was conducted in five centers and Experiment B, in one center, it is more likely that sampling bias was present and a type I error was committed in Experiment A rather than in Experiment B.

94. The answer is D. *(Microbiology)*

The induction of disseminated intravascular coagulation (DIC) is among the many pathophysiologic effects induced by lipopolysaccharide (LPS). LPS, also known as endotoxin, activates the first step in the intrinsic clotting cascade by interacting with factor XII (Hageman factor). Important results are the conversion of fibrinogen to fibrin, formation of plasmin (a proteolytic enzyme), and hemorrhagic necrosis due to occlusion of small blood vessels. DIC is a frequent complication of gram-negative bacteremia. Heparin can sometimes minimize the pathological effects associated with DIC.

When freed from the bacterial cell wall, LPS binds to circulating proteins, which then interact with receptor molecules on macrophages and monocytes. These cells respond to the stimulus with the production of interleukin-1 (IL-1), tumor necrosis factor (TNF), and other cytokines. IL-1 induces fever in addition to promoting T lymphocyte-mediated responses. TNF has numerous biological effects. LPS is among the most potent inducers of TNF that has ever been identified.

LPS is a good activator of the alternative complement pathway. Consequences of complement activation include the generation of anaphylatoxins (C3a, C4a, C5a), chemotaxis of leukocytes, and membrane damage.

Mycobacterium tuberculosis, Brucella species, and *Legionella* species are all prime examples of bacteria that can survive within phagocytic cells. However, this ability is not due to LPS. The mechanisms are variable and include lack of entry into phagolysosomes, prevention of phagosome–lysosome fusion, and resistance to lysosomal enzymes.

95. The answer is B. *(Behavioral science)*

As with child abuse, if there is a suspicion of elder abuse, the physician's first responsibility is to protect the patient by contacting a social service agency. This 75-year-old woman is probably a victim of such abuse, which is a growing problem in the United States. You do not have to tell the daughter that you believe the mother is being abused, nor do you have to inform the daughter that you are contacting a social service agency. If necessary, the agency will contact the police. Sending the elderly patient home with her daughter and instructing her to come back in one week puts the mother at risk for further abuse. Instructing the daughter on how to reduce her own stress may be addressed after the immediate problem of danger to the mother.

96. The answer is D. *(Pathology)*

Carcinoembryonic antigen (CEA) is produced by cancerous colorectal cells in the majority of patients with the disease. After treatment, a rising CEA level may indicate recurrence. This marker also may be elevated in several other types of cancers, including those of the pancreas, lung (e.g., small cell carcinoma), and breast. In healthy adults, CEA is detectable in trace amounts. During embryogenesis, CEA is produced by normal cells in the fetal gut, thus the term oncofetal antigen. Increased expression of CEA can also be detected in individuals with nonmalignant conditions, such as colitis and pancreatitis, so its usefulness lies mostly in monitoring disease status after therapy.

CEA is a secreted glycoprotein, measured in serum, and the best characterized marker for solid tumors. It is classified as a member of the immunoglobulin superfamily because of its chemical and structural similarities with other members of that group. CEA complexed with CEA antibodies can deposit in the glomeruli and produce membranous glomerulonephritis (nephrotic syndrome).

High levels of antibody light chains (Bence Jones protein) may be found in the serum and urine of patients with multiple myeloma, a malignant plasma cell disorder. The Bence Jones protein contributes to kidney failure because of its toxicity for renal tubular cells or its precipitation at low pH.

α-Fetoprotein (AFP) is a commonly used marker for monitoring liver tumors (e.g., hepatocellular carcinoma) and germ cell tumors (e.g., yolk sac tumors).

AFP is normally secreted by fetal liver and yolk sac cells.

Human chorionic gonadotropin is found at high levels in women with trophoblastic tumors, such as hydatidiform moles and choriocarcinoma.

Prostate specific antigen (PSA) is elevated in the majority of men with prostate cancer. However, high levels of PSA may also be present in benign prostatic hyperplasia, thus, it lacks specificity.

97. The answer is E.   *(Microbiology)*

In bacteria, related enzymes are often encoded by genes that lie next to each other and are regulated as one unit (an operon). Regulation is frequently at the level of transcription initiation. One long, polycistronic messenger RNA molecule is produced, which carries information for all of the enzymes encoded in the operon. Translation of this single message leads to the coordinate production of all enzymes of the pathway.

Only a fraction of enzymes in bacteria are expressed constitutively (i.e., at the same level at all times). Size, cofactor requirements, and ability to be regulated by feedback inhibition have nothing to do with expression or synthesis of the enzyme molecules.

98. The answer is B.   *(Biochemistry)*

Ribonucleotide reductase is an enzyme that supplies the need for deoxyribonucleotides for DNA synthesis by reducing ribonucleoside diphosphates to their corresponding deoxyribonucleoside diphosphates. Any base may be present, but the nucleotide must be at the diphosphate level in order for the enzyme to work. Therefore, uridine diphosphate is the only possible answer. Adenosine monophosphate and guanosine triphosphate are nucleotides, adenine is a base, and inosine is a nucleoside.

99. The answer is C.   *(Pharmacology)*

Levamisole, a compound originally tested as an antihelminthic drug, is probably the best known chemical immunomodulator. It is not cytotoxic and has little or no effect in healthy individuals. Although its exact mechanism of action is unknown, it appears to act as a nonspecific enhancer of immune responsiveness. For example, it can reverse postviral anergy in persons with measles or influenza. In addition, the survival time of

patients with colon cancer is increased when levamisole is combined with 5-fluorouracil.

Cyclophosphamide is a powerful cell cycle-specific immunosuppressant that is cytotoxic to both B and T lymphocytes. The inactive parent drug is metabolized in the liver to phosphoramide mustard and other alkylates. Thus, cyclophosphamide is an alkylating agent that binds to and produces cross-links in DNA chains. This eventually results in death of the target cell. Before the discovery of cyclosporine A, the drug was used extensively for prolongation of allograft survival.

Methotrexate is one of the earliest drugs used for cancer therapy. It inhibits dihydrofolate reductase, which is needed for conversion of folic acid to tetrahydrofolate. The result is the inhibition of DNA synthesis. Methotrexate can inhibit both humoral and cell-mediated immune responses. This agent is used for preventing graft versus host reactions in allogeneic bone marrow transplantation and in the treatment of severe rheumatoid arthritis and other autoimmune diseases.

Prednisone is among the most commonly used corticosteroids. Corticosteroids are potent inhibitors of inflammatory responses and can be toxic to lymphocytes when given systemically. Prednisone, together with one or more drugs, is often used to overcome acute episodes of graft rejection. However, prolonged use of corticosteroids can result in numerous unwanted side effects (e.g., weakness of bone, atrophy of adrenal glands, increased incidence of infections).

Lymphocytes are extremely susceptible to ionizing radiation, which interacts with DNA. Total lymphoid irradiation consists of administering low doses of radiation over a period of time. The T-helper cells appear to be most affected, and a reversal of the T-helper cell:T-suppressor cell ratio is noted in the peripheral blood. The technique has been successfully used in some patients with intractible rheumatoid arthritis and severe lupus-related nephritis. It is also being tested in organ transplantation as an adjunctive form of immunosuppression.

100. The answer is B.   *(Microbiology)*

Escherichia coli is the most common organism isolated from urinary tract infections. In young women, *E. coli* is involved in approximately 90% of these cases.

The organisms are also the most common cause of gram-negative sepsis.

Nephrotoxigenic *Escherichia coli* usually produce hemolysin and possess P pili, both of which are considered virulence factors. Nephrotoxigenic *E. coli* can be quickly identified by a zone of hemolysis around colonies on a blood agar plate, its colonial morphology, a positive spot indole test, and an iridescent "sheen" on differential media (e.g., eosin-methylene blue, EMB, agar). P pili bind specifically to galactose-containing moieties on epithelial cells within the urinary tract.

NPEC can infect any portion of the urinary tract. Pyelonephritis (infection of the kidney) can be very painful and is among the most serious consequences of urinary tract infection. Virtually 100% of NPEC isolates from cases of pyelonephritis have P pili.

There is no single antibiotic that is effective for *E. coli*, and susceptibility testing is critical. Sulfonamides, ampicillin, chloramphenicol, cephalosporins, and other antibiotics are effective against many of the enteric organisms, but variability is great. Resistance to multiple drugs can be passed (even among different genera) via plasmids.

Proteus vulgaris is also a relatively common cause of urinary tract infections in patients with kidney stones or calculi (staghorn calculi). *Klebsiella pneumoniae* is an occasional cause. *Serratia marcescens* and *Pseudomonas aeruginosa* generally are associated with complicated urinary tract infections (i.e., patients with structural abnormalities of the urinary tract) and other types of hospital-acquired infections.

101. The answer is B. *(Microbiology)*
Enterotoxigenic *Escherichia coli* (ETEC) produces a heat-labile toxin. This toxin is an exotoxin of 80,000 molecular weight that is encoded by a gene in a plasmid and is made up of A and B subunits. The B subunit attaches to the GM_1 ganglioside of epithelial cells in the small intestine and assists entry of the A subunit. The A subunit, which is the active portion of the toxin, promotes adenylate cyclase activity. This results in a dramatic increase in cyclic adenosine monophosphate and hypersecretion of water and chlorides into the intestinal lumen.

Some strains of ETEC produce a heat-stable toxin (ST). The ST enhances guanylate cyclase activity, which results in increased cyclic guanosine monophosphate and excessive fluid secretion.

Site of infection	Toxins and other important factors	Comments
Intestinal tract		
Enteropathogenic *Escherichia coli* (EPEC)	O55 antigen O111 antigen	Watery diarrhea, especially in infants
Enterotoxigenic *E. coli* (ETEC)	LT, ST enterotoxins Pili	"Travelers diarrhea"
Enterohemorrhagic *E. coli* (EHEC)*	Verotoxin O157:H7 serotype	Hemorrhagic colitis (raw hamburgers; diarrhea and hemolytic uremic syndrome; acute renal failure)
Enteroinvasive *E. coli* (EIEC)	Have ability to penetrate epithelial cells in intestinal mucosa	Dysentery-like disease
Urinary tract		
Nephropathogenic *E. coli* (NPEC)	Hemolysin Capsule P pili	Lower and upper (pyelonephritis) urinary tract infections
Central nervous system		
E. coli	K1 antigen in capsule (similar to group B streptococcus)	Meningitis, especially in infants

* The verotoxin is so named because of its ability to kill Vero cells (a cell line of African green monkey kidney cells) in culture. EHEC has been recently isolated from outbreaks of severe disease due to ingestion of undercooked hamburger at fast-food restaurants.

102. The answer is E. *(Biochemistry)*
Both an electron donor and a phosphate acceptor must be present for oxidative phosphorylation to occur. Electron transport and phosphorylation will occur with added succinate and adenosine diphosphate (ADP). Using this method, two adenosine triphosphates (ATP) are synthesized for each succinate used (per electron pair transported or atom of oxygen used). However, in order to make ATP, protons must pass through complex V, thus limiting the rate of oxidative phosphorylation. When adding 2,4-dinitrophenol with the succinate, this latter process is unnecessary, and the rate of oxidation is increased. Because this compound avoids phosphorylation, ADP is no longer required, and electron transport becomes uncoupled from phosphorylation.

103. The answer is D. *(Microbiology)*
HIV type 1 (HIV-1) binds to the CD4 molecule, which is found in relatively large numbers on T-helper lymphocytes. More specifically, HIV-1 binds at the V1 region of the CD4 protein.

The molecule of attachment on the virus is a glycoprotein known as gp120 (glycoprotein with a molecular weight of 120 kD). The virus infects the cells by fusing its envelope with the cytoplasmic membrane of the cell.

The CD4 molecule appears to be present on cell types other than the T-helper lymphocytes but probably at a much lower density. Monocyte–macrophage, microglial, and endothelial cells in the brain, Langerhans cells, follicular dendritic cells, immortalized B cells, mucosal cells of the colon, and cells of the retina are all susceptible to HIV-1 infection.

HIV-1 does not bind to the T-cell antigen receptor, human leukocyte antigen (HLA) class I, HLA class II, or CD8 molecules.

104. The answer is A. *(Microbiology)*
Identification of the HIV type 1 (HIV-1) genome in the infant's cells is strong evidence for infection. The polymerase chain reaction is used to amplify virus-specific nucleotide sequences. Other procedures that can be done include a culture of the virus from tissues or cells and a demonstration of the presence of HIV-1 antigens.

Maternal immunoglobulin G can cross the placenta. HIV-1 can infect the fetus by crossing the placenta (vertical transmission) or be transmitted to the newborn by breast-feeding. Studies show that the incidence of transmission from mother to offspring ranges from 15% to 30%. Passively-acquired HIV-1 antibodies may give positive results in serological assays for as long as 15 months. High antibody titer is not always seen in HIV-1 infected newborns. Panhypogammaglobulinemia, a low level of all antibody classes, may be present. It is not known if immunoglobulin M antibodies specific to the virus are useful in a diagnosis of the infant.

Low birth weight (small for gestational age) could be caused by a range of different conditions.

An infant's immune system does not respond well to bacterial polysaccharides. This finding would not necessarily indicate HIV-1 infection.

105. The answer is D. *(Microbiology)*
The A and B antigens are carbohydrates. These antigens are used to classify an individual's erythrocytes into one of four groups: A, B, AB, and O.

Erythrocytes of virtually all individuals have a common oligosaccharide chain (the H antigen) protruding from the cytoplasmic membrane. The H antigen is not antigenic in humans, but other animal species produce antibodies against it. The specific blood group is determined by single terminal sugar residues, which may or may not be present on the common H-antigen stem. Although the A and B antigens differ in only one sugar residue, there is no cross-reactivity. A few rare individuals have erythrocytes that do not produce the H antigen. These erythrocytes are Bombay type; this type was first discovered in Bombay.

106. The answer is C. *(Microbiology)*
The three genes that determine ABO blood groups code for enzymes that function to attach sugar moieties to the H-antigen stem. The H gene codes for fucosyl transferase, which adds fucose to precursor chains and completes the H-antigen stem. The A gene codes for a transferase, which transfers the terminal *N*-acetylglucosamine to the completed H-antigen stem. The B gene codes for a transferase, which transfers the terminal galactose to the completed H-antigen stem.

Unlike proteins, carbohydrates are not encoded in genes.

The A and B antigens are expressed on cells other than erythrocytes. These antigens exist on most endothelial cells, which line the walls of blood vessels, and on many epithelial cells.

Although the mechanisms of genetic control of the Rh antigens are not clear, it is known that these mechanisms are different from those of the ABO system.

107-108. The answers are: 107-B, 108-A. *(Pathology)*
The case history suggests that the infant has X-linked hypogammaglobulinemia (Bruton's disease). X-linked diseases appear only in males. Infections in infants with the condition usually begin at about 5 to 6 months of age, when maternal immunoglobulin G (IgG) falls below a protective level. Recurrent bacterial (rather than viral, fungal, or protozoal) infections are typical of B-cell (antibody) deficiencies. *Haemophilus influenzae* is among the most common agents.

An extremely low serum antibody titer is not consistent with selective immunoglobulin A (IgA) deficiency. IgA is normally low in serum and is present primarily in secretions. The low serum antibody level indicates that all immunoglobulin classes are deficient. IgA deficiency is the most common of the selective immunoglobulin deficiencies.

Thymic aplasia (DiGeorge syndrome) is a T-cell deficiency. The most common infectious agents are viruses, fungi, and protozoans. Infants with the disease have significant congenital and other abnormalities not mentioned in this case history.

Ataxia-telangiectasia, a T-cell and B-cell deficiency, is characterized by muscle incoordination, dilatation of small blood vessels, and IgA deficiency.

Wiskott-Aldrich syndrome is a T-cell and B-cell deficiency accompanied with bleeding due to thrombocytopenia and lack of a normal immunoglobulin M response to polysaccharide bacterial capsules.

Therapy for Bruton's disease primarily consists of intravenous infusion of γ-globulin, which contains mostly IgG and may also be given intramuscularly. These latter types of solutions are similar to the intravenous preparations but do not require chemical treatments to prevent aggregation or complement activation. Most preparations, regardless of the intended route of administration, contain small amounts of nonantibody proteins.

The γ-globulin is obtained from randomly selected donors and is screened for infectious agents before administration. The pooled antibodies have a wide range of specificities and, therefore, are likely to be protective against many foreign agents. The γ-globulin must be given every 3 to 4 weeks, because its half-life in the serum is only about 1 month. Anaphylactoid reactions are rare, and continuous prophylactic use of broad-spectrum antibodies may be necessary in some cases. A few patients with the disease have survived for 20 to 30 years.

A thymus transplantation is used for T-cell and combined T-cell and B-cell immunodeficiencies.

A blood transfusion would have little or no lasting effect and could result in complications.

Immunization with attenuated vaccines would not significantly increase the immunoglobulin level because the individuals have no B lymphocytes.

Bacteria, not fungi, are the major infectious agents implicated in B-cell deficiencies.

109. The answer is C. *(Pathology)*
Infants with severe combined immunodeficiency disease (SCID) have severely depressed immunologic function, lymphopenia, and no detectable T-lymphocyte or B-lymphocyte responses. Early indications of the disease include those listed in the brief case history. There may also be failure to thrive and sepsis. Infections with virtually all types of infectious agents (bacteria, viruses, fungi, and protozoa) are common.

Deficiency in adenosine deaminase is seen in some patients. Lack of this enzyme results in the accumulation of adenosine triphosphate and deoxyadenosine triphosphate, both of which are more toxic to lymphocytes than to most other cells. B lymphocytes are either absent or markedly reduced in number. During the first 5 to 6 months, maternal immunoglobulin G provides protection, and diagnosis may initially be difficult. The skin rash at birth is most likely due to a graft versus host reaction. Maternal lymphocytes that reach the fetus during gestation become activated by fetal antigens and attack; the fetus is unable to fend off the attack.

Ataxia-telangiectasia is the only other T-cell and B-cell deficiency listed. The deficiency stems from defective DNA repair. The immune system is affected because of abnormalities in the genes, which code for antibody light and heavy chains and the T-cell antigen receptor.

Hereditary angioedema is C1 esterase inhibitor deficiency in which recurrent attacks of subcutaneous and submucosal swelling occurs. Deficiencies have been noted in virtually all major and minor components of the complement system.

Chronic granulomatous disease, an X-linked recessive disease, is the most important deficiency of phagocytic cells. The disease is due to a deficiency of reduced nicotinamide adenine dinucleotide phosphate oxidase, which is an enzyme needed for the respiratory burst.

Chédiak-Higashi syndrome is a phagocytic cell deficiency characterized by giant cytoplasmic granular inclusions in leukocytes, abnormal neutrophil chemotaxis, and decreased intracellular killing of microorganisms.

110. The answer is A. (Pathology)

A mesothelioma, derived from serosal cells lining body cavities, is an example of a malignant tumor of mesenchymal origin. These tumors arc strongly associated with exposure to asbestos. Hemangiomas, chondromas, rhabdomyomas, and meningiomas are also of mesenchymal origin, but they are benign.

Tumors of mesenchymal origin include those derived from connective tissue (fibrosarcoma), muscle (leiomyoma), hematopoietic cell (leukemias), endothelial, and other lining cells (lymphangioma, synovial sarcoma).

111. The answer is C. (Pathology)

An ABO mismatch involving an A patient receiving a B heart transplant results in a hyperacute rejection. The immunoglobulin M antibodies of the patient attack the B antigens on the surface of the endothelial cells in the graft. Complement is activated, vessel injury occurs, and vessel thrombosis produces ischemia in the graft with eventual rejection. This is a type II hypersensitivity reaction.

Recipient testing for a potential transplant typically involves determining the patient's ABO blood group, screening for human leukocyte antigen (HLA) antibodies, HLA testing of the patient's lymphocytes, and reacting the patient's lymphocytes against donor lymphocytes. ABO compatibility and the absence of preformed HLA antibodies prevent hyperacute reactions

in liver, kidney, and heart transplant patients. Normally, HLA antibodies should not be present in a recipient unless they have been exposed to foreign HLA antigens, such as with a previous pregnancy (fetal–maternal bleed) or blood transfusion. These antibodies are identified by taking the recipient's plasma and reacting it against a potential donor's lymphocytes (lymphocyte crossmatch) or reacting plasma against test lymphocytes of known HLA makeup.

112. The answer is B. (Pathology)

The patient developed a graft versus host (GVH) reaction due to a transfusion of antigenically active lymphoid cells into a patient with no cellular immunity.

The DiGeorge syndrome (thymic hypoplasia) is characterized by failed development of the third and fourth pharyngeal pouches with subsequent absence of the parathyroid glands and thymus, which is required to generate T cells. If transfusions are necessary, the blood should be irradiated to destroy the donor lymphocytes and prevent the graft versus host reaction, as well as cytomegalovirus (CMV) pneumonitis (CMV infects lymphocytes).

113. The answer is B. (Pathology)

The patient has selective immunoglobulin A (IgA) deficiency, which occurs in 1 out of 500 individuals and is the most common hereditary immunodeficiency. IgA deficiency has a heterogeneous hereditary pattern (autosomal recessive, autosomal dominant). There is an intrinsic defect in the differentiation of B cells committed to synthesizing IgA or failure of IgA production secondary to a defect in T cells. IgA is second to immunoglobulin G (IgG) in concentration. IgG has a J chain attached to secretory IgA. IgA prevents microorganisms and pollens from binding to epithelial cells. Clinical manifestations of IgA deficiency include sinopulmonary infections (most common), diarrhea (*Giardia*), increased incidence of allergies, and increased autoimmune disease (Hashimoto's thyroiditis, vitiligo). Patients with IgA antibodies are at increased risk for an anaphylactic reaction if they receive blood components containing IgA.

Laboratory findings include decreased serum IgA and salivary IgA, normal IgG, and normal immunoglobulin M. Many of these patients have selective IgG_2 and IgG_4 subclass deficiencies.

Most patients do well with antibiotic therapy. Treatment must avoid using blood products (e.g., γ-globulin) because patients frequently develop an anaphylactic reaction.

114. The answer is C. *(Pathology)*
The patient has C1 esterase inhibitor deficiency. This deficiency (hereditary angioedema) is an autosomal-dominant disease that results in the excessive release of C4- and C2-derived kinins. These kinins increase vessel permeability resulting in the sudden onset of edema of the extremities, intestine (painful), face, or oropharynx (the most common cause of death). These clinical findings can last for 24 to 72 hours. Laboratory studies reveal reduced levels of C1 esterase inhibitor (confirmatory test), decreased C4 (best screen), decreased C2, and normal C3. Synthetic androgen (stanozolol) prevents attacks by increasing the synthesis of inhibitor. Maintenance of the upper airway is imperative. Fresh frozen plasma also contains the inhibitor.

There is no abnormality in the serum immunoglobulin E levels because it is not a type I hypersensitivity reaction. The presence of autoantibodies against the C3 complement component describes type II membranoproliferative glomerulonephritis or dense deposit disease.

115. The answer is D. *(Pathology)*
The patient has DiGeorge syndrome. This syndrome is characterized by failure of the third and fourth pharyngeal pouches to develop with subsequent absence of the parathyroid glands and thymus. There is no distinct genetic predisposition. Patients have low-set ears, small jaws, and major cardiac vessel abnormalities (e.g., truncus arteriosus). The clinical presentation usually relates to cardiac failure from the vessel abnormalities and/or tetany from hypoparathyroidism, which is the first clinical sign. These patients have a variable susceptibility to infection (e.g., septicemia), chronic candidiasis, and *Pneumocystis*. Laboratory studies reveal an absent thymic shadow, peripheral T-cell lymphocyte deficiency, and defective T-cell function. If transfusions are necessary, the blood should be irradiated to prevent the graft versus host reaction.

Severe combined immunodeficiency syndrome (SCID) is a heterogeneous group of conditions with both B-cell and T-cell deficiencies. SCID is more common in females. Clinical findings include protracted diarrhea, vomiting and cough (usually *Pneumocystis*), and a candida diaper rash. Laboratory studies reveal an absent thymic shadow, hypogammaglobulinemia, and no T-cell mitogen response. A bone marrow transplant offers the best chance for cure.

Ataxia-telangiectasia is an autosomal-recessive disease with cerebellar ataxia developing between 2 and 5 years of age, prominent arteriolar telangiectasias around the eyes and on the skin, and severe sinopulmonary disease. Respiratory tract infections are the most common cause of death.

Bruton agammaglobulinemia is a sex-linked recessive disease due to a failure of pre-B cells to differentiate into B cells. Patients are particularly susceptible to *Streptococcus pneumoniae* infections or other encapsulated bacteria but do well against viruses (except echoviruses) and most fungi. Respiratory infections (e.g., sinusitis, pneumonia, and otitis media) and skin infections (e.g., cellulitis, abscesses) predominate usually after 4 months when maternal immunoglobulins have subsided.

116. The answer is E. *(Pathology)*
In a pure B-cell deficiency state, such as Bruton agammaglobulinemia, an absence of isohemagglutinins in the serum is expected because isohemagglutinins represent immunoglobulin M (IgM) antibodies. Recall that IgM synthesis only begins shortly after birth.

The other choices are tests for T-cell function. Skin testing with common antigens involves cellular immunity. The antigens used are those to which most people are commonly exposed, such as streptokinase/streptodornase, dermatophytin, mumps, and *Trichophyton*. The absence of an immune response (no redness and induration) indicates anergy.

An abnormal phytohemagglutinin mitogen assay indicates a defect in cellular immunity. Mitogen assays provoke the division of T cells and B cells, the latter detected by an increased uptake of tritiated thymidine by the stimulated cells. Phytohemagglutinin and concanavalin A specifically activate T cells. Group A staphylococcus specifically activates B cells. Pokeweed is a T-cell dependent B-cell mitogen.

Plasma cells are absent in the lymph nodes of patients with Bruton agammaglobulinemia, but these cells are present in a pure T-cell immunodeficiency state. Patients with pure T-cell immunodeficiency, such as DiGeorge syndrome, have an absent paracortical area in the lymph nodes and an absent mantle zone in the white pulp in the spleen.

An antibody response to routine immunizations is normal for most patients. However, in transient hypogammaglobulinemia where infants are unable to synthesize immunoglobulins until 9 to 15 months of age, infants can host an antibody response to their immunizations and synthesize isohemagglutinins, despite low immunoglobulin G levels.

117. The answer is C. *(Pathology)*

Because the contact dermatitis associated with poison ivy is a type IV hypersensitivity reaction, a skin reaction against nickel is most closely related to this reaction. Contact dermatitis is a common inflammatory disorder of the skin that is associated with exposure to various antigens and irritating substances.

Sensitivity to nickel and poison ivy are examples of allergic contact dermatitis. Three conditions are required to produce this reaction: a genetic predisposition, absorption of sufficient antigen through the skin surface, and a competent immune system. Antigenic substances of low molecular weight penetrate the skin, are phagocytized by Langerhans cells, and are transported to regional lymph nodes where they are presented to T lymphocytes. These T lymphocytes release cytokines that are responsible for the inflammatory response in the area of the tissue that is involved. Antigenic substances include rhus (poison ivy, poison oak), nickel (earrings, hair dyes), potassium dichromate (household cleaners, leather, cement), formaldehyde (cosmetics, fabrics), ethylenediamine (dyes, medications), mercaptobenzothiazole (rubber products), and paraphenylenediamine (hair dyes, chemicals in photography).

118. The answer is A. *(Physiology)*

Hyperkalemia is a stimulus for the immediate release of stored insulin.

Insulin has a biphasic release pattern, which means that there is an immediate release of insulin from stored levels followed by a protracted release from synthesis of new insulin. Immediate release of insulin is impaired in early diabetes mellitus. This disorder is detected by infusing glucose and collecting insulin levels minutes apart. Other stimuli for insulin release include hyperglycemia (both phases), caffeine (immediate phase only), and sulfonylurea compounds (immediate phase only).

Factors that impair insulin release include hypokalemia and the counteraction of insulin by growth hormone. This is the pathogenesis of the "dawn effect" in insulin-dependent diabetics. Because growth hormone is usually released around 5 A.M., the counteraction of insulin at this time can result in high glucose at 7 A.M. Other hormones that antagonize insulin include adrenocorticotrophic hormone, cortisol, catecholamines, somatostatin, glucagon, and thyroxine.

119-120. The answers are: 119-B, 120-B. *(Biochemistry)*

The following abbreviated schematic depicts the metabolism of glucose and production of adenosine triphosphate (ATP).

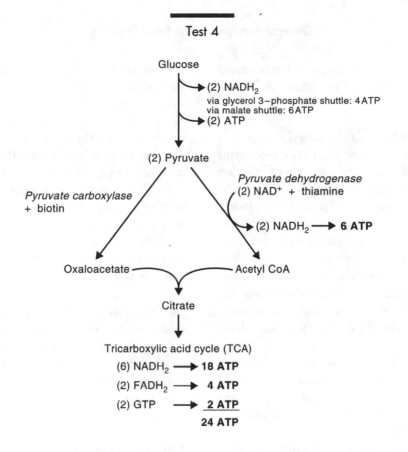

Note that in aerobic glycolysis, there is a net gain of 2 ATPs. The 2 NADH are converted in the oxidative phosphorylation pathway of the mitochondria into 4 ATPs or 6 ATPs, depending on the shuttle used to transport NADH into the mitochondria. The conversion of 2 pyruvates into acetyl CoA in the mitochondria produces another 2 NADHs, which accounts for an additional 6 ATPs. A total of 24 ATPs are generated in the tricarboxylic acid cycle (TCA cycle). Because the question only asks for the number of ATPs from pyruvate through the TCA cycle, 30 ATPs are formed per glucose molecule. If the ATP count begins with glucose, the total number ranges from 36 to 38 ATPs.

Note that the only ATP that is generated without the use of oxidative phosphorylation are the 2 ATPs directly produced by glycolysis and the conversion of 2 guanosine 5-triphosphates (GTPs) in the TCA cycle into 2 ATPs, for a total of 4 ATPs.

121. The answer is B. *(Microbiology)*
The cytoplasmic membrane, or cell membrane, of bacteria is a typical unit membrane composed of a bilayer of phospholipids and proteins. The major functions of the cytoplasmic membranes are selective permeability and transport of solutes; electron transport and oxidative phosphorylation in aerobic species; excretion of hydrolytic exoenzymes; containing the enzymes of biosynthesis of DNA, cell wall polymers, and membrane lipids; and bearing receptors for chemotactic systems.

Cell walls, composed of peptidoglycan only in gram-positive bacteria and peptidoglycan and outer membrane (endotoxin) in gram-negative bacteria, provide a rigid support and protect against osmotic pressure.

Ribosomes exist in the cytoplasm and serve as the mechanism to translate messenger RNA into proteins.

Capsules and glycocalyx layers are extracellular polymers of polysaccharides that would be present as soluble substances in the supernatant from centrifugation.

122. The answer is B. *(Behavioral science)*
Patients rarely deliberately misuse medication. Common reasons for noncompliance with medical advice include oral rather than written instructions for taking medication, failure to understand the instructions for

taking the medication, dislike of a physician perceived as cold or unapproachable, and an illness that has few or no symptoms.

123. The answer is C. *(Microbiology)*
Staphylococcus aureus does produce a variety of toxins and enzymes that aid in the establishment of infection in tissues. Catalase converts hydrogen peroxide to water and oxygen, and coagulase clots citrated plasma. Other tissue-destroying enzymes include hyaluronidase, staphylokinase, proteinases, lipases, and beta-lactamases. Exotoxins hemolyze red blood cells, and leukocidin can kill white blood cells. Exfoliative toxin, toxic shock toxin, and enterotoxins cause specific disease patterns. There is little or no evidence, however, that an IgA protease is produced that facilitates colonization.

On the other hand, IgA proteases are well characterized from the four remaining organisms listed in the question. The two *Neisseria* bacteria produce enzyme that splits and inactivates IgA1, a major mucosal immunoglobulin of humans.

Pneumococci produce immunoglobulin-degrading extracellular proteases. Proteases that degrade secretory IgA, IgG, and IgM have been found in large numbers of isolates from acutely ill patients and from symptomless carriers. The production of these extracellular proteases is thought to be an important mechanism for establishing bacterial colonization on mucosal surfaces.

Haemophilus influenzae is known to produce IgA proteases. These enzymes have the unique ability to hydrolize the human IgA1 heavy chain as the only known substrate. *H. influenzae* is the only member of the genus that produces this enzyme. As with the other organisms, such an ability promotes more effective colonization of the mucous membranes.

124. The answer is A. *(Biochemistry)*
The α-carbon of all the common amino acids except glycine is asymmetric (attached to four different chemical groups). The α-carbon of glycine is linked to two hydrogens. Thus, all the amino acids except glycine are optically active. The amino acids found in proteins are all of the L configuration.

125. The answer is E. *(Pathology)*
Central nervous system tumors, such as glioblastoma multiforme, are usually highly vascular and necrotic.

Because the brain tissue lacks fibroblasts, tumor cells are not able to evoke a fibroblastic response of the stroma, which gives the tissue a scirrhous (indurated, hardened) texture. Scirrhous cancers are more commonly seen in the breast and pancreas. Secondary descriptors are useful because they further classify the morphology of the tumor.

Papillary cancers are common in the bladder, endometrium, ovary, and thyroid. These tumors usually have a fibrovascular core.

Medullary implies a soft tumor. This is a characteristic feature of a medullary carcinoma of the breast, which is soft and bulges on the cut surface.

Mucinous tumors imply the presence of mucin in glands and stroma. These tumors are commonly seen in the ovary, pancreas, colon, and breast.

Comedo refers to necrotic material resembling a comedone or pimple. Comedocarcinoma of the breast is a classic example of this tumor type. It portends a poor prognosis.

126. The answer is C. *(Pathology)*
Activation of cytotoxic T cells by tumor antigens is expected to counteract tumor cell growth. Thus, this is not a good way for tumor cells to escape immune defenses.

Immunoselection is the ability of less immunogenic tumor variants to survive an attack by the immune system. Cells within a tumor often display considerable heterogeneity in surface proteins. Those cells that are only slightly immunogenic are most likely to survive because the less immunogenic a cell, the greater its chances are of being "selected" out.

Tolerance can be induced by very small or very large doses of antigen. When a cell initially becomes malignant, the amount of tumor antigen that exists is small and may not evoke a response from the immune system.

Many types of tumors shed at least some of their antigens. These soluble, released antigens can bind to tumor-specific receptor molecules on cytotoxic T lymphocytes, thereby "blinding" them (i.e., the cells are no longer able to "see" or bind to the antigen on the tumor cell surface).

Shed tumor antigens can form soluble immune complexes with tumor antibodies. This prevents the antibodies from reaching the tumor cell itself.

127. The answer is E.   *(Pathology)*
Patch testing involves applying a substance (e.g., nickel, formaldehyde) to the skin, taping over it, and then examining the patch for evidence of an eczematous reaction. This reaction signifies the presence of a contact dermatitis, which is a type IV hypersensitivity reaction analogous to poison ivy or a positive purified protein derivative skin test.

Type I hypersensitivity refers to immediate hypersensitivity reactions involving the production of immunoglobulin E (IgE) antibodies against an allergen. Subsequently, inflammation occurs from the activation of mast cells and basophils and the release of chemical mediators. Upon first exposure to the allergen, IgE antibodies are formed either locally or regionally in the lymph nodes draining that area. IgE antibodies have an affinity for mast-cell and basophil membranes but must be activated by subsequent exposure to allergens or other mechanisms, such as the anaphylatoxins C3a and C5a, drugs (e.g., codeine and morphine), or warm water. Degranulation of mast cells, caused by an antigen bridging two subjacent IgE antibodies, causes the release of preformed primary mediators including histamine, serotonin, neutral proteases, and chemotactic factors for neutrophils and eosinophils. This release reaction triggers phospholipase in the cell membrane and the synthesis of arachidonic acid metabolites (late phase reaction). Included in this late phase reaction are prostaglandins (vasodilators, increased mucous secretions, bronchoconstrictors) and leukotrienes C_4, D_4, E_4, which increase vessel permeability and are potent bronchoconstrictors. The late phase reaction potentiates the initial allergic response. Eosinophils attracted to the inflamed area release arylsulfatase, which neutralizes leukotrienes, and histaminase, which neutralizes histamine. They are excellent markers of an allergic reaction. Pollens, which constitute one of the most important groups of allergens, include ragweed, grasses, trees, molds, house dust (specifically an allergy to the dust mite), danders in animals, animal hairs, and feathers. Cats are the most highly allergenic of the animals.

128. The answer is B.   *(Microbiology)*
Viral meningitis is more common and less severe than bacterial meningitis. Only meningeal and ependymal cells are involved, and recovery is usually complete.

A patient with aseptic (viral) meningitis presents with headache, fever, neck stiffness (nuchal rigidity), and possibly vomiting and photophobia. A lumbar puncture reveals a clear cerebral spinal fluid (CSF) under slightly increased pressure with near normal glucose concentrations. The white cell count may range from normal ($< 10/mm^3$) to more than $1000/mm^3$ but is usually 30 to $300/mm^3$. Lymphocytes predominate after the first 24 hours. Protein elevation is moderately higher (0.50 mg/dl) than normal because of increased vessel permeability, and the glucose content is usually normal, in contrast to the reduced CSF sugar content in bacterial meningitis. CSF glucose levels must be considered in relation to blood glucose levels. Normally, the CSF glucose level is 20 to 30 mg/dl lower than blood glucose level or 50% to 70% of the blood glucose normal value.

Bacterial CSF infections produce a cloudy spinal fluid and polymorphonuclear leukocytes predominate.

129. The answer is E.   *(Pathology)*
Host CD8 cytotoxic T cells do not use an antibody-dependent, cell-mediated cytotoxicity involving antibodies. Instead, these cells recognize class I antigens on donor cells and destroy them by emitting perforin, which damages the donor cell membrane.

The following process describes the cellular immune response that leads to the graft destruction. Antigen-presenting cells in the graft (macrophages) have foreign class I antigens to which host CD8 cytotoxic T cells react, as well as foreign class II antigens to which host CD4 T-helper cells react. The foreign antigen-bearing macrophages release interleukin-1, which causes further proliferation of host CD4 T-helper cells. The CD4 T-helper cells release lymphokines (in response to the foreign class II antigens) and interleukin-2 (IL-2). Lymphokines stimulate B-cell production of antibodies against the graft. IL-2 further augments the proliferation of CD4 cells, promotes B-cell differentiation, and causes the differentiation and proliferation of CD8 cytotoxic T cells.

In order to prevent the destruction of the graft, immunosuppressive therapy is utilized. Adverse effects include an increased incidence of cervical cancer, malignant lymphomas (immunoblastic), and basal and squamous cell carcinomas of the skin (the most common overall malignancies). Other major complications are infection and bone marrow suppression.

130. The answer is C. *(Pharmacology)*
Tetracyclines are drugs of choice for rickettsial infections, chlamydial infections, cholera, and brucellosis. These drugs are useful in treating syphilis and gonorrhea in patients who are allergic to penicillin. Tetracyclines are also used in the treatment of acne. Legionnaires disease, caused by *Legionella pneumophila* is treated with a macrolide (erythromycin), ciprofloxacin, or trimethoprim–sulfamethoxazole).

131. The answer is E. *(Behavioral science)*
In the United States, approximately 50% of children live with parents who both work. The nuclear family commonly includes parents and their dependent children. While most of the population marries at some time, approximately half of the marriages will end in divorce. Only 10% to 15% of couples are childless; about half of these by choice.

132. The answer is B. *(Microbiology)*
All streptococci (including the pneumococci) are catalase negative. Along with other laboratory characteristics, this test easily distinguishes streptococci from staphylococci. Red blood cells in blood agar plates provide catalase, which aids in the growth of the laboratory organisms.

Streptococcus pneumoniae (pneumococcus) causes pneumonia, bacteremia, meningitis, and infections of the upper respiratory tract, such as otitis and sinusitis. Pneumococci are pathogenic due to the presence of well-defined polysaccharide capsules that prevent phagocytosis. Bile solubility distinguishes these organisms from other α-hemolytic streptococci. Another laboratory characteristic that is clinically useful is that pneumococcal growth is inhibited by optochin.

133. The answer is A. *(Behavioral science)*
Hypnotic capability is not related to an individual's intelligence. The hypnotic capability of a person can be ranked on a scale of 1 to 5, with 5 being the easiest individual to hypnotize. Hypnotic capability is an innate characteristic that can be increased only marginally with training. The effects of hypnosis are commonly short term. Subjects under hypnosis can disregard suggestions made by the hypnotist.

134-135. The answers are: 134-B, 135-E. *(Anatomy)*
The Golgi complex is composed of stacked, flattened, membranous cisternae and is usually situated near the nucleus or its surrounding. There may be 3 to 10 membranes. The other two components of the Golgi are numerous small vesicles, which are seen in the figure budding from the membrane sides, and larger vacuoles, which are near the top of the figure. The flattened membranes are smooth and receive vesicles, seen budding in the figure, from the rough endoplasmic reticulum.

Microtubules are hollow, linear organelles that are not constructed as pictured.

Annulate lamellae are structures derived from and resemble the nuclear membrane. These organelles are evident in oocytes and rapidly dividing cells. Nuclear, pore-like structures are visible along the membranes of annulate lamellae.

Rough endoplasmic reticulum is a network of flattened membranes with ribosomes attached.

Smooth endoplasmic reticulum is a network of membranes without ribosomes. The membranes are more tubular and interconnected than in the Golgi complex. Smooth endoplasmic reticulum occupies a broader area of the cell.

Detoxification enzymes are found on the membranes of smooth endoplasmic reticulum. This function occurs in the liver where certain hormones and noxious substances are detoxified.

136. The answer is D. *(Behavioral science)*
Problems with erection are often seen in diabetic men and may be the first sign of diabetes. Amphetamines have a stimulating effect on sexual activity through a direct action on the brain. Antihypertensive medication, alcohol, and antidepressant medication commonly have negative effects on sexual performance.

137. The answer is B. *(Pathology)*
Some tumor antigens induce an immune response strong enough to reject a tumor. This has been demonstrated with certain types of transplantable syngeneic animal tumors. Immunization of an animal with nonviable tumor cells can induce protective immunity against a challenge dose of viable tumor cells. These antigens are referred to as tumor-associated transplantation antigens.

Oncofetal antigens, which are normally expressed in large amounts by fetal cells during embryogenesis, are either not present or present in very small amounts in the healthy adult. However, they may reappear on neoplastic cells. Carcinoembryonic antigen and α-fetoprotein are common examples of oncofetal antigens.

Tumor antigens found on cells transformed by a particular oncogenic virus are often cross-reactive, even when beginning with different cell types. The antigens may be either products of the virus itself or products of cellular genes that are characteristically activated by the virus.

Tumor antigens expressed by cells transformed with carcinogenic chemicals (e.g., polycyclic aromatic hydrocarbons) are often unique, even when starting out with cells of the same type. Physical agents, such as chemicals and ionizing radiation, interact randomly with cell DNA to produce mutations, chromosomal rearrangements, and other abnormalities. This can result in the production of a variety of different proteins.

138. The answer is A. *(Pathology)*

Cell-mediated immunity is considered to be more important in controlling tumor progression than production of tumor antibodies. If the tumor antibodies are blocking antibodies, they may enhance the growth of the tumor.

According to the theory of immune surveillance, every individual develops many neoplastic cells during a lifetime, but these cells are destroyed when the immune system recognizes them as foreign. Although this concept is controversial, immune surveillance may operate against uncommon types of human cancers (i.e., leukemias and lymphomas). However, immune surveillance either does not exist or is somehow limited in preventing the occurrence of the more common cancers (i.e., lung, colon, breast, and prostate). The major cell type thought to be responsible for immune surveillance is the natural killer (NK) cell. NK cells are likely to represent a first-line defense against tumors.

Cytotoxic T lymphocytes are capable of killing tumor cells. However, as with virally-infected cells, they are highly specific and require antigen presentation in the context of major histocompatibility complex (MHC) class I molecules.

T-helper cells function in immune defense against tumors in the same way as against other recognized foreign cells. They secrete helper factors after tumor antigen is presented in the context of MHC class II molecules.

Resting macrophages do not attack tumor cells. However, once activated by macrophage-activating factors produced by T lymphocytes, they are capable of tumor cell lysis and can infiltrate into solid tumors. Interferon-γ is a major macrophage activator.

139. The answer is C. *(Biochemistry)*

Attenuation is a mechanism for the regulation of certain operons coding for the production of amino acid biosynthetic pathways in bacteria. Regulation is achieved through the formation of alternate secondary structures in the messenger RNA produced from the operon as it is being transcribed. The rate of movement of the ribosome, which is translating the message even as it is being transcribed, influences the formation of the alternate secondary structures. If a structure called the "attenuator" forms, transcription will prematurely terminate, and the structural genes encoding the enzymes will not be transcribed. This mechanism only works in bacteria because it requires that transcription and translation occur simultaneously. Eukaryotes have a nuclear membrane that separates transcription from translation in both time and space.

140. The answer is E. *(Pathology)*

Administration of antitumor immunoglobulin is not part of the adoptive immunotherapy procedure for cancer.

Immunity conferred by transfer of cells (not antibody) is called adoptive transfer or adoptive immunization. In animals, adoptive immunotherapy is done by transfering lymphoid cells between genetically identical or highly inbred subjects. In humans, adoptive immunotherapy uses a patient's own cells after they are treated in vitro. Currently, this approach to treatment is used only for cancer.

In adoptive immunotherapy, peripheral blood is collected from a cancer patient, and the mononuclear cells are isolated and treated in vitro with interleukin-2 for several days. This produces lymphokine-activated killer (LAK) cells, most of which appear to be activated natural killer cells. Then, the LAK cells are infused into the same patient. In order to ensure continued cell activation, interleukin-2 injections (usually in high doses) are given. Partial, as well as complete, tumor responses have been reported. This technique has been most successful in cases of renal cancer and malignant melanoma, with the most serious side effect, vascular leak syndrome, attributed to the high doses of interleukin-2.

141. The answer is E.   *(Biochemistry)*
Each transfer RNA (tRNA) molecule becomes covalently attached to a specific amino acid and carries that amino acid to the ribosome, where it becomes incorporated into the growing polypeptide chain during protein synthesis. The anticodon portion of the tRNA molecule binds to the complementary codon on the messenger RNA molecule. Transfer RNA characteristically contains many modified bases as a result of post-transcriptional modifications. Each tRNA molecule is specific for only one amino acid, so that a family of tRNAs is necessary in order to carry all of the 20 possible amino acids.

142. The answer is C.   *(Microbiology)*
Patients with AIDS have a low CD4$^+$:CD8$^+$ cell ratio. A normal ratio is approximately 1.8:1.0. HIV type 1 infects the CD4$^+$ T lymphocytes because they express a relatively large amount of the CD4 protein (the attachment molecule for the virus). The ratio declines progressively as the CD4$^+$ T cells die.

How the infected CD4$^+$ T cells are killed is not fully understood. The destruction of the cells could be due to an accumulation of virus materials, an attack by T-cytotoxic lymphocytes (viral proteins are expressed by the infected cell), or a combination of these and other possibilities.

143. The answer is B.   *(Immunology)*
Neutralizing antibodies generated against HIV type 1 (HIV-1) are directed against the gp120 (glycoprotein with a molecular weight of 120 kD) surface glycoprotein of the virus that protrudes from the viral envelope. These antibodies prevent infection because attachment of the gp120 to the CD4 molecule on target cells leads to virus entry. Individuals with neutralizing antibodies can clear the virus from circulation, reduce the rate of infection of new cells, and may remain asymptomatic.

Unfortunately, relatively low titers of neutralizing antibodies are found in HIV-1–infected patients.

The virus has a high mutation rate and, therefore, exhibits great antigenic variation. A variant may multiply to relatively large numbers before an effective immune response is waged. The virus may eventually outrun the ability of the immune system to control infection with continued appearance of new variants.

Most latently infected cells do not transcribe viral RNA and do not express viral proteins. Thus, the immune system is unable to detect the presence of the virus.

Soon after infection, the cytotoxic activity of CD8$^+$ T lymphocytes against HIV-1 is often high. However, with time this level declines moderately. Natural killer-cell activity also becomes impaired because of decreased ability to bind to the HIV-1 infected target cells.

The number of HIV-1–infected cells in organs such as the lymph nodes is thought to be higher than what is seen in the peripheral blood, where approximately 1 in 10 CD4$^+$ T lymphocytes is infected. Disruption of lymph nodes and other lymphoid organs in patients with AIDS becomes increasingly severe with time.

144. The answer is B.   *(Pathology)*
Although esophageal cancer is common in Russia, hepatocellular carcinoma is not.

Squamous cell carcinoma of the bladder is common in Egypt because of the presence of *Schistosoma haematobium*. The adult worms locate in the bladder where they lay eggs that induce squamous metaplasia of the overlying transitional epithelium. This progresses into dysplasia, carcinoma in situ, and invasive cancer. Hematuria is the first sign of the disease.

Burkitt lymphoma due to Epstein-Barr virus and Kaposi sarcoma, possibly related to HIV, are common in Africa.

145. The answer is E.   *(Biochemistry)*
The pathogenesis of peripheral neuropathy involves osmotic damage rather than nonenzymatic glycosylation. In addition, osmotic damage from sorbitol is invoked in the genesis of cataracts, retinal microaneurysms, and nephropathy. The following biochemical reaction is involved.

$$\text{Glucose} + \text{NADPH} + \text{H}^+ \xrightarrow{\text{aldolase reductase}} \text{Sorbitol} + \text{NADP}^+$$

When glucose is inside cells containing aldolase reductase, it is converted into sorbitol. Sorbitol is osmotically active and draws water into: the lens, producing cataracts; Schwann cells, resulting in a sensorimotor peripheral neuropathy; mesangium in the glomeruli, which contributes to glomerulosclerosis; pericytes in retinal vessels, which weakens the vessels and allows the formation of microaneurysms. Drugs that inhibit aldolase reductase are useful in reversing osmotic damage.

146. The answer is E. *(Microbiology)*

Actinomyces israelii is a gram-positive anaerobe that can cause oral or facial abscesses with "sulfur granules" that may drain through sinus tracts in skin. These anaerobes are branching organisms that tend to fragment into bacteria-like pieces.

Mycobacteria have a high-lipid content cell wall that resists entry of the Gram stain reagents. Mycobacteria are acid-fast, which refers to an alternative staining procedure that uses heat to drive the carbol fusion dye through the cell wall. Bacteria that stain with the Gram procedure would destain with the acid-fast protocol and take up the color of the counter stain.

Mycoplasma organisms have no cell wall and cannot retain the crystal violet–iodine complex of the Gram stain. They would appear only as gram negative.

Chlamydae are intracellular parasites that are quite small. Because chlamydae stain gram-negative or variable on Gram stain, this procedure is not useful in the identification of these agents. They are most often detected with monoclonal antibodies in fluorescence staining procedures.

Treponema are essentially too thin to be visualized, but can be visualized by darkfield microscopy or fluorescent techniques.

147-151. The answers are: 147-C, 148-A, 149-E, 150-B, 151-D. *(Pharmacology, Microbiology)*

Traditionally, chloroquine has been used for prophylaxis and treatment of malaria. However, many strains are now resistant to chloroquine, so mefloquin is often used. Mebendazole is a broad spectrum antihelmintic for nematode infections including whipworm and pinworm. Praziquantel is used for trematode infections including all forms of schistosomiasis. Pentamidine is an alternative to trimethoprim sulfamethoxazole for the prophylaxis and treatment of *Pneumocystis* infections. Metronidazole treats several protozoal infections (e.g., amebiasis, trichomoniasis, and giardiasis).

152-153. The answers are: 152-A, 153-C. *(Microbiology)*

Escherichia coli, *Enterobacter*, and *Klebsiella* ferment lactose resulting in the production of acid and gas (i.e., they are lactose positive). *Proteus* ferments lactose very slowly, if at all, and *Pseudomonas* is lactose negative. *Escherichia coli* and *Enterobacter* have peritrichous flagella scattered over the body of the organisms and are almost always motile, whereas *Klebsiella* is never motile. *Pseudomonas* and especially *Proteus*, which can "swarm" all over the surface of an agar plate, are motile. *Escherichia coli* and *Enterobacter* are differentiated on the basis of indole production from tryptophan.

Klebsiella species produce an unusually large polysaccharide capsule that helps identify the organisms in the laboratory. On solid media, the capsule gives the colonies a striking mucoid or gelatinous appearance. *Klebsiella pneumoniae* can be found not only in the feces and urine, but also in the respiratory tract of approximately 5% to 10% of healthy individuals. The other four organisms are much less likely to be isolated from the respiratory tract of healthy persons.

154-158. The answers are: 154-D, 155-A, 156-C, 157-E, 158-B. *(Behavioral science)*

O'Connor v. *Donaldson* determined that patients who were judged to be mentally ill but who were not dangerous to themselves or to others could not be held against their will without treatment. In the Tarasoff decision, the court found that therapists must warn the intended victims of significant threats issued by their patients. In the doctrine of *parens patriae*, the court decided that the state can make decisions for persons who cannot take care of themselves or who may harm themselves. *Rouse* v. *Cameron* found that patients who are hospitalized involuntarily have a right to treatment. In the Good Samaritan statute, liability is limited for physicians who provide emergency medical care outside of their usual practice.

159-163. The answers are: 159-G, 160-D, 161-I, 162-A, 163-E. *(Pharmacology)*

New drug development in the United States requires preclinical toxicology studies followed by three phases of clinical testing. Phase I examines safety and pharmacokinetics in healthy volunteers; phase II determines safety and efficacy in a small group of patients with the disease being treated, and phase III is a large clinical trial to provide statistical evidence of efficacy and safety.

The drug developer submits an IND application after completing short-term preclinical studies. The IND application contains proposed protocols for human testing. After completing human testing, the developer submits an NDA. An abbreviated NDA (ANDA) can be submitted for generic equivalents of approved brand-name products. The ANDA includes the results of a bioequivalence study comparing the generic and brand-name formulations.

Orphan drugs are developed for diseases with fewer than 200,000 patients in the United States. Special incentives encourage manufacturers to produce orphan drugs.

The Controlled Substances Act establishes schedules for drugs that have abuse potential. Schedules I and II contain drugs with high potential for abuse. Those drugs in schedule I have no approved medical use, while those in schedule II may be prescribed by physicians. Schedule IV drugs have a low risk of causing physical addiction.

164-165. The answers are: 164-A, 165-E. *(Microbiology)*

The tourist is most likely to have been infected with *Vibrio cholerae*. Following an incubation period of approximately 1 to 4 days, the onset of symptoms (nausea, vomiting, diarrhea, and abdominal cramps) is abrupt. Stools, which contain large numbers of vibrios, epithelial cells, and flecks of mucus, have the appearance of rice water (i.e., the grayish-white stool in the case history). In severe cases, massive amounts of fluid, sometimes 15 to 20 liters per day, can be lost, which leads to profound dehydration, electrolyte imbalance, anuria, and circulatory collapse.

V. cholerae is not invasive. After ingestion, it attaches to the microvilli of the brush border of the intestinal tract and secretes the cholera toxin. The mechanism of action of the toxin is like that of the heat-labile toxin of *Escherichia coli*. It increases the intracellular level of cyclic adenosine monophosphate (cAMP).

The El Tor biotype of *V. cholerae* generally causes less severe disease than the classic biotype but is able to persist longer in the body, as well as in the environment. Both the El Tor and the classic cholera biotypes have the O1 antigen and cause epidemics. Non-O1 *V. cholerae* cause only sporadic cases or are non-pathogenic.

The O1 *V. cholerae* reappeared in the western hemisphere in 1991 (for the first time in nearly 100 years) and has since spread to many South American countries, as well as Mexico. *V. cholerae* are spread by direct contact with an infected person and by contaminated water, food, and flies. The organisms are naturally pathogenic only for humans.

Helicobacter pylori is a comma-shaped, gram-negative rod that is now strongly associated with the development of duodenal (peptic) ulcer disease and gastric ulcers. Although direct evidence that the organisms cause the disease is lacking, clinical trials have shown that effective antimicrobial therapy eradicates the organisms and also greatly improves the duodenal disease. After triple therapy with metronidazole, bismuth subsalicylate, and amoxicillin, the organisms are eradicated and the disease resolves. On the other hand, *H. pylori* may exist in the stomach and cause no symptoms. Approximately 40% to 60% of persons who are 60 years of age and older have *H. pylori* in the gastric mucosa. The route of transmission is primarily person-to-person (fecal–oral route). There is no known animal reservoir.

H. pylori survives the acidity of the stomach by embedding itself deep into the epithelium so that it is protected by a layer of gastric mucus. This mucus has a strong buffering capacity and is relatively impermeable by acid. A protease enzyme secreted by the organisms modifies the mucus to further reduce its acid permeability.

166-170. The answers are: 166-C, 167-A, 168-E, 169-D, 170-B. *(Pharmacology)*

Ampicillin produces a maculopapular rash in a high percentage of patients with viral infections, particularly mononucleosis. Erythromycin estolate is the form of erythromycin that usually is associated with reversible cholestatic jaundice. Tetracyclines may deposit in growing teeth and cause permanent discoloration. Ototoxicity, including both vestibular and auditory, may be caused by aminoglycosides (e.g., gentamicin). Certain third-generation cephalosporins, such as moxalactam and cefoperazone, may cause platelet dysfunction and bleeding. These cephalosporins are also associated with disulfiram-like reactions when administered with ethanol.

171-175. The answers are: 171-F, 172-C, 173-B, 174-A, 175-I. *(Biochemistry)*

Hartnup disease is a genetic dysfunction of the transporter system. This system is responsible for the absorption of neutral amino acids with aromatic or hydrophobic side chains from the gut and the renal tubules. The clinical symptoms are associated with a deficiency of the relevant essential amino acids and nicotinamide. Although nicotinamide is considered a vitamin, it is also synthesized from tryptophan.

Enteropeptidase (formerly enterokinase) is a protease produced by duodenal epithelial cells. It cleaves a hexapeptide from trypsinogen to produce trypsin. Trypsin then autocatalytically converts additional trypsinogen molecules to form more active trypsin. Also, trypsin catalytically activates the other pancreatic proenzymes to form active chymotrypsin, elastase, and carboxypeptidase.

Pinocytic absorption of proteins is active in neonates. In this process, the small intestine absorbs intact proteins. This is important in the transfer of maternal antibodies to the offspring. Persistence of this process beyond the immediate neonatal period can also result in transfer of other proteins and the production of antibodies against these proteins. This process is responsible for the initiation of at least some food allergies and perhaps autoimmune conditions.

Pepsins are a group of proteolytic enzymes that are liberated from pepsinogen under acidic conditions. At pH values less than 5, the proenzyme is cleaved. The active pepsin is characterized by having a very low pH optimum. After initial activation, further cleavage occurs via autocatalysis. The active enzyme breaks ingested proteins into large peptide fragments as well as some free amino acids. These proteolytic products act as stimulants of cholecystokinin release by cells in the duodenum. Then, the cholecystokinin induces the release of the pancreatic enzymes involved in protein digestion.

As with pepsin, rennin is secreted in gastric juice as an inactive precursor (prorennin) and is activated by HCl. However, it is activated and operates at a slightly higher pH value than pepsin. This is important in neonates whose stomach juices are not as acidic as adults. Rennin's main function is to initiate the digestion of milk proteins. Rennin should not be confused with renin, a protease (not a hormone) that forms angiotensin I.

176-180. The answers are: 176-D, 177-B, 178-G, 179-A, 180-C. *(Pharmacology)*

β_1-Adrenergic and histamine H_2 are the primary receptors mediating cardiac stimulation, which includes increased heart rate and/or contractility. α_1-Adrenergic, β_2-adrenergic, histamine H_1, and serotonin receptors have minor roles in mediating cardiac stimulation.

Vasodilation is primarily mediated by β_2-adrenergic and cholinergic muscarinic receptors. Serotonin may also induce vasodilation in skeletal muscle via $5HT_2$ receptors, whereas other vascular beds are constricted.

Vasoconstriction is mediated by α_1-adrenergic and serotonin $5HT_{1D}$ receptors.

Bronchoconstriction is primarily mediated by histamine H_1 and muscarinic receptors, whereas α_1-adrenergic and serotonin $5HT_2$ receptors have smaller roles in producing bronchoconstriction. The role of serotonin is usually not important, except in carcinoid syndrome when elevated levels of the amine may cause bronchoconstriction.

Gastrointestinal motility may be increased by activating muscarinic and serotonin $5HT_2$, $5HT_3$, and $5HT_4$ receptors. Severe diarrhea may occur in patients with carcinoid syndrome. Cisapride increases motility by activating $5HT_4$ receptors.

SUBJECT ITEM INDEX

ANATOMY

Test 1 : 88, 101, 104, 112, 115, 136, 153, 155, 156, 176, 177, 178, 179, 180.
Test 2 : 79, 94.
Test 3 : 90, 98, 118.
Test 4 : 87, 134, 135.

PHYSIOLOGY

Dx Test : 26.
Test 1 : 31, 93, 96, 109, 120, 174, 175.
Test 2 : 128.
Test 4 : 84, 118.

PATHOLOGY

Dx Test : 3, 28, 32, 34, 37.
Test 1 : 5, 8, 10, 14, 17, 21, 106, 107, 108, 110, 113, 114, 118, 127, 128, 159, 172, 173.
Test 2 : 7, 11, 15, 19, 25, 27, 31, 35, 37, 112, 113, 114, 115, 116, 117, 118, 119, 120, 123.
Test 3 : 10, 17, 19, 21, 23, 25, 27, 29, 31, 33, 35, 37, 65, 113, 117, 119, 126, 130, 153, 159.
Test 4 : 5, 11, 13, 15, 17, 19, 31, 89, 93, 96, 107, 108, 109, 110, 111, 112, 113, 114, 115, 116, 117, 125, 126, 127, 129, 137, 138, 140, 144.

PHARMACOLOGY

Test 1 : 27, 34, 38, 49, 58, 60, 64, 66, 70, 72, 74, 76, 78, 85, 94, 97, 135, 163, 164, 165, 166.
Test 2 : 62, 66, 71, 161, 162, 163, 164, 165, 166, 167, 168, 169, 170.
Test 3 : 41, 52, 56, 64, 68, 71, 73, 75, 77, 131, 135, 139, 143, 145, 172, 173, 174, 175, 176.
Test 4 : 23, 30, 44, 49, 53, 59, 72, 86, 99, 130, 147, 148, 149, 150, 151, 159, 160, 161, 162, 163, 166, 167, 168, 169, 170, 176, 177, 178, 179, 180.

BEHAVIORAL SCIENCE

Dx Test : 5, 10, 12, 14, 18, 22, 23, 41, 42.
Test 1 : 1, 23, 40, 42, 46, 48, 50, 52, 54, 55, 56, 57, 59, 61, 62, 63, 65, 67, 69, 71, 75, 79, 80, 81, 82, 83, 86, 91, 98, 99, 100, 111, 123, 124, 125, 126, 139, 141, 143, 145, 147, 149, 151, 167, 168, 169, 170, 171.

Test 2 : 1, 3, 4, 40, 42, 48, 52, 56, 58, 60, 63, 65, 67, 69, 70, 72, 73, 74, 78, 80, 82, 84, 85, 86, 87, 88, 90, 92, 107, 124, 125, 137, 139, 142, 144, 145, 146, 147, 148, 150, 155.

Test 3 : 1, 5, 7, 9, 11, 13, 15, 26, 36, 45, 50, 54, 58, 62, 66, 69, 72, 78, 80, 82, 84, 85, 87, 89, 91, 93, 95, 97, 99, 101, 103, 105, 107, 109, 111, 114, 122, 124, 137, 141, 147, 157, 160.

Test 4 : 1, 27, 32, 36, 38, 39, 43, 45, 47, 55, 58, 60, 62, 64, 66, 68, 70, 74, 75, 78, 80, 95, 122, 131, 133, 136, 154, 155, 156, 157, 158.

MICROBIOLOGY

Dx Test : 7, 8, 16, 20, 25, 27, 29, 31, 33, 35, 39, 40, 43, 44, 45, 46, 47, 48, 49, 50.

Test 1 : 2, 4, 6, 12, 19, 25, 29, 33, 35, 37, 39, 41, 43, 45, 47, 51, 53, 89, 95, 102, 105, 122, 130, 132, 134, 137, 140, 142, 144, 146, 150, 152, 154, 157, 158, 161, 162.

Test 2 : 2, 6, 8, 10, 12, 14, 16, 18, 20, 22, 23, 29, 33, 38, 44, 46, 50, 54, 81, 91, 96, 97, 98, 99, 100, 101, 102, 103, 104, 105, 106, 108, 109, 110, 111, 122, 126, 129, 130, 132, 133, 135, 136, 138, 140, 141, 143, 151, 152, 154, 171, 172, 173, 174.

Test 3 : 2, 4, 14, 20, 24, 28, 32, 39, 43, 47, 49, 51, 53, 55, 57, 59, 61, 63, 67, 92, 94, 100, 104, 108, 112, 121, 123, 128, 132, 134, 136, 138, 140, 142, 144, 146, 148, 150, 152, 154, 156, 158, 161.

Test 4 : 2, 4, 6, 8, 9, 21, 25, 34, 41, 46, 48, 50, 52, 54, 56, 77, 81, 82, 83, 90, 92, 94, 97, 100, 101, 103, 104, 105, 106, 121, 123, 128, 132, 142, 143, 146, 152, 153, 164, 165.

BIOCHEMISTRY

Dx Test : 1, 2, 4, 6, 9, 11, 13, 15, 17, 19, 21, 24, 30, 36, 38.

Test 1 : 3, 7, 9, 11, 13, 15, 16, 18, 20, 22, 24, 26, 28, 30, 32, 36, 44, 68, 73, 77, 84, 87, 90, 92, 103, 116, 117, 119, 121, 129, 131, 133, 138, 148, 160.

Test 2 : 5, 9, 13, 17, 21, 24, 26, 28, 30, 32, 34, 36, 39, 41, 43, 45, 47, 49, 51, 53, 55, 57, 59, 61, 64, 68, 75, 76, 77, 83, 89, 93, 95, 121, 127, 131, 134, 149, 153, 156, 157, 158, 159, 160, 175, 176, 177, 178, 179, 180.

Test 3 : 3, 6, 8, 12, 16, 18, 22, 30, 34, 38, 40, 42, 44, 46, 48, 60, 70, 74, 76, 79, 81, 83, 86, 88, 96, 102, 106, 110, 116, 120, 125, 127, 129, 133, 149, 151, 155, 162, 163, 164, 165, 166, 167, 168, 169, 170, 171, 177, 178, 179, 180.

Test 4 : 3, 7, 10, 12, 14, 16, 18, 20, 22, 24, 26, 28, 29, 33, 35, 37, 40, 42, 51, 57, 61, 63, 65, 67, 69, 71, 73, 76, 79, 85, 88, 91, 98, 102, 119, 120, 124, 139, 141, 145, 171, 172, 173, 174, 175.